Blueprints

CLINICAL CASES
PEDIATRICS

Check Out all the Titles in This Great Series!

Blueprints Clinical Cases in Emergency Medicine, 2e
Blueprints Clinical Cases in Family Medicine, 2e
Blueprints Clinical Cases in Medicine, 2e
Blueprints Clinical Cases in Neurology, 2e
Blueprints Clinical Cases in Obstetrics & Gynecology, 2e
Blueprints Clinical Cases in Psychiatry, 2e
Blueprints Clinical Cases in Surgery, 2e

Blueprints

CLINICAL CASES

SECOND EDITION

PEDIATRICS

Vedang A. Londhe, MD
Assistant Professor of Pediatrics
Division of Neonatology and Developmental Biology
David Geffen School of Medicine at UCLA
Los Angeles, California

Andrea K. Marmor, MD
Assistant Professor of Pediatrics
University of California, San Francisco
San Francisco General Hospital
San Francisco, California

Abhay S. Dandekar, MD
Associate Director
UCLA Tri-Campus Pediatric Residency Training Program
Cedars-Sinai Medical Center
Assistant Professor of Pediatrics
David Geffen School of Medicine at UCLA
Los Angeles, California

Aaron B. Caughey, MD, MPP, MPH (Series Editor)
Assistant Professor in Residence
Department of Obstetrics, Gynecology, and Reproductive Sciences
University of California, San Francisco
San Francisco, California

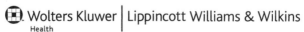
Wolters Kluwer | Lippincott Williams & Wilkins
Health
Philadelphia · Baltimore · New York · London
Buenos Aires · Hong Kong · Sydney · Tokyo

Acquisitions Editor: Nancy Anastasi Duffy
Managing Editor: Stacey L. Sebring
Marketing Manager: Jennifer Kuklinski
Associate Production Manager: Kevin P. Johnson
Creative Director: Doug Smock
Compositor: International Typesetting and Composition
Printer: R.R. Donnelley & Son's

Printed in the United States of America

First Edition, 2002 Blackwell Publishing

Library of Congress Cataloging-in-Publication Data

Londhe, Vedang A.
    Blueprints clinical cases in pediatrics / Vedang A. Londhe,
Andrea K. Marmor, Abhay S. Dandekar.—2nd ed.
        p. ; cm.—(Blueprints. Clinical cases)
    Includes bibliographical references and index.
    ISBN-13: 978-1-4051-0492-0
    ISBN-10: 1-4051-0492-9
    1. Pediatrics—Case studies.   I. Marmor, Andrea K.   II. Dandekar,
Abhay S.   III. Title.   IV. Title: Clinical cases in pediatrics.   V. Series.
    [DNLM: 1. Pediatrics—Case Reports.   2. Pediatrics—Examination
Questions.   WS 18.2 L847b 2007]
RJ58.B58 2007
618.92'00076—dc22

                                                2006026471

*The publishers have made every effort to trace the copyright holders for borrowed material.
If they have inadvertently overlooked any, they will be pleased to make the necessary
arrangements at the first opportunity.*

Dedication

For my daughter, Anisa, her brother, Shaan, and their mom, Anjali.
Ved

My portion of this book is dedicated to the many people who have inspired me to learn and to teach every day of my life. From the patients, students, and physicians who constantly challenge me to become a better doctor, to my friends and family who are my teachers in life, I extend to each of you credit for this book, my warmest thanks, and the joy of lifelong learning.
Andi

I would like to thank my wife, Aparna, and our daughter, Vaidehi, for their unwavering love and support. I also offer my most heartfelt thanks to the students who have helped me teach, and the teachers who have helped me learn. To all who are dedicated to providing compassionate care for children, I am grateful that this cycle of inspiration has provided us with a continuous source of intellectual stimulation and energy!
Abhay

We would all like to thank the staff at Blackwell Publishing and LWW. We would also like to thank our family, friends, and colleagues, including the residents and faculty in the Departments of Pediatrics and Obstetrics and Gynecology at UCSF, Kaiser Oakland, and UCLA. I dedicate this book to my parents, Bill and Carol, who have had an immeasurable effect on the children they have cared for throughout their careers.
Aaron

Preface

Blueprints Clinical Cases in Pediatrics, Second Edition, was developed to enrich and supplement the clinical experience of the medical student or sub-intern rotating through pediatrics. We have designed and written these problem-based scenarios to emphasize the most common and important childhood illnesses, as well as to hit hot topics that will appear on in-service examinations, on rounds, and on Boards. This second edition includes revisions of the 50 cases from the first edition, 10 new cases, and a new section with 100 Board-format questions and detailed explanations of the answers. We have also incorporated a new section providing evidence-based resources for each case to promote additional reading.

The cases reflect the special challenges of the diagnosis and treatment of illness in children. As you know, children are not simply small adults, and many of the diseases and conditions that affect infants and children are unique. In addition, the unusual and often subtle presentation of disease in pediatric patients demands patience and attention to details such as vital signs, growth parameters, and the interaction between the parent and child.

Case-based learning is fun and effective, but requires substantial motivation from the student for maximum benefit. The cases are designed to take you through the clinical thought process, beginning with the patient's complaint; proceeding through history, examination, and diagnostic tests; and ending with diagnosis and management. As you work through the cases, focus on improving your skills in assessment of the sick child, as well as making the diagnosis and learning about the specific illness. The following are suggestions on how to get the most out of these pediatric cases.

1. *Approach the cases as you would approach your patients.* Read the information carefully, pay attention to details, and think about what you would ask or do next.
2. *Write down your answers to the Thought Questions before moving on.* This is a key step in maximizing your learning from the cases. In the interest of space, we have presented only pertinent positives and negatives. If a portion of the history or physical exam that you are interested in is not presented, assume it to be normal or

noncontributory.(It should still be a part of your complete history and physical, however!)

3. *Note the elements of the history that are unique to pediatrics.* These include the birth history, immunization history, and developmental history. This information is presented when relevant to the case, and should be carefully reviewed. Social and family histories are also important in pediatrics, because children depend on their caretakers for adequate nutrition, injury prevention, and other health maintenance behaviors.

4. *Pay special attention to the vital signs and growth parameters in each case.* Since children often cannot communicate to us about discomfort or distress, abnormal vital signs are an important clue to the etiology of illness, and may be the only abnormalities on physical exam. The vital signs presented are normal for age unless a range of values appears after them, and percentiles are given for all growth parameters.

5. *Assess the nutritional status and hydration of the child.* Plot each child's height and weight on growth charts. Look for evidence of hydration status on history and physical exam, such as fluid intake, urine output, tachycardia, mucous membranes, skin color, and capillary refill.

6. *Answer the multiple choice questions at the end of each case and at the end of the book.* These questions and answers provide additional important information about the case diagnosis and address additional conditions in the differential diagnosis that are worth knowing about.

7. *Read about topics that you want to know more about in* Blueprints in Pediatrics, *in a pediatric textbook, or by referring to the additional resources listed at the end of each case.* You can also do a literature search to find out about recent discoveries and current therapy for topics that interest you.

8. *Remember that pediatrics, like all of medicine, is a constantly changing field.* Check with the pediatricians with whom you are working to find out the latest information on diagnosis and treatment.

We hope that you find the pediatric cases fun and interesting, and a good complement to your experience in the pediatric clinic, nursery, and ward. Keep your eyes and ears open; children have a lot to teach us all!

Vedang A. Londhe
Andrea K. Marmor
Abhay S. Dandekar
Aaron B. Caughey

Contents

Abbreviations/Acronyms

ABC	airway, breathing, circulation
ABD	abdomen
ABG	arterial blood gas
AFO	anterior fontanel open
AIDS	acquired immunodeficiency syndrome
All	allergies
ALL	acute lymphocytic leukemia
AN	anorexia nervosa
ANA	antinuclear antibody
AP	anteroposterior
ARF	acute rheumatic fever
ASD	atrial septal defect
BP	blood pressure
BUN	blood urea nitrogen
C	Celsius
CAH	congenital adrenal hyperplasia
CBC	complete blood count
CCAM	congenital cystadenomatous malformations
C/C/E	cyanosis/clubbing/edema
CC/ID	chief complaint/identification
CDC	Centers for Disease Control and Prevention
CM	costal margin
CMV	cytomegalovirus
CNS	central nervous system
CPAP	continuous positive airway pressure
CRP	C-reactive protein
CRT	capillary refill time
CSF	cerebrospinal fluid
CT	computerized tomography
CTA(B)	clear to auscultation (bilaterally)
CV	cardiovascular
CXR	chest x-ray
DevHx	developmental history
DKA	diabetic ketoacidosis
DMSA	dimercaptosuccinic acid
DOL	day of life

DTaP	diphtheria, tetanus toxoids, and acellular pertussis (vaccine)
DTR	deep tendon reflex
EBV	Epstein-Barr virus
ECG/EKG	electrocardiogram
ED/ER	emergency department (room)
EEG	electroencephalogram
EOMI	extraocular movements intact
ESR	erythrocyte sedimentation rate
Ext	extremities
F	Fahrenheit
FHx	family history
FRC	functional residual capacity
FTT	failure to thrive
GA	gestational age
GAS	group A streptococci
GBM	glomerular basement membrane
GBS	Guillain-Barré syndrome
GERD	gastroesophageal reflux disease
GI	gastrointestinal
GN	glomerulonephritis
GU	genitourinary
Hct	hematocrit
HEENT	head, eyes, ears, nose, throat
HHV	human herpesvirus
HIV	human immunodeficiency virus
HLA	human leukocyte antigen
HR	heart rate
HPI	history of present illness
HSP	Henoch-Schönlein purpura
HSV	herpes simplex virus
IBD	inflammatory bowel disease
ICH	intracranial hemorrhage
ICN	intensive care nursery
ICP	intracranial pressure
IDDM	insulin-dependent diabetes mellitus
ITP	idiopathic thrombocytopenic purpura
IV	intravenous
IVIG	intravenous immunoglobulin
IVP	intravenous pyelogram
JRA	juvenile rheumatoid arthritis
KUB	kidney, ureters, bladder (radiograph)
LLQ	left lower quadrant
LP	lumbar puncture

LR	Lactated Ringer's solution
LUQ	left upper quadrant
LVH	left ventricular hypertrophy
MAP	mean arterial pressure
MCD	minimal change disease
MMR	measles, mumps, rubella (vaccine)
MRI	magnetic resonance imaging
MS	musculoskeletal
NABS	normal active bowel sounds
NAD	no acute distress
NCAT	normocephalic atraumatic
ND	nondistended
NHL	non-Hodgkin lymphoma
NICU	neonatal intensive care unit
NKDA	no known drug allergy
NL	normal
NS	normal saline
NSAID	nonsteroidal anti-inflammatory drug
NSVD	normal spontaneous vaginal delivery
NT	nontender
OP	oropharynx
OR	operating room
OTC	over-the-counter
P	pulse
PE	physical exam
PERRLA	pupils equal, round, reactive to light and accommodation
PICU	pediatric intensive care unit
PID	pelvic inflammatory disease
PMHx	past medical history
PPD	purified protein derivative
PPHN	persistent pulmonary hypertension
PRN	as needed
PSGN	poststreptococcal glomerulonephritis
PSHx	past surgical history
PT/PTT	prothrombin time/partial thromboplastin time
RA	room air
RAD	reactive airway disease
RBC	red blood cell
RDS	respiratory distress syndrome
Resp	respiratory/respirations
RLQ	right lower quadrant
ROS	review of systems
RR	respiratory rate
RR&R	regular rate and rhythm

RSV	respiratory syncytial virus
RUQ	right upper quadrant
RVH	right ventricular quadrant
SCFE	slipped capital femoral epiphysis
SHx	social history
SLE	systemic lupus erythematosus
STD	sexually transmitted disease
SVD	spontaneous vaginal delivery
SVT	supraventricular tachycardia
T	temperature
TAPVR	total anomalous pulmonary venous return
TGA	transposition of the great arteries
TM	tympanic membrane
TORCH	toxoplasmosis, other (syphilis, HIV, EBV), rubella, CMV, herpes
UA	urinalysis
UC	ulcerative colitis
U/S	ultrasound
URI	upper respiratory infection
UTD	up to date
UTI	urinary tract infection
VCUG	voiding cystourethrogram
VDRL	Venereal Disease Reference Laboratory (test)
VS	vital signs
VSD	ventricular septal defect
WBC	white blood cell
WNL	within normal limits
WPW	Wolff-Parkinson-White (syndrome)
Wt	weight

I

Cases
Presenting with
Fever

Fever and Fussiness

CC/ID: 16-month-old girl brought in by her mother for fussiness and fever.

HPI: D.C. has had a cold for 3 days, with runny nose and cough, and last night she developed a fever and increased fussiness. She refuses to eat and only wants her bottle. Last night D.C. woke up crying and was inconsolable until she was given ibuprofen for fever and was finally able to go back to sleep. Mother says she acted like this 3 months ago when she had an ear infection, and she is worried that she has one again.

PMHx: Ear infection 4 months ago; resolved with treatment.

Meds: Ibuprofen for fever

All: None

Immun: Up to date (UTD)

THOUGHT QUESTIONS

- In addition to middle ear infection (acute otitis media, or AOM), what illnesses are likely based on this child's presentation?
- What findings will you look for in this child's ear to confirm the diagnosis of AOM?

DISCUSSION

Fever, runny nose, and cough are common signs of a viral upper respiratory infection. However, you must always consider a more serious infection such as pneumonia or meningitis in the febrile, irritable young child. Careful evaluation of the ill child's hydration and overall appearance and examination of the lungs, skin, joints, and nervous system will help identify signs of serious bacterial infection. If no source of fever can be found in the child aged 3 to 36 months, consider the child's risk for occult infection such as bacteremia or urinary tract infection (UTI). In the older child who complains of ear pain, consider otitis externa ("swimmer's ear") or an otic foreign body in the differential.

The ear exam is one of the most challenging parts of the pediatric physical examination. You should look at as many normal eardrums as you can to facilitate recognizing the abnormal findings that suggest AOM. A normal tympanic membrane (TM) appears smooth, pearly, and translucent, with a sharp light reflex, and the bones of the inner ear are visible through it. An infected TM is hyperemic and irregular or bulging in appearance, with an abnormal or absent light reflex, and bony landmarks are obscured. Occasional findings include pus behind the eardrum or fluid in the ear canal, the latter of which suggests a perforated drum or otitis externa.

 CASE CONTINUED

VS: Temp 38.9°C (102°F), HR 130, RR 32; Weight 12 kg (80%)

PE: *Gen:* fussy but consolable girl who is crying tears and drinking from her bottle. *HEENT:* mucous membranes are moist and clear, crusting rhinorrhea is noted, and pharynx is unremarkable. The left TM is slightly injected, but light reflex and landmarks are clearly visible. The right TM is opaque and red, and has an irregular surface with disturbed light reflex. Bony landmarks are not visualized (Fig. 1-1). Shotty anterior cervical adenopathy is noted, greater on the right than on the left. No nuchal rigidity or

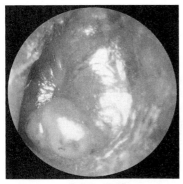

Otitis media

FIGURE 1-1.
Signs of otitis media, illustrated here, include a bulging red tympanic membrane, dullness and loss of sharp light reflex, and decreased mobility. Infection of the middle ear in children is often secondary to upper respiratory infections, which cause partial or complete blockage of the pharyngotympanic tube due to inflammation and swelling of the mucous membrane lining the tympanic cavity.

photophobia. *Lungs:* clear; no signs of respiratory distress. The remainder of the exam is within normal limits.

THOUGHT QUESTIONS

- This patient's exam and history suggests AOM. What organisms are the most likely cause?
- How will you treat her?

DISCUSSION

Acute otitis media is a common childhood infection, accounting for more physician visits than any other pediatric illness. The peak age of incidence is 6 to 36 months. About 30% to 50% of cases of AOM in this age group are caused by viruses; the remainder are bacterial in origin. The most common bacterial cause is *Streptococcus pneumoniae* (50%), followed by nontypeable *Haemophilus influenzae* (30%) and *Moraxella catarrhalis* (10% to 15%).

Uncomplicated AOM is usually treated with a 7- to 10-day course of high-dose oral amoxicillin, a safe and inexpensive medication with good coverage against *S. pneumoniae*. Recent recommendations include the option to manage symptomatically for 48 hours in children who appear well, adding antibiotics only if symptoms do not resolve. Treatment of resistant or recurrent otitis media may require a change in antibiotics, or preventive measures such as daily antibiotic therapy or ear tubes.

QUESTIONS

1-1. In addition to oral antibiotics, this patient with AOM should be treated with
- A. Antibiotic ear drops
- B. Tympanocentesis (drainage of fluid from the middle ear)
- C. Prophylactic antibiotics to prevent future episodes
- D. Medications for control of pain and fever

1-2. The most common complication of AOM is
- A. Ear pits
- B. Conductive hearing loss
- C. Mastoiditis
- D. Otitis externa

1-3. Which of the following is considered a risk factor for otitis media?

A. Family history of deafness
B. Caretaker smoking
C. Age <6 months
D. Breastfeeding

1-4. Otitis externa in the healthy child is typically caused by

A. *Staphylococcus* and *Streptococcus* species, and *Pseudomonas*
B. *Staphylococcus* and *Streptococcus* species, and fungus (e.g., *Candida*)
C. Viruses
D. *S. pneumoniae, H. influenzae,* and *M. catarrhalis*

ANSWERS

1-1. **D.** The only additional management strategy indicated in this patient with uncomplicated AOM is pain and fever control. Antibiotic otic drops (such as ciprofloxacin or Polysporin) are effective treatment for otitis externa and are often recommended for perforated AOM, but are not indicated in uncomplicated otitis media. If a child shows signs of systemic toxicity or intracranial spread of infection, admission for IV antibiotics, supportive care, and tympanocentesis for diagnostic or therapeutic purposes could be indicated. Recurrent otitis media (more than four episodes in a year, or three in 6 months) may be an indication for prophylactic antibiotics or therapeutic myringotomy (ear tubes). Otitis media that fails to respond to the initial antibiotic choice may respond to amoxicillin-clavulanic acid or a cephalosporin, which are options with additional coverage against *H. influenzae* and *M. catarrhalis.*

1-2. **B.** Conductive hearing loss is the most common complication of otitis media. Hearing loss is usually reversible with relief of negative pressure within the middle ear. If it is significant and occurs during the years in which language is developing, it may affect language acquisition and cognitive development. Additional complications include mastoiditis and chronic otitis media. Mastoiditis is an infection of the mastoid air cells, characterized by posterior auricular swelling over the mastoid process, which may displace the ear laterally. It is a potentially serious infection that should be treated with parenteral antibiotics, and imaging should be considered to document the extent of the infection. Chronic otitis, caused by anatomic predisposition to middle ear effusion or difficult-to-treat organisms, can be managed by the insertion of tubes or by prophylactic antibiotic therapy. Other rare but serious complications of otitis media include meningitis, brain abscess, and lateral sinus thrombosis. Ear pits, a congenital anomaly consisting of tiny holes anterior to the tragus that are occasionally associated with renal anomalies, are *not* a complication of otitis media.

Perforation of the TM, although relatively common, is not considered a complication of otitis media because it is usually self-resolving and does not require specific treatment. In fact, perforation is often accomplished intentionally in cases of chronic or recurrent otitis by the insertion of tympanostomy tubes.

1-3. B. Caretaker smoking is the only option that is a recognized risk factor for otitis media. Bottle feeding, especially in the horizontal position, day-care attendance, chronic middle ear effusion, lower socioeconomic status, male gender, and Native American or Eskimo ethnicity are other recognized risk factors. Breastfeeding is actually considered a protective factor against otitis media.

1-4. A. Otitis externa (OE) can be thought of as a cellulitis of the external ear canal. The usual organisms recovered are grampositive skin organisms (*Staphylococcus* and *Streptococcus* species) as well as *Pseudomonas*, which has a predilection for moist environments. For this reason, OE is usually treated with antibiotic ear drops with coverage against these organisms, such as ciprofloxacin or Polysporin otic solutions. These otic preparations often include a corticosteroid as well, which helps symptomatically with inflammation and discomfort. Although fungus can be found in the external ear canal in immunosuppressed patients or those with chronic otitis externa, it is not a typical pathogen.

 ## SUGGESTED ADDITIONAL READING

American Academy of Pediatrics Subcommittee on Management of Acute Otitis Media. Diagnosis and management of acute otitis media. *Pediatrics*. 2004;113(5):1451–1465.

McCormick DP, Chonmaitree T, Pittman C, et al. Nonsevere acute otitis media: a clinical trial comparing outcomes of watchful waiting versus immediate antibiotic treatment. *Pediatrics*. 2005;115:1455–1465.

Fever and Vomiting

CC/ID: 2½-year-old girl, brought in by her babysitter because of fever and vomiting.

HPI: A.D. developed a fever last night to 103°F, ate poorly, and vomited after dinner. This morning she vomited twice and continued to be febrile, although the fever came down temporarily with ibuprofen. Her babysitter brought her in because she is "lethargic" and complaining of a "tummy ache," and the fever has returned. She has not had diarrhea or constipation, cough or upper respiratory infection (URI) symptoms, difficulty breathing, or rash. A.D. has not complained of pain on urination, per her babysitter.

PMHx: None

Meds: None

All: NKDA

Immun: UTD

SHx: Noncontributory

FHx: Noncontributory

VS: Temp 38.9°C (102°F), HR 120, RR 25; Weight 17 kg (50%)

PE: *Gen:* a nontoxic but tired and uncomfortable-appearing girl. *HEENT:* mucous membranes are moist; oropharynx clear; no rhinorrhea; TMs normal. *Abdomen:* diffuse mild tenderness to palpation in the lower quadrants, without rebound or involuntary guarding. No focal areas of tenderness of the abdomen. Normal active bowel sounds; no hepatosplenomegaly. *GU:* normal prepubertal female genitalia, with no discharge or rashes. On percussion of the left flank, the child squirms and cries. Remainder of exam is within normal limits.

THOUGHT QUESTIONS

- What conditions are in your differential diagnosis at this point for this girl with fever, vomiting, and abdominal pain?
- What laboratory tests or studies would you obtain?

DISCUSSION

This child presents with fever, vomiting, and abdominal pain, a constellation of symptoms that suggests a wide variety of diagnoses. Briefly, the differential diagnosis should include infections of the GI and GU system, as well as obstructive and surgical conditions of those systems. Keep in mind that infections in other locations, such as pneumonia and streptococcal pharyngitis, can also present this way in a child.

Because the abdominal exam does not suggest an acute abdominal process, and the remainder of the exam is normal, serious infections or operative diagnoses are less likely. However, this history and the left flank pain are consistent with pyelonephritis (urinary tract infection, or UTI, involving the upper urinary tract), so a useful screening study at this point would be a urinalysis (UA). Urine specimens may be obtained by catheterizing the bladder, attaching a bag for collection, or by midstream clean catch, depending on the child's age and the urgency for diagnosis. UA may suggest UTI, but the gold standard for diagnosis is urine culture. Urine should be sent for culture when the history or UA suggests UTI, to confirm the diagnosis and identify the organism.

CASE CONTINUED

Urine is collected by bag, and the urinalysis shows the following: specific gravity of 1.020, 1+ blood, 1+ nitrites and 3+ leukocyte esterase; otherwise it is negative. A microscopy of the urine reveals 5 to 10 RBCs and 50 to 100 WBCs, as well as bacteria. The urine sample is sent for culture.

THOUGHT QUESTIONS

- What does this patient have?
- How would you manage her?

DISCUSSION

This patient's UA findings (leukocyte esterase, nitrites, 50–100 WBCs) suggest UTI. The clinical findings of flank pain and fever suggest pyelonephritis. UTI is the most common bacterial cause of fever without localizing signs in infants and children. Although children and adolescents with UTI may complain of dysuria, infants do not typically manifest this symptom and are more likely to present with nonspecific symptoms such as fever, poor feeding, vomiting, or abdominal pain. Infants are also more likely to have pyelonephritis with UTI.

The bacterial causes of urinary tract infections in children, similar to those in adults, are primarily fecal organisms, the most common being *Escherichia coli*. The goals of treatment of UTI are to eradicate the infecting organism and identify any conditions that may predispose the infant to serious or recurrent UTI. Uncomplicated UTI/pyelonephritis in the nontoxic child older than 3 months may be treated with a 10- to 14-day course of oral antibiotics; in the toxic or very young child, admission for intravenous therapy is recommended.

In high-risk infants and those with recurrent UTI, imaging of the urinary tract with ultrasound or voiding cystourethrogram (VCUG) or both is recommended to evaluate for anatomic abnormalities or vesicoureteral reflux (VUR) (Fig. 2-1). Severe VUR or anatomic abnormalities may predispose to recurrent UTI and possible renal scarring. The American Academy of Pediatrics (AAP) recommends imaging of the urinary tract in *all* infants younger than 2 years with their first UTI, but these guidelines are somewhat controversial because the evidence behind them is weak.

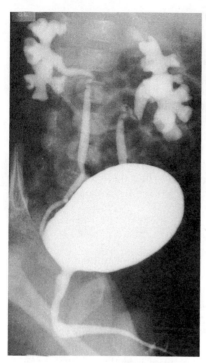

FIGURE 2-1.
Severe bilateral vesicoureteral reflux on voiding cystourethrogram. (*From Rudolf M, Levene M. Paediatrics and Child Health. Oxford: Blackwell Science; 1999:113, with permission.*)

QUESTIONS

2-1. If left untreated, recurrent pyelonephritis may result in
A. Renal scarring
B. Vesicoureteral reflux
C. Ureterocele
D. Neurogenic bladder

2-2. In addition to the proper antibiotic therapy, this patient's management should include
A. Close follow-up for subsequent UTI
B. Voiding cystourethrogram (VCUG)
C. An intravenous pyelogram (IVP)
D. Prophylactic antibiotics for 1 year

2-3. Typical findings on urinalysis that suggest UTI include
A. Ketones, glucose, and urobilinogen
B. Specific gravity greater than 1.025
C. pH less than 5.0
D. Leukocyte esterase and nitrites

2-4. You are taking care of a 5-week-old uncircumcised male infant who has a fever and no other symptoms. A catheterized urine specimen is cloudy, and the microscopy shows 100 to 200 WBCs. As you are discussing the likely diagnosis of pyelonephritis with the family, the infant becomes unarousable, his breathing seems shallow, his skin looks mottled with poor capillary refill, and his temperature reads 40.1°C. Your first priority should be to
A. Obtain blood and CSF for culture
B. Administer broad-spectrum antibiotics
C. Assess and stabilize ABCs (airway, breathing, and circulation)
D. Treat the fever to prevent a febrile seizure

ANSWERS

2-1. A. Renal scarring is a complication of untreated or recurrent pyelonephritis, which can lead to renal failure in severe cases. In patients in whom renal scarring is suspected, a nuclear study, the 2,3-dimercaptosuccinic acid (DMSA) scan, can be performed to document the presence of renal scarring. Renal abscesses and hypertension are other complications of untreated or recurrent UTI. These consequences are rare in isolated bladder infections, but increase in likelihood with recurrence and severity of infection, as well as with the presence of anatomic or functional abnormalities of the urinary tract. Vesicoureteral reflux, the most common functional urinary tract abnormality, is *not* a complication of UTI. It can occur from many causes and is associated with increased renal scarring in the setting of recurrent UTI. Because of the risk of recurrent and damaging UTI in children with urinary tract abnormalities and VUR, current guidelines recommend consideration of imaging to screen for these problems in selected populations (see AAP guidelines). Ureterocele and neurogenic bladder may both predispose an individual to UTI, but they are not considered consequences of UTI.

2-2. A. Renal imaging is not routinely recommended for girls older than 2 years with the first UTI. Although controversial, current guidelines recommend renal imaging after the first UTI in infants younger than 2 years. Imaging should also be considered in the setting of recurrent UTIs in all boys and in nonadolescent girls. The goal of renal imaging is to recognize structural or functional urinary tract abnormalities that could lead to further UTIs or renal damage. Ultrasound of kidneys, ureters, and bladder is an inexpensive, noninvasive study that demonstrates most structural abnormalities. Voiding cystourethrogram is a fluoroscopic study in which contrast is instilled into the bladder. Although more invasive than ultrasound, it is also more sensitive and specific for functional urinary tract anomalies, such as vesicoureteral reflux. Patients with documented VUR or anatomic abnormalities should be treated with prophylactic antibiotics and referred to a urologist for further management.

An IVP is not a recommended imaging modality for screening for urinary tract abnormalities in children. Prophylactic antibiotics would be indicated only in the setting of recurrent UTI, or if VUR were documented.

2-3. D. Leukocyte esterase and nitrites are the most sensitive and specific signs, respectively, of UTI on urinalysis. The microscopy often shows white cells and bacteria, and sometimes red cells. It is important to keep in mind that in young infants with UTI these urinalysis findings may not be present, because babies empty their bladders so quickly that the urine may not accumulate sufficient inflammation to turn the test positive. In addition, since these young infants are at such high risk of UTI, urine culture should always be sent to confirm the diagnosis, regardless of UA results. A catheter specimen is always preferable for this purpose, because it is less likely to contain contamination with bacteria or white cells found on the perineum that can affect the urinalysis and culture. However, in older children it is reasonable to obtain a clean catch or bag specimen first to avoid the trauma of bladder catheterization, and then consider catheterization if the urinalysis reveals numerous epithelial cells, suggesting contamination.

2-4. C. The described changes in the infant's appearance and vital signs suggest that the infant has developed urosepsis and is going into shock. Young infants are at especially high risk of this complication of pyelonephritis. Your first priority in this situation is to assess and stabilize the infant's airway, breathing and circulation (ABCs). This may include intubating to control the airway, obtaining additional intravenous access, and administering fluids and medications to stabilize blood pressure. These lifesaving measures should be prioritized above all other interventions. Although administration of antibiotics and obtaining of cultures should be done as soon as possible, these actions should not interfere with or prevent the control of the ABCs. Fever control is primarily for comfort and for decreased metabolic demands. Although febrile seizures are relatively common in infants, they are not a reason to emergently treat fever in an unstable patient.

SUGGESTED ADDITIONAL READING

Hoberman A. Oral versus initial intravenous therapy for urinary tract infections in young febrile children. *Pediatrics*. 1999;104 (1 pt 1):79–86.

Roberts KB. The AAP practice parameter on urinary tract infections in febrile infants and young children. American Academy of Pediatrics. *Am Fam Physician*. 2000;62(8):1815–1822.

Febrile Infant

CC/ID: 2-month-old boy is brought in by his parents for poor feeding and sleepiness.

HPI: T.J. had been well until yesterday, when he was noted to be sleepier than usual, and today he felt warm to the touch. Although usually a vigorous breastfeeder, he has been feeding only small amounts and vomited once. Today T.J. was difficult to arouse for feeds; his parents also note that the infant seems to be breathing quickly. The parents deny any history of runny nose, cough, rash, or diarrhea.

PMHx: Unremarkable birth history; no previous illnesses or hospitalizations.

Meds: None

All: NKDA

Immun: First set of shots (DTaP, Hib, HepB and pneumococcal vaccine) 4 days ago

SHx: 4-year-old brother and 6-year-old sister at home; both attend school and are healthy.

FHx: No family history of metabolic or cardiac disorders, or infant death.

VS: Temp 39.2°C (102.5°F), BP 75/40, HR 177 (110–150), RR 48 (25–40); Weight 6.1 kg (50%); O_2 saturation 99% on RA

PE: *Gen:* nontoxic but sleepy, somewhat pale infant who cries appropriately when you examine him. *HEENT:* fontanelle is soft but slightly sunken; no rhinorrhea; oropharynx and TMs normal. *Lungs:* tachypneic; lungs clear to auscultation bilaterally; no retractions or grunting. *CV:* tachycardic; no murmur; pulses 2 throughout; extremities are cool and pink, with capillary refill of 3 seconds. *Abdomen:* soft, without masses or tenderness. *GU:* circumcised male.

Skin: no rashes, jaundice, or petechiae. Remainder of exam is within normal limits.

THOUGHT QUESTIONS

- What diagnoses are you most concerned about in this febrile infant?
- What diagnostic workup would you pursue at this time?

DISCUSSION

This infant is well appearing ("nontoxic") but has a fever without an apparent source on physical exam (FWS). His tachycardia and tachypnea, which are important early signs of illness in an infant, may also be due to fever or dehydration. While performing the diagnostic workup, you can try to correct these conditions, which will help you to assess the infant's level of illness.

Although most fevers in young infants are caused by harmless viral infections or recent immunizations, studies have shown that even well-appearing young infants with FWS have a small but appreciable risk of pyelonephritis or serious bacterial infection (SBI). Pyelonephritis is far more likely than SBI and should be considered in all young infants with FWS. An individual infant's risk for SBI (which includes bacteremia and meningitis) can be stratified by age, immunization status, and total WBC count. For example, this 2-month-old infant's risk for SBI is about 3% to 6%. A WBC count >15 or <5 increases his risk to around 10%, whereas a normal WBC decreases it to around 1%. *Streptococcus pneumoniae* is the major cause of SBI in infants older than 1 month. Since immunization against this organism decreases the risk of SBI to <1%, a CBC is less likely to affect management in immunized infants. However, this infant is not considered immunized, since his vaccines were given too recently for him to have mounted an immune response. Lumbar puncture is recommended in all neonates and in any infant in whom meningitis is suspected based on history or examination.

CASE CONTINUED

A CBC and blood culture are sent, and urine is obtained by catheter for urinalysis and urine culture. While obtaining the blood, you decide to give the infant an intravenous bolus of normal saline (NS) and a dose of acetaminophen, after which the tachycardia and tachypnea resolve, and he appears pinker, smiles, and begins to breastfeed. The CBC comes back with a WBC count of 20,000 with 7% bands, 75% neutrophils, and 15% lymphocytes. The platelets, hemoglobin (Hb), and hematocrit (Hct) are within normal limits. The urinalysis is negative. Blood and urine cultures are pending.

THOUGHT QUESTIONS

- Which laboratory results raise the likelihood of SBI in this infant?
- How would you manage this infant?

DISCUSSION

The laboratory result of most concern is the elevated WBC count with left shift (75% neutrophils with bandemia). Febrile infants with a high WBC count are considered at higher risk of SBI. Based on his young age, well appearance, and high WBC count, current guidelines recommend the empiric treatment of this infant with broad-spectrum antibiotics with close follow-up until the final results of all cultures are obtained. In infants younger than 3 months, in whom clinical signs of meningitis may be subtle or absent, a lumbar puncture is highly recommended prior to starting antibiotics.

CASE CONTINUED

CSF is obtained and sent for culture. The CSF results shows 1 RBC, 0 WBC, glucose of 70 and protein of 32. Based on this reassuring result, you treat the infant with a nonmeningitic dose of ceftriaxone. The infant goes home, and returns to clinic the next day for a second dose of ceftriaxone. Later that day his blood culture grows a few colonies of *S. pneumoniae.* A repeat blood culture is performed in clinic, a third dose of ceftriaxone is given, and the patient is given a 10-day course of oral amoxicillin to treat his asymptomatic bacteremia. The second blood culture and the urine and CSF cultures remain negative, and the patient makes a complete recovery.

QUESTIONS

3-1. The most likely organisms to cause SBI in infants older than 1 month are
   A. *Streptococcus pneumoniae, Haemophilus influenzae* type b, *Neisseria meningitidis*
   B. *S. pneumoniae, Staphylococcus aureus, Staphylococcus epidermidis*
   C. Group B streptococcus, *Escherichia coli, Listeria monocytogenes*
   D. Group B streptococcus, *S. aureus, S. epidermidis*

3-2. You are evaluating a 6-month-old girl with a fever without a source. Which of the following is associated with an *increased* risk of SBI in this febrile child?
   A. Female gender
   B. Fever >40°C
   C. Presence of a profusely runny nose and cough
   D. Lower socioeconomic status

3-3. The 6-month-old child in Question 3-2 has received all three doses of the seven-valent pneumococcal vaccine. Her parents want to know how this vaccination affects her rate of infection. You can tell them that
   A. The vaccine is expected to reduce her risk of SBI by about 90%.
   B. The vaccine is expected to reduce her risk of SBI and pyelonephritis by about 90%.
   C. The vaccine is expected to reduce her risk of SBI and otitis media by about 90%.
   D. Although at decreased risk of SBI from pneumococcus, she is at increased risk of SBI from other organisms.

3-4. Sepsis can be differentiated from bacteremia by the presence of
   A. Fever >40°C
   B. A WBC count greater than 20,000 on CBC
   C. Hemodynamic instability and/or toxic appearance in the patient
   D. Presence of bacteria on Gram stain of blood

ANSWERS

3-1. A. The most likely organisms recovered from blood cultures in well-appearing infants with occult bacteremia are *S. pneumoniae*, *H. influenzae* type b, and *N. meningitidis*. Currently, *S. pneumoniae* accounts for the vast majority of cases, although its prevalence has decreased due to the recent initiation of routine vaccination of children older than 2 months against this organism. In neonates (younger than 1 month) with bacteremia or sepsis, group B streptococci, *E. coli*, and *L. monocytogenes* are the organisms most often recovered from blood cultures. Most cases of occult bacteremia with *S. pneumoniae* resolve spontaneously in 24 to 48 hours, but there is a 3% risk of developing meningitis.

3-2. B. Factors increasing the likelihood of SBI include higher fever, WBC count >15 (and <5 in young infants), and lack of immunization. Having an apparent source for fever, especially a named viral infection or distinct viral syndrome, decreases the likelihood of SBI. No particular ethnic, geographic, or socioeconomic factor has been found to correlate with higher risk of SBI.

3-3. A. Large prelicensure studies of efficacy of the seven-valent pneumococcal vaccine showed a decrease in invasive pneumococcal disease of 90% to 98% (Black et al., 2000). Postlicensure studies have supported these data. The incidence of otitis media in the vaccinated population is only slightly decreased (7% to 10%), because strains of pneumococci that cause this relatively benign infection were not included in the vaccine. The vaccine does not protect against pyelonephritis, since pneumococcus is not a major cause of this infection. There has not been an increase in invasive disease by nonvaccine serotypes, or by other organisms, since the vaccine was introduced.

3-4. C. Sepsis is defined as an invasion of the intravascular compartment by bacteria. This invasion results in excessive release of endogenous mediators, leading to the clinical features of sepsis: circulatory collapse (shock) and multiorgan system involvement. Blood cultures often remain negative, and the absence of a causative organism should not preclude the diagnosis. High fever and elevated white blood cell count often accompany sepsis, but they also occur in occult bacteremia and many viral infections. Sepsis is a medical emergency, and it must be identified and treated early to prevent mortality. It is important to keep in mind that children often compensate well for early shock with tachycardia and vasoconstriction, so the appearance of these signs in a febrile or ill-appearing child should alert the clinician to the possibility of sepsis. The most common causes of sepsis in the child aged 3 to 36 months are the same as those responsible for SBI.

 SUGGESTED ADDITIONAL READING

Baraff LJ. Management of fever without source in infants and children. *Ann Emerg Med*. 2000;36(6):602–614.

Black SB, Shinefield HR, Fireman B, et al. Efficacy, safety and immunogenicity of heptavalent pneumococcal conjugate vaccine in children. *Pediatr Infect Dis J*. 2000;19:187–195.

Fever and Adenopathy

CC/ID: 16-year-old girl comes into the clinic with a lump on her neck.

HPI: E.L. has been feeling sick and tired with a "flu" for about a week. She complains of chills and a very sore throat, and has been staying home from school. The sore throat makes it difficult to swallow, but she is able to keep down fluids. The lump showed up a few days ago and is tender. She is otherwise healthy, and no one at home is ill.

PMHx: Unremarkable

Meds: Ibuprofen for fever/pain

All: NKDA

Immun: UTD

SHx: Junior in high school; has a boyfriend but is not sexually active; denies drug use; wants to be an engineer. No significant family or travel history.

VS: Temp 39°C (102.2°F), BP 118/80, HR 92, RR 15; Weight 65 kg (80%)

PE: *Gen:* tired-appearing teen, slightly obese, with visible swelling on the left side of her neck. *HEENT:* Multiple 0.5- to 1-cm slightly tender lymph nodes are palpable bilaterally in the anterior cervical area. Among them on the left is a 2.5-cm mass that is soft, mobile, tender, and nonsuppurative. Oropharynx is remarkable for tonsillar injection with whitish exudate (Fig. 4-1). There is no nuchal rigidity, photophobia, or sinus tenderness, and no further lymphadenopathy is noted on exam. *Abdomen:* soft and nontender, without masses except for a palpable and slightly tender spleen tip on the left. Remainder of exam is within normal limits.

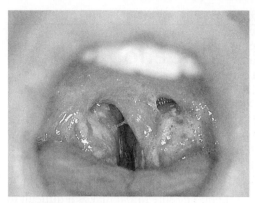

FIGURE 4-1.
Exudative tonsillitis, as might be seen in this patient. (*From Rudolf M, Levene M. Paediatrics and Child Health. Oxford: Blackwell Science; 1999:104, with permission.*)

THOUGHT QUESTIONS

- What is your differential diagnosis at this point?
- What laboratory tests or studies would you consider to help with your diagnosis?

DISCUSSION

This patient is a teen with fever and pharyngitis and an acutely enlarged and tender cervical mass, likely a lymph node. Mild cervical adenopathy is a common and usually benign finding in children, because the cervical nodes enlarge in reaction to many viral illnesses. However, asymmetric, hard, painful, or generalized adenopathy deserves further investigation, since the cause may be infection, malignancy, or a systemic illness. Most acute lymphadenopathy in children is infectious in origin. The most common causes are viruses, including Epstein-Barr virus (EBV), cytomegalovirus (CMV), adenovirus, and human immunodeficiency virus (HIV). Bacterial adenitis (suppurative infection of the lymph node) is most common in young children and is usually caused by Group A *Streptococcus* or *S. aureus* instead of gram-positive bacteria. Although subacute or chronic lymphadenopathy is also likely to be infectious in origin, noninfectious causes of neck masses, such as malignancy, autoimmune disease, and congenital malformations, should be more strongly considered in these cases.

In considering the differential diagnosis, it is important to take into account the age of the child, the acute versus chronic nature of the adenopathy, and whether the adenopathy is local or generalized. Associated findings such as rash, hepatosplenomegaly, and a history of recent illness or weight loss are also important to elicit. Laboratory tests and studies should be guided by the patient's presentation and by the suspicion of an infectious or noninfectious cause. This teen has symptoms suggestive of an acute viral illness, in particular, infectious mononucleosis. Other viral infections, bacterial adenitis, group A streptococcus (GAS) pharyngitis, and malignancy should also be considered. A CBC is a good initial screening tool for this broad differential, because it will identify signs of inflammation and basic immune function, both helpful in this case. More specific diagnostic tests include the Monospot, a heterophile antibody test for EBV infection that is available in most centers, and a throat swab for rapid GAS test and culture.

 ## CASE CONTINUED

Labs: CBC reveals WBC of 20,000 with 70% lymphocytes (15% atypical lymphs), Hct 38, and platelets 175. A Monospot test is positive; rapid GAS test is negative.

 ## THOUGHT QUESTIONS

- What does this patient have?
- How will you manage her?

 ## DISCUSSION

This patient's clinical picture and laboratory results support a diagnosis of acute infectious mononucleosis (IM) syndrome, usually caused by infection with EBV. Although EBV infection acquired in early childhood is usually subclinical, infection in adolescence or adulthood results in the classic IM syndrome of fever, exudative pharyngitis, and local or generalized lymphadenopathy. Profound malaise and fatigue often accompany the syndrome and may last for weeks to months. Treatment of IM is generally supportive, consisting of pain and fever control. In this patient, who has an enlarged and tender spleen, avoidance of contact sports should be advised.

QUESTIONS

4-1. E.L's mother wants to know how long she should stay out of soccer practice. You can answer her that E.L. should avoid contact sports until

A. Her Monospot test is negative
B. Her fever has resolved
C. She no longer has an enlarged and tender spleen
D. She is no longer suffering from fatigue

4-2. The most common reason for hospital admission due to EBV infection is

A. Splenic rupture
B. Neutropenia
C. Acute suppurative adenitis
D. Airway obstruction

4-3. A teen with symptoms similar to E.L is treated with amoxicillin by a physician who thinks she has strep throat. Several days later she develops a blanching, erythematous maculopapular rash over her trunk that is mildly pruritic. A subsequent Monospot test is positive. This rash is *most* likely to be

A. An allergic reaction to amoxicillin
B. A toxin-mediated rash caused by group A streptococcus
C. A viral exanthem typically seen during EBV infection
D. Caused by antipenicillin antibodies produced during EBV infection

4-4. A previously healthy 2-year-old child presents with a 2-day history of a painful, red, swollen cervical lymph node. What is the most likely cause?

A. Group A streptococcus
B. Tuberculosis
C. Anaerobic organisms
D. Catscratch disease (*Bartonella henselae*)

ANSWERS

4-1. C. In patients with IM syndrome who have an enlarged and tender spleen, avoidance of contact sports is advised because of the rare but serious complication of splenic rupture. This avoidance should be continued until the spleen is no longer enlarged and tender.

4-2. D. Complications of EBV infection are relatively common, but most are transient and relatively benign. Airway obstruction is the most common cause for hospital admissions related to EBV infection. This complication is of particular concern in young children because their already small airways are more susceptible to obstruction by swollen pharyngeal tissue. Hematologic complications, which include neutropenia, thrombocytopenia, and hemolytic anemia, are quite common and are usually transient. Steroids have been shown to be helpful in treating hematologic and airway obstructive complications. Splenic rupture is a rare but serious complication of EBV or CMV infection, so contact sports should be avoided as a preventive measure in patients with an enlarged or tender spleen. Hepatitis, usually asymptomatic with elevated transaminases, is another common but usually transient complication. Immunosuppressed individuals, especially after transplant surgery, are at risk of reactivation of dormant EBV, which contributes to lymphoproliferative disorder. Other rare complications include encephalitis, cerebellitis, and cranial neuritis.

4-3. D. The rash is most likely an antibody-mediated reaction to amoxicillin that occurs in up to 100% of older IM patients receiving penicillins. A transient increase in penicillin-specific IgM antibodies during EBV infection is likely responsible. A viral exanthem can also occur with IM in patients *not* receiving antibiotics, but is much less common.

4-4. A. Unilateral suppurative adenitis in young children is usually bacterial in origin, and the most common organisms are *Streptococcus pyogenes* and *Staphylococcus aureus*. In older children, anaerobes (often arising from dental or periodontal disease) and mycobacteria, as well as *Toxoplasma gondii* and *Bartonella henselae*, become the more likely organisms. Suspected staphylococcal or streptococcal adenitis in a nontoxic child should be treated with a course of oral first-generation cephalosporin, such as cephalexin, or another antibiotic with good staphylococcal and streptococcal coverage. Incision and drainage may be necessary if the node is very large or does not respond to appropriate oral therapy.

SUGGESTED ADDITIONAL READING

Junker AK. Epstein-Barr virus. *Pediatr Rev.* 2005;26(3):79–85.
Peters TR, Edwards KM. Cervical lymphadenopathy and adenitis. *Pediatr Rev.* 2000;21:399–405.

Yeh B. Evidence-based emergency medicine/systematic review
    abstract. Should sore throats be treated with antibiotics?
    Ann Emerg Med. 2005;45(1):82–84.

High Fever in a Toddler

 CC/ID: 15-month-old girl is brought in by her mother for a fever and refusal to drink.

HPI: J.M. was well until last night, when she felt hot to the touch and refused her bottle. After some acetaminophen, she seemed better and drank well. Mom also noticed "spots" on her hands and a diaper rash. Since this morning J.M. has been pushing away her bottle and has been fussy. Mom measured her temperature at 104°F rectally and gave another half dose of acetaminophen. Although the child "doesn't seem sick," Mom brought her in because she was concerned about giving so much medicine.

PMHx: Normal birth history; no prior hospitalizations or serious illnesses.

Meds: Tylenol for fever

All: NKDA

Immun: UTD to 1 year

SHx: Lives with single mother; attends day care. No current sick contacts at home.

FHx: 6-year-old brother has asthma.

THOUGHT QUESTIONS

- What will you look for on the examination of this patient?
- How can you evaluate her hydration status, since she has not been drinking well?

DISCUSSION

This child appears well but has a high fever, so you must try to establish an identifiable viral or bacterial source for the fever, and consider the possibility of occult infection or bacteremia. Many viral syndromes may be identified by subtle findings hidden in the mouth or on the skin (including palms and soles), so your search for a fever source should include careful examination of these areas as well as the ears, throat, and lungs.

Assessment of hydration status includes a thorough history of fluid intake and output. For example, to get 60% of fluid needs, a child should take a minimum of 2 oz/kg/day orally for the first 10 kg of weight, an additional 1 oz/kg/day for the next 10 kg, and an additional ½ oz/kg/day for weight over 20 kg. Infants and children should urinate at least every 6 to 8 hours. Intake or output below these minimums should raise concern for dehydration. Physical exam for hydration should include assessment of mucous membranes, tear production, skin turgor and perfusion, and vital signs.

CASE CONTINUED

J.M has urinated twice in the last 12 hours, and she has had one normal stool. Her total intake in the last 24 hours has been two 8-oz bottles of milk and 6 oz of juice, but no solids.

VS: Temp 39.9°C (104°F), HR 140, RR 30; Weight 12 kg (80%)

PE: *Gen:* fussy but consolable girl, drooling and occasionally mouthing her bottle, then pushing it away. *HEENT:* TMs clear bilaterally; crying tears; moist mucous membranes. The oropharynx is remarkable for several shallow grayish vesicles on posterior oropharynx, and one on the base of the tongue. There are no lip lesions. *Lungs:* CTA(B); no stridor, grunting, flaring, or retracting. *Skin:* Capillary refill is brisk, <3 seconds, and the skin is well-perfused. Careful examination of hands and feet reveals several shallow, linear gray vesicles on the fingers of both hands, and one on the left sole (Fig. 5-1). The perineum is remarkable for a diffuse mildly erythematous maculopapular rash.

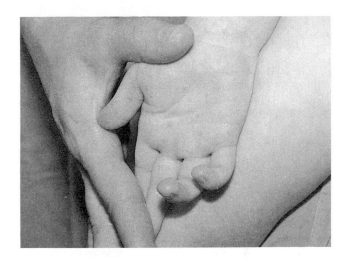

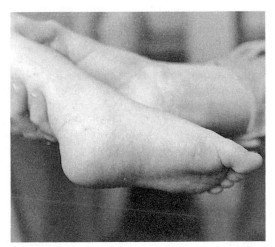

FIGURE 5-1. Appearance of lesions on this patient's extremities. (*From Banniser B, Begg N, Gillespie S. Infectious Disease. 2nd ed. Oxford: Blackwell Science; 2000:plate 5.10, with permission.*)

THOUGHT QUESTIONS

- What is your differential diagnosis and most likely diagnosis?
- What is the most likely morbidity from this condition, and how will you manage it?

DISCUSSION

The differential diagnosis in this case should include several common viral illnesses associated with rash and/or oral findings, including parvovirus (fifth disease), human herpesvirus 6 (roseola), herpes simplex virus (HSV), measles, and varicella. Nonviral illnesses in the differential diagnosis include Kawasaki syndrome and toxic shock syndrome. This patient, however, has the classic findings of infection by coxsackie virus A, otherwise known as hand-foot-and-mouth disease.

Most prevalent in the spring and summer, infection with coxsackie virus causes a prodrome of high fever and oral pain ("herpangina"). Typical skin and oral findings follow, which include painful, shallow, linear grayish or whitish vesicles on the posterior oropharynx and posterior third of the tongue, and similar but usually painless lesions on the palms and soles. The presentation may include some or all of these findings. The diagnosis of this infection is clinical and can be easily missed without a thorough physical examination. The primary morbidity from hand-foot-and-mouth disease is dehydration.

QUESTIONS

5-1. The most appropriate intervention to make at this time for this patient is
   A. Recommend oral and/or topical pain medications
   B. Prescribe antiviral medication
   C. Administer IV fluids
   D. Admit for observation

5-2. A "slapped-cheek" rash is classically seen with infection by
   A. Measles virus
   B. Rubella virus
   C. HHV-6 (roseola)
   D. Parvovirus B19 (fifth disease)

5-3. Although varicella (chickenpox) is usually self-limited in children, the most common complication is
A. Bacterial infection of skin lesions
B. Disseminated varicella infection
C. Encephalitis
D. Pneumonia

5-4. The routine childhood viral vaccinations include MMR, polio, hepatitis A and B, and
A. Herpes simplex virus (HSV)
B. Parvovirus
C. Varicella
D. HHV-6 (roseola)

ANSWERS

5-1. A. Pain and fever control and ensuring adequate hydration are the mainstays of management of hand-foot-and-mouth syndrome. Adequate doses of oral antipyretics/analgesics such as acetaminophen or ibuprofen are usually quite effective against pain. Aspirin should be avoided because of the association between viral illnesses and Reye syndrome. Some practitioners prescribe a topical mixture of Benadryl, Maalox, and viscous lidocaine ("magic mouthwash"), which may be swabbed onto the mouth prior to feeding to help with pain. Parents should encourage hydration with cool liquids and soft foods, and be taught how to identify signs of dehydration. Antivirals are not effective against coxsackie virus infections. Although dehydration is the most common complication of this syndrome, this child is not currently clinically dehydrated, so IV hydration would not be indicated. Most patients with this syndrome can be managed as outpatients with good supportive care.

5-2. D. Parvovirus B19 (i.e., erythema infectiosum, slapped-cheek rash, fifth disease) is a usually mild viral syndrome consisting of a low-grade fever followed by a rash that evolves in three stages. The first stage is marked erythema of the cheeks (a slapped-cheek appearance), which may be accompanied by circumoral pallor. The second is a maculopapular rash that begins on the arms and spreads to the trunk and legs and may take on a reticulated or livedo appearance. The third stage lasts several weeks and consists of fluctuations in the appearance and severity of the rash, often in relation to light or heat exposure. Although self-limited in healthy children, parvovirus infections may cause a hemolytic anemia, which can precipitate an aplastic crisis in patients with sickle cell disease, and cause fetal hydrops if acquired during pregnancy.

Human herpesvirus 6 (i.e., HHV-6, roseola, exanthem subitum, sixth disease), one of the most common viral exanthems of childhood, consists of a prodrome of 1 to 5 days of high fever, followed on day 3 to 4 by a rose-colored macular rash that begins on the trunk and spreads to the periphery. Appearance of the rash is accompanied by resolution of the fever. The illness is benign but may be associated with febrile seizures due to the rapid rise of the fever.

Measles (rubeola) virus causes a clinical syndrome that occurs in three stages: (1) *Prodrome* consists of fever and the three Cs (cough, coryza, conjunctivitis). (2) *Koplik spots* (pathognomonic, white, 1- to 2-mm macules on an erythematous base), often with bluish flecks, are found on the buccal mucosa 2 to 3 days after the onset of fever, and 2 days before the rash. (3) *Rash*, which starts on the forehead or behind the ears, consists of discrete erythematous papules that coalesce and spread downward, lasting 6 to 7 days and potentially undergoing desquamation. Although measles is now uncommon in the United States due to vaccination practices, sporadic epidemics still occur. The illness is usually self-limited, but complications include pneumonia, laryngitis, myocarditis, pericarditis, and thrombocytopenic purpura.

5-3. A. Varicella (i.e., chickenpox, zoster) is generally a self-limited viral infection in healthy children. The most common complication is bacterial superinfection of the skin, usually with *Staphylococcus* and *Streptococcus* species. Severe bacterial infections of the skin can rarely lead to disseminated varicella infection or necrotizing fasciitis. Disseminated infection can occur in immunocompromised children or those on immunosuppressive drugs. Varicella pneumonia is a rare complication in children, with 90% of cases occurring in the adult population. Central nervous system complications, including encephalitis, Guillain-Barré syndrome, and acute cerebellar ataxia, have been reported, but are rare. Other rare complications include hepatitis, thrombocytopenia, and myocarditis.

Treatment with acyclovir is recommended for immunocompromised children, those with chronic severe skin conditions such as atopic dermatitis, newborns, and teenagers because these groups are at risk for more severe infection and complications.

Clinically, infection with varicella virus is followed in 7 to 10 days by a mild fever and malaise accompanied by crops of characteristic pruritic vesicles, beginning on the trunk and spreading peripherally. The lesions begin as red papules, develop a clear vesicle with a "teardrop on a rose petal" appearance, and then become cloudy, break, and become excoriated to form crusts or scabs. Lesions in various stages of development are typically present (Fig. 5-2). The vesicles may occur on mucous membranes as well, including the cornea. Patients are infectious from 24 hours prior to the onset of the rash until all of the lesions are crusted.

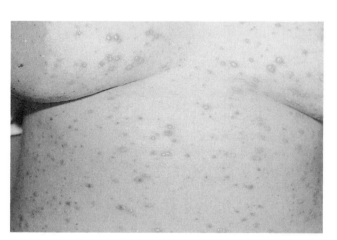

FIGURE 5-2. Typical vesicular rash of varicella infection. (*From Banniser B, Begg N, Gillespie S. Infectious Disease. 2nd ed. Oxford: Blackwell Science; 2000:plate 11.10, with permission.*)

5-4. C. Varicella is the only listed virus that is part of the routine childhood immunization schedule (Table 5-1). The most current childhood vaccination schedule can be found online at http://www.cdc.gov/nip/recs/child-schedule.htm.

TABLE 5-1 Example of Childhood Immunization Schedule[a]

Age	Hepatitis B (HepB)[b]	Diphtheria, Tetanus, Acellular Pertussis (DTaP)	Haemophilus influenza Type b (Hib)	Inactivated Polio Vaccine (IPV)	Seven-valent Pneumococcal Conjugate Vaccine (PCV-7)	Measles, Mumps, Rubella (MMR)	Varicella (Var)
Birth	HepB						
2 mo	HepB	DTaP	Hib	IPV	PCV-7		
4 mo		DTaP	Hib	IPV	PCV-7		
6 mo		DTaP	Hib		PCV-7		
6–18 mo	HepB			IPV			
12–15 mo			Hib		PCV-7	MMR	Var[c]
15–18 mo		DTaP					
4–6 y		DTaP		IPV		MMR	

[a]This schedule may vary depending on timing of visits and use of combination vaccines (e.g., HepB/Hib and HepB/IPV/DTaP).
[b]In some states, hepatitis A vaccine is also given routinely. It is given in two doses, starting at age 2 years.
[c]MMR and varicella must be given together, or at least 1 month apart.

SUGGESTED ADDITIONAL READING

Nguyen HQ, Jumaan AO, Seward JF. Decline in mortality due to varicella after implementation of varicella vaccination in the United States. *N Engl J Med.* 2005;352(5):450–458.

Fever and Irritability

CC/ID: 6-month-old boy brought in to the clinic for fever and crying for 3 hours.

HPI: B.C., who had been previously healthy, vomited after feeding this morning and since then has been inconsolable. He refused feeds the rest of the day, vomited twice more, and has been crying "as if something is hurting him." Just before taking him to the clinic, his mother noticed that his face felt hot, but that his hands and feet were cold. B.C. has had "a cold" for a couple of days, but has been otherwise well.

PMHx: Normal birth history; no complications; no illness or hospitalizations.

Meds: None

All: NKDA

Immun: Parents have elected not to immunize their three children, who have "always been healthy."

SHx: 3-year-old brother had an ear infection recently; otherwise, the family is healthy.

VS: Temp 40.1°C (104.1°F), HR 180 (110–130), RR 56 (30–40), BP 60/40

PE: *Gen:* lethargic male infant who is very irritable when touched or moved, arching his back with a shrill cry. He is not consolable. *HEENT:* anterior fontanelle bulging and firm; mucous membranes slightly dry; oropharynx clear; no lymphadenopathy. *Lungs:* tachypneic; lungs are clear. *CV:* tachycardic; no murmurs; extremities cool, with capillary refill 4–5 seconds. *Skin:* mottled appearance; no rashes or petechiae. *Neuro:* nonfocal exam; symmetric in tone and strength.

THOUGHT QUESTIONS

- What diagnoses are you most concerned about in this infant?
- What would be your initial approach to this patient's diagnosis and management?

DISCUSSION

In this febrile, irritable, and toxic-appearing infant you should be most concerned about meningitis, sepsis, or another serious invasive bacterial infection. Meningitis in particular is suggested due to the bulging fontanelle and irritability. Nuchal rigidity is difficult to assess and rarely presents in infants because of their short necks and open fontanelle. This infant's presenting signs and symptoms can also be seen in nonbacterial (aseptic) meningitis, toxic ingestion, and conditions causing increased ICP, such as an intracranial hemorrhage, abscess, or mass.

As in any ill-appearing infant, your first concern should be the ABCs (airway, breathing, and circulation). Thus, measures should be taken immediately to ensure adequate ventilation and hemodynamic stability. Further workup and treatment should occur in a timely fashion following stabilization of the patient. Because you are primarily concerned about infection, a CBC and cultures of blood, urine, and CSF should be obtained, preferably before the administration of antibiotics. Recent evidence suggests that corticosteroids, when given prior to antibiotics, may help improve the outcome of bacterial meningitis in infants and children.

CASE CONTINUED

After ensuring that the infant's airway and breathing are secure, you obtain IV access quickly and administer a bolus of normal saline (NS) and a dose of dexamethasone. This improves the infant's perfusion and blood pressure. Meanwhile, you draw a CBC and blood culture, obtain urine by catheter, and perform a lumbar puncture. Immediately after obtaining all cultures, you give the patient a dose of IV ceftriaxone and vancomycin for broad-spectrum coverage against gram-positive and gram-negative organisms. Soon afterward, the lab calls with the results of the lumbar puncture: the

WBC count is 700 with 95% neutrophils, and the RBC count is 2, with a total protein of 150 and glucose of 25 (Table 6-1). Gram-positive diplococci are seen on Gram stain of the CSF.

TABLE 6-1   Acceptable Normal Range of CSF Values in Infants and Children

Age	WBC/mm³	Protein	Glucose
Preterm neonate	0–10	<120	>60% of serum
Neonate (0–4 wk)	0–20	<100	>60% of serum
Infant/child (>4 wk)	0–5	<45	>50% of serum

THOUGHT QUESTIONS

- What does this patient have?
- How will you manage him?

DISCUSSION

This patient's clinical and CSF findings are consistent with acute bacterial meningitis (Fig. 6-1). The most likely cause is *Streptococcus pneumoniae*, based on the Gram stain results. This dangerous infection, with a mortality of 1% to 8% after the neonatal period, occurs when invasive bacteria gain access to the CSF. Risk factors for meningitis include otitis media, sinusitis, CSF leak (e.g., from skull fracture), and immunodeficiency (e.g., sickle cell disease, AIDS). The prognosis with early diagnosis and treatment is good, but as many as 50% of patients will have some neurodevelopmental sequelae. The seven-valent pneumococcal vaccine, which is now part of the routine vaccination schedule, has reduced the incidence of pneumococcal meningitis in infants and children.

Patients with acute bacterial meningitis should be hospitalized for IV antibiotic therapy and observation for increased intracranial pressure, seizures, or other neurologic sequelae. Audiologic testing should be performed prior to discharge and on follow-up evaluations. For meningitis caused by *Haemophilus influenzae* or *Neisseria meningitidis*, prophylaxis of family members and close contacts is indicated.

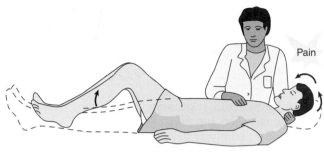

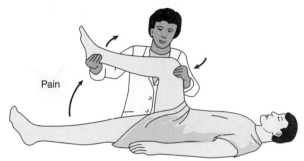

FIGURE 6-1. In the older child, signs of meningeal irritation include nuchal rigidity and positive Brudzinski's and Kernig's signs. **A:** Brudzinski's sign: With patient supine, flex the head upward, stretching the meninges. Resulting flexion of hips, knees, and ankles indicates meningeal irritation. **B:** Kernig's sign: With patient supine, flex one hip and flex knee to 90 degrees, and then slowly extend the lower leg, stretching the meninges. Resistance to further extension indicates meningeal irritation.

 QUESTIONS

6-1. The most common causes of bacterial meningitis in children over 1 month old are

A. *S. pneumoniae, N. meningitidis*, and *H. influenzae* type B

B. *Escherichia coli*, group B streptococcus, and *Listeria*

C. *S. pneumoniae*, nontypeable *H. influenzae*, and *Moraxella catarrhalis*

D. *S. pneumoniae, S. aureus*, and *Pseudomonas aeruginosa*

6-2. The most common significant sequela of meningitis in children is
- A. Sensorineural hearing loss
- B. Mental retardation
- C. Seizures
- D. Paralysis

6-3. Lumbar puncture is contraindicated in an infant who
- A. Is younger than 1 month
- B. Has focal neurologic deficits on exam
- C. Has a bulging fontanelle on exam
- D. Has already been treated with antibiotics

6-4. The primary cause of aseptic (nonbacterial) meningitis in children is
- A. Varicella-zoster virus (VZV)
- B. *Cryptococcus*
- C. Enterovirus
- D. Herpes simplex virus (HSV)

ANSWERS

6-1. A. The most common bacterial causes of meningitis in the infant or child are *S. pneumoniae*, *N. meningitidis*, and *H. influenzae* type B. Immunizations for all three exist, but only *H. influenzae* and *S. pneumoniae* are currently part of the routine immunization schedule. The pneumococcal vaccine has been routine since August 2000 and has already caused a significant reduction in pneumococcal meningitis. The bacteria listed in option B are the most common causes of meningitis in the neonate, and those listed in C are causes of otitis media. Although not listed, tuberculous meningitis is an indolent form of bacterial meningitis that must be suspected in a child who does not respond as expected to appropriate therapy.

6-2. A. Sensorineural hearing loss is the most common significant sequela of meningitis in children, occurring in as many as 30% of patients with pneumococcal meningitis. Severe neurodevelopmental disability (e.g., seizures, mental retardation) occurs in 10% to 20% of patients. As many as 50% may have some mild neurobehavioral morbidity, which may include subtle changes such as language delay and behavioral issues. Several recent studies suggest that corticosteroids, when administered prior to or concomitantly with antibiotics in the acute phase, may reduce mortality and neurodevelopmental morbidity in children with *S. pneumoniae* and *H. influenzae* meningitis.

6-3. B. Lumbar puncture is contraindicated in an patient suspected of having a mass-occupying lesion in the brain. Mass shift caused by an expanding mass can predispose the patient to herniation with lumbar puncture. Therefore, any patient with focal neurologic deficits or a clinical picture suggestive of an intracranial mass should have a head CT done before lumbar puncture to exclude mass shift. Other contraindications include hemodynamic instability and skin infection over the lumbar puncture site.

6-4. C. Enterovirus is the primary cause of aseptic meningitis in children. Other viruses, including HSV, VZV, mumps, EBV, and arboviruses, can all infect the central nervous system and cause meningitis or encephalitis. Cryptococcal meningitis is uncommon in immunocompetent children, but can occur in those with HIV, malignancy, or other forms of immunosuppression. The long-term prognosis of aseptic meningitis depends on the cause of the infection and the health of the child, but is generally more favorable than that of bacterial meningitis. Acute complications such as increased intracranial pressure and seizures occur in about 10% of children with enteroviral disease. As with bacterial meningitis, audiologic and neurodevelopmental evaluation should be part of routine follow-up examinations.

 SUGGESTED ADDITIONAL READING

Chaudhuri A. Adjunctive dexamethasone treatment in acute bacterial meningitis. *Lancet Neurol.* 2004;3(1):54–62.

Prolonged Fever

CC/ID: 33-month-old boy brought in for a fever that "won't go away."

HPI: T.R. is a previously healthy toddler whose father brought him in because he has had a fever for the last 7 days and now is refusing to eat or drink. Initially his parents thought he had "the flu" and were treating the fever with acetaminophen, but it keeps coming back. Dad was concerned because now his lips look very dry and he has been "crying all the time." He also is wondering if his hands hurt because they look swollen. Dad reports that the child has taken only 2 ounces of juice since this morning and has urinated once, a small amount.

PMHx: No major illnesses; usually a healthy and active boy.

Meds: Acetaminophen for fever

All: Peanuts

Immun: UTD

THOUGHT QUESTIONS

- What categories of illness are you concerned about in this toddler with a persistent fever?
- What additional historical physical or lab findings will you seek to help you in your diagnosis?

DISCUSSION

In any child with an acute febrile illness, <u>infection</u> is the most common etiology. However, other categories of illness, such as <u>malignancy</u> and <u>rheumatologic disease</u>, can cause <u>inflammation or</u>

immune dysregulation that can cause fever. Noninfectious causes of fever become more likely with longer duration of fever, and with the involvement of multiple organ systems. A fever of unknown origin is defined as fever without clear etiology for more than 14 days.

When noninfectious causes for fever are suspected, a careful physical exam can help to localize stigmata of various disease entities. Certain patterns of involvement of joints, lymph nodes, skin, and internal organs (spleen, liver) can suggest malignancy or rheumatologic/autoimmune disease. For example, rheumatologic disease often presents with joint involvement, whereas malignancy is often suggested by generalized lymphadenopathy. Other important historical findings include weight loss, decrease in energy or appetite, pattern of fever, and family history. Laboratory tests that confirm inflammation, such as elevated ESR or WBC count, are supportive but nonspecific. When the cause of prolonged fever remains unclear, laboratory testing should be targeted toward the etiologies most suggested by the history and physical exam.

 CASE CONTINUED

On further history, Dad says that before this illness T.R. had been feeling well. The fever is persistent, recurring whenever the acetaminophen wears off, and typically reaching 103°F. There is a family history of migraine headaches and adult-onset diabetes.

VS: Temp 39.8°C (103.5°F), HR 165, RR 32; Weight 15 kg (75%)

PE: *Gen:* fussy and crying when touched; somewhat consolable. *HEENT:* bilateral conjunctivitis, sparing a ring around the iris; no eye discharge. Lips are dry, cracked. Tongue red, inflamed; no other oropharyngeal lesions. Neck is supple; bilateral shotty cervical adenopathy with one 2-cm node noted on the right. *Abdomen:* soft, nontender; no masses. *Skin:* well-perfused with brisk capillary refill; blanching, maculopapular rash noted on trunk and perineum. *Ext:* hands and feet appear edematous and erythematous. No joint redness, swelling, or pain.

Labs: *CBC:* WBC 17.4, Hb 11.4, Hct 34, Plat 675. *Lytes:* All WNL, except albumin of 2.2 (low). *Urine:* 50–100 WBC; no bacteria; no blood. *ESR:* 36 (NL: 5–15).

THOUGHT QUESTIONS

- What is this child's most likely diagnosis?
- What is the most serious complication of this child's illness, and how will you prevent it?

DISCUSSION

This child meets the clinical criteria for Kawasaki disease (KD). KD is a vasculitis of unknown etiology, affecting primarily medium-sized arteries. It occurs almost exclusively in the pediatric population. Diagnosis is by clinical criteria: fever for 5 or more days, plus four of five additional criteria (rash, mucous membrane involvement, unilateral cervical adenopathy, nonpurulent conjunctivitis, and swollen hands and feet). Other common clinical findings are seen in Figure 7-1. Typical lab findings include hypoalbuminemia, thrombocytosis, and elevated ESR. The primary morbidity of Kawasaki disease is its cardiac complications, which include coronary vasculitis and aneurysm formation leading to arrhythmias, infarction, congestive heart failure, and even death. KD is the leading cause of acquired heart disease in children in the United States and Japan. Treatment of the syndrome with high-dose aspirin and 1 to 2 days of intravenous immunoglobulin (IVIG) significantly reduces the risk of cardiac complications.

Fever for ≥ 5 days
plus:

4/5 {
Rash
Mucous membrane involvement (strawberry tongue)
Unilateral cervical LA
Nonpurulent conjunctivitis
Swollen hands/feet
}

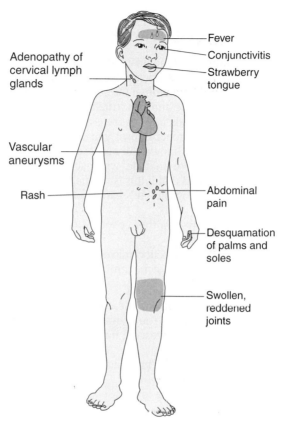

FIGURE 7-1. Some clinical findings associated with Kawasaki disease.

QUESTIONS

7-1. T.R. is admitted to the hospital and receives 2 g/kg of IVIG and high-dose aspirin. An echocardiogram reveals a normal heart with no evidence of inflammation of the coronary arteries. With treatment, T.R. becomes afebrile and less irritable, his rash fades, his lips begin to heal, and his hands and feet return to near-normal appearance. At discharge, his parents inform you that they are moving to another state, and want to know if he needs any particular follow-up care. You should tell them that he will need an echocardiogram 1 week after discharge and that if this is normal, then

    A. T.R. has been completely treated, and only routine care is needed.

    B. T.R. should have another echocardiogram 6 to 8 weeks after discharge.

    C. T.R. should have an echocardiogram with every febrile illness.

    D. T.R. should have an echocardiogram once per year for the rest of his life.

7-2. T.R.'s nurse asks you if there are any discharge medications you would like to order. You should tell him that

    A. Since T.R. has defervesced, no outpatient medications are needed.

    B. T.R. will need to take low-dose aspirin daily for at least 6 to 8 weeks.

    C. T.R. will need to take low-dose aspirin daily for the rest of his life.

    D. T.R. will need monthly infusions of IVIG for 1 year.

7-3. You become interested in vasculitides of childhood, and read about one called Henoch-Schönlein purpura (HSP). This syndrome affects mostly small vessels, and classically presents with abdominal pain, hematuria, and a rash best described as

    A. Painful, linear vesicles of the palms and soles

    B. A rough, pruritic, sandpaperlike rash over the trunk and extremities

    C. Nonblanching purplish macules and papules over the buttocks and lower extremities

    D. Pinpoint, nonblanching macules over the face and trunk

7-4. The primary morbidity of HSP is
  A. Vascular necrosis in the distal extremities
  B. Superinfection of skin lesions
  C. Glomerulonephritis, rarely progressing to renal failure
  D. A chronic, relapsing course

ANSWERS

7-1. B. In patients who are not known to have coronary artery disease, current recommendations include an echocardiogram at 1 week after discharge, and another in 6 to 8 weeks. If these are negative, some patients are still followed by a cardiologist for about 1 year. However, development of coronary artery disease after a normal echocardiogram 6 to 8 weeks postdischarge is rare.

7-2. B. KD is associated with thrombocytosis, usually occurring after the first week of illness, so low-dose aspirin is recommended as an antiplatelet agent after discharge until coronary artery disease is ruled out. This therapy is usually continued for a minimum of 6 to 8 weeks, and discontinued when the platelet count is normal, follow-up echocardiogram is negative, and no further signs of inflammation remain. Patients with documented coronary disease should remain on low-dose aspirin for the rest of their lives. IVIG has not been shown to have utility after the initial febrile period of illness, and should not be given monthly to KD patients with no complications.

7-3. C. The rash of HSP consists of palpable or flat purpuric lesions occurring primarily on the buttocks and lower extremities (Fig. 7-2). The rash is quite recognizable and is present in nearly 90% of cases of HSP. Painful, linear vesicles of the palms and soles occur with coxsackie virus infection. A sandpaperlike rash is associated with streptococcal scarlet fever. Pinpoint nonblanching macules of the face and trunk are consistent with petechiae, which can be traumatic (from coughing or vomiting) but are also an important sign of infection or platelet dysfunction/thrombocytopenia.

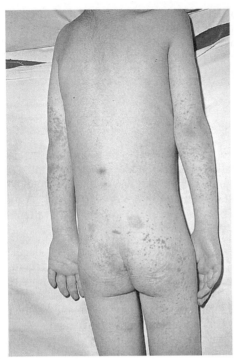

(a)

FIGURE 7-2.
Typical palpable, nonblanching rash of Henoch-Schönlein purpura (HSP). (*From Rudolf M, Levene M. Paediatrics and Child Health. Oxford: Blackwell Science; 1999:200, with permission.*)

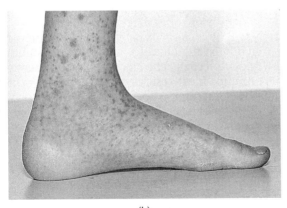

(b)

7-4. C. HSP is primarily a self-limited illness that does not usually cause long-term sequelae. Most cases resolve completely. Glomerulonephritis, which can rarely progress to renal failure, is the primary complication. Severity of renal involvement is the primary predictor of morbidity. Since multiple systems are involved in this systemic vasculitis, rare complications can occur from inflammation in other organ systems. One example is the GI tract, where inflammation of the bowel wall can act as a lead point for intussusception.

 SUGGESTED ADDITIONAL READING

Dedeoglu F. Vasculitis in children. *Pediatr Clin North Am.* 2005;52(2):547–575, vii.

Newburger JW, Takahashi M, Gerber MA, et al. Diagnosis, treatment, and long-term management of Kawasaki disease: a statement for health professionals from the Committee on Rheumatic Fever, Endocarditis, and Kawasaki Disease, Council on Cardiovascular Disease in the Young, American Heart Association. *Pediatrics.* 2004;110(17):2747–2771.

Oates-Whitehead RM, Baumer JH, Haines L, et al. Intravenous immunoglobulin for the treatment of Kawasaki disease in children. *Cochrane Database Syst Rev.* 2003;(4):CD004000.

II

Cases Presenting with Respiratory Distress

Infant with Cough

CC/ID: 15-month-old boy with cough and difficulty breathing is brought in by his mother.

HPI: B.B. presents with a 4-day history of rhinorrhea, low-grade fever, and mild cough. His mother states that the cough has progressively become worse over the last 36 hours and now sounds "terrible." His mother was concerned that he was having difficulty catching his breath and was breathing very fast, and she subsequently brought him to see you. He has refused to eat or drink today. The mother states that he attends day care and "one of the older children may have a throat infection."

PMHx: SVD at term with no complications, no hospitalizations, and no chronic illnesses.

Meds: Over-the-counter decongestant/cough suppressant, acetaminophen

All: NKDA

Immun: Received 2-, 4-, 6-, and 12-month vaccines.

SHx: Lives with parents; no smokers, no pets in household.

ROS: As above; no vomiting or diarrhea; no rash.

VS: Temp 37.9°C (100.3°F), BP 100/55, HR 130, RR 42; pulse oximetry 97% on room air, decreases to 90% during coughing episode

PE: *Gen:* alert, nontoxic appearing, comfortable while supine in mother's lap but crying as you approach, with audible hoarseness and inspiratory stridor and a "barking" cough. *HEENT:* mild nasal flaring with inspiration; TMs erythematous but otherwise clear. Oropharynx erythematous with no exudate; mucosa moist. *Lungs:* sternal and mild supraclavicular retractions; no crackles; rhonchi audible in middle fields; no audible wheezing. *CV:* RR&R; no murmur; capillary refill time <2 seconds; strong pulses throughout.

THOUGHT QUESTIONS

■ What is in this patient's differential diagnosis?

■ What components of this history and physical should help in your diagnosis?

■ What additional studies may aid in making a diagnosis?

DISCUSSION

The differential diagnosis for this patient includes the various causes of upper airway obstruction in this age group: acute laryngotracheitis (croup), epiglottitis, pneumonia, foreign body aspiration, bacterial tracheitis, underlying laryngotracheomalacia, retropharyngeal or peritonsillar abscess, or ingestion of caustic agents. Previous history of intubation may lead to inclusion of subglottic stenosis.

On history and physical examination, the course of presentation, with mild but progressive upper respiratory tract symptoms, characteristic barking, seal-like cough, and inspiratory stridor, is suggestive of croup. The initial visual evaluation of the child's appearance, along with the physical examination, is the most helpful diagnostic resource in helping to distinguish croup from other entities, such as epiglottitis (Table 8-1). This patient is comfortable while supine, is

TABLE 8-1   Croup and Epiglottitis

	Croup	Epiglottitis
Pathogenesis	Inflammation of the subglottic tissues (laryngotracheobronchitis)	Inflammation and edema of the epiglottis and aryepiglottic folds
Etiology	Parainfluenza virus (most common); also influenza, RSV	*Haemophilus influenzae* type b previously most common (prior to vaccine)
Peak age	3 months to 3 years	3 to 5 years
Clinical features	Prodrome of low-grade fever, rhinorrhea; stridor and hoarse voice	Fever, ill or toxic appearance, sore throat, stridor; drooling
Imaging	"Steeple" sign on AP neck film	"Thumbprinting" on lateral neck film
Treatment	Supportive care, oxygen/mist; corticosteroids, racemic epinephrine	Emergent airway management, parenteral antibiotics; fluids

not drooling, is nontoxic appearing, and is not distressed or apprehensive, all of which lessen the likelihood of epiglottitis.

Traditionally, croup is a clinical diagnosis, but some tools can be used to support your initial findings. Lateral plain films of the neck may reveal narrowing of the air column in the subglottic area, known as the "steeple" sign. The CBC may reveal leukocytosis. Pulse oximetry is generally normal, but may be decreased during coughing episodes and with superimposed lower airway involvement.

CASE CONTINUED

The patient is initially treated with cool mist aerosol while sitting on his parent's lap. After initially responding with decreased stridor and cough, his symptoms return and he develops an audible stridor with slightly worse retractions. His pulse oximetry is 97% on room air.

QUESTIONS

8-1. At this time, the next likely step in management should be
   A. A trial of nebulized albuterol
   B. A trial of nebulized racemic epinephrine
   C. Endoscopic evaluation of the child's airway in a controlled setting
   D. Intravenous antibiotics
   E. More cool mist and comfort

8-2. The likely organism involved in this disease process is
   A. *Haemophilus influenzae*
   B. Respiratory syncytial virus (RSV)
   C. *Streptococcus pneumoniae*
   D. Parainfluenza virus species
   E. Epstein-Barr virus

8-3. Which of the following is most appropriate in the management of croup?
  A. The majority of children with viral croup are symptomatic enough to prompt hospitalization.
  B. Children with respiratory distress may benefit from nebulized racemic epinephrine.
  C. Beta-agonist therapy should be initiated rapidly.
  D. Evaluation for foreign body aspiration in toddlers is useful only with a noted history of choking.
  E. Children with suspected croup should initially receive parenteral antibiotics.

8-4. For a child with suspected epiglottitis, which of the following is an appropriate first step in management?
  A. Observation and administration of cool mist and other supportive measures
  B. Lateral neck films, which may show a "thumbprint" sign
  C. Epiglottitis is an acute airway emergency and requires controlled airway management.
  D. Administration of the *Haemophilus influenzae* type b vaccine
  E. None of the above

ANSWERS

8-1 B, 8-2 D, 8-3 B, 8-4 C. For croup, the disease process involves obstruction and edema of the upper airways. Although the majority of patients are toddlers, croup also can affect older children. The majority of patients have symptoms that usually resolve on their own. Viral croup usually begins with upper respiratory tract infection symptoms generally lasting 2 to 3 days, followed by stridor and barking cough. Stridor can often be worse at night and in periods of agitation. Initial care should involve supportive care with cool mist and fluids. For the patient in respiratory distress who has not responded to these measures, racemic epinephrine should be administered. Its effect primarily lies in stimulation of alpha-adrenergic receptors and a decrease in laryngeal mucosal edema. A child who responds to this treatment can safely be discharged from care after careful observation and an examination that reveals no stridor at rest, no color changes, and adequate air entry. Corticosteroids are often used to treat airway edema and can benefit patients with noted stridor at rest. Nebulized albuterol has not been shown to be effective in the management of croup. Wheezing after cool mist therapy may be found in the child whose croup involves the larger airways, but it is uncommon in children with croup. The most likely pathogens associated with croup are parainfluenza viruses, followed by influenza viruses, RSV, and adenoviruses. Spasmodic croup, which is not related to a primary infectious cause, can occur in older children but usually is self-limiting.

Suspicion of epiglottitis warrants emergent, careful, and controlled management of the airway. In the ill-appearing child with imminent upper airway obstruction, this should be done most preferably in the operating room with airway support readily available. Epiglottitis traditionally is caused by *H. influenzae* type b (Hib), but streptococcal species have increasingly been implicated since introduction of the Hib vaccine. The onset of symptoms in epiglottitis is generally much quicker than croup, and can result in obstruction of the airway within several hours. The advent of routine vaccination has helped decrease the incidence over the last 5 years. Antibiotics are indicated for the child in whom epiglottitis or another bacterial process (bacterial tracheitis, pneumonia, abscess) is suspected; a clinical examination should support the diagnosis (Figs. 8-1 and 8-2).

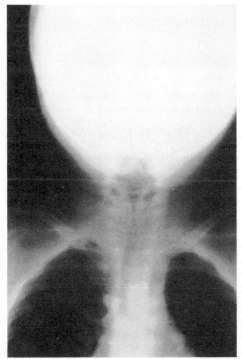

FIGURE 8-1.
Croup in a 3-year-old child. Note the "steeple" sign indicative of subglottic narrowing. (*From Marino B, Snead K, McMillan J. Blueprints in Pediatrics. 2nd ed. Malden, MA: Blackwell Science; 2001:157, with permission.*)

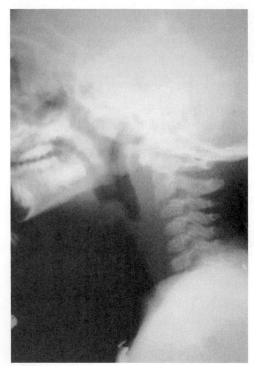

FIGURE 8-2.
Epiglottitis in a 4-year-old child, with massive edema of the epiglottis, thickened aryepiglottic folds, and effacement of the valleculae. (*From Marino B, Snead K, McMillan J. Blueprints in Pediatrics. 2nd ed. Malden, MA: Blackwell Science; 2001:158, with permission.*)

SUGGESTED ADDITIONAL READING

Malhotra A, Krilov LR. Viral croup. *Pediatr Rev.* 2001;22:5–12.
Rafei K, Lichenstein R. Airway infectious disease emergencies. *Pediatr Clin North Am.* 2006;53(2):215–242.

Wheezing

CC/ID: 2-year-old boy with a 1-day history of cough and "noisy," difficult breathing.

HPI: A.T. was previously well, but his father noticed this morning that he had "noisy" breathing. He seemed to have some difficulty, which was temporarily relieved by steam mist. He has been coughing and has some audible wheezing. He has no fever or runny nose. He has not had any vomiting or diarrhea, nor has he had any rash. The child has refused feeding today, is more irritable, and has been less active. His father says he was worried because he noticed a faster rate of breathing and that the child was having more difficulty breathing. He tried administering albuterol from a previous prescription, without any success.

PMHx: Hospitalized for bronchiolitis at 6 months of age; born at term without complications.

Meds: Albuterol as above

All: NKDA

SHx: Lives with father and 5-year-old sibling; no smokers; no household pets.

VS: Temp 37.5°C (99.5°F), HR 135, RR 45; pulse oximetry 88% on room air

PE: *Gen:* sitting in father's lap; tachypneic; visible intercostal retractions, appears in moderate respiratory distress. *HEENT:* oropharynx is slightly erythematous, but otherwise clear. *Lungs:* intermittent mild coughing; decreased expiratory breath sounds on right side, with expiratory wheezes at bases (R>L); fine crackles heard at right base. Rest of exam is within normal limits.

THOUGHT QUESTIONS

- What is in the differential diagnosis?
- What additional history may be helpful in this case?
- What diagnostic and therapeutic evaluations are indicated for this child?

DISCUSSION

The differential diagnosis for wheezing includes asthma, bronchiolitis, pneumonia and other causes of lower respiratory tract infection, gastroesophageal reflux disease, cystic fibrosis, anatomic abnormalities (vascular rings, pulmonary cysts), and extrapulmonary causes (cardiac failure, poisonings or ingestions, thoracic cage defects). Anaphylactic reactions must also be considered.

Although the age and possibility of aspirating a small object or the toy of a nearby toddler are suggestive on their own, it is unlikely that a given history of observed aspiration of a foreign body will lead to the diagnosis. Signs and symptoms suggesting the diagnosis of foreign body aspiration depend on the location and type of foreign body, and may include the acute onset of inspiratory stridor or respiratory distress, unilateral auscultatory findings and an abnormal chest x-ray. Due to its course and natural continuity with the upper airways, the right mainstem bronchus is the most common site for foreign bodies to be found. A chest x-ray that reveals hyperinflation of one lung (usually the right) that persists during films obtained during expiration and in the lateral decubitus position suggests air trapping and a possible "ball valve" mechanism of obstruction secondary to a likely partial foreign body obstruction. If a foreign body aspiration is suspected, the definitive diagnosis is made with bronchoscopy, which can also be used to remove the foreign object.

CASE CONTINUED

A chest x-ray is obtained, which reveals hyperinflation of the right lung. A.T. is admitted to the hospital for rigid bronchoscopy. During the procedure a peanut is discovered and removed from the right mainstem bronchus. After the procedure, the child is discharged home after a discussion of aspiration precautions with his parents.

QUESTIONS

9-1. Which of the following may be an early sign or symptom related to foreign body aspiration?
A. Retractions
B. Stridor
C. Wheezing
D. Cough
E. All of the above

9-2. What is the most likely age at presentation for a foreign body aspiration?
A. 6 to 36 months
B. 4 to 5 years
C. 0 to 6 months
D. 6 to 11 years
E. 11 to 15 years

9-3. Expiratory chest x-ray in a complete right mainstem bronchus obstruction should demonstrate
A. Left lung hyperinflation with mediastinal shift toward right
B. Left lung atelectasis with heart drawn to left side
C. Right lung atelectasis with heart drawn to right side
D. Right lung hyperinflation with mediastinal shift toward left

9-4. Which of the following may be suspected in patients who present with recurrent bouts of wheezing?
A. Retained foreign body
B. Asthma
C. Immunoglobulin deficiency
D. Gastroesophageal reflux disease
E. All of the above

ANSWERS

9-1. E. All of the mentioned symptoms are generally early indications of a lodged foreign body in the trachea and mainstem bronchus. Later manifestations may include blood-tinged sputum and possible pneumothorax.

9-2. A. It is also important to be aware of foreign body aspiration in the developmentally delayed patient at any age.

9-3. C. For a complete obstruction, the affected side will have a unilateral atelectasis with a shift of the heart to the affected side. In contrast, a partial obstruction allows a "ball-valve" mechanism for air-trapping on the affected side and a shift of the mediastinal structures away from the affected side (Fig. 9-1).

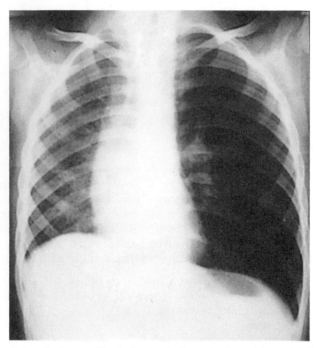

FIGURE **9-1.**   Expiratory film in foreign body aspiration with partial obstruction. The obstructed left lung is hyperinflated, whereas the heart (and mediastinum) is shifted to the right. (*From Marino B, Snead K, McMillan J. Blueprints in Pediatrics. 2nd ed. Malden, MA: Blackwell Science; 2001:10, with permission.*)

9-4. E. Chronic and recurrent wheezing may indeed be a long-term result of a retained aspirated foreign body. The differential diagnosis for chronic wheeze and cough also includes asthma, cystic fibrosis, immunodeficiencies, anatomic lesions (tracheoesophageal fistula, mediastinal tumors), ciliary dyskinesia, and chronic exposure to irritants (tobacco smoke, aspirated contents from gastroesophageal reflux disease).

SUGGESTED ADDITIONAL READING

Rovin JD, Rodgers BM. Pediatric foreign body aspiration. *Pediatr Rev*. 2000;21:86–90.

Cough and Runny Nose

CC/ID: 2½-year-old girl with 2 days of cough, runny nose, vomiting, and irritability.

HPI: B.G. is brought into the emergency room after having had a cough, vomiting, and diarrhea for nearly 2 days. The parents note that she had started having a runny nose and fever 2 days ago. She subsequently began vomiting a clear, nonbilious fluid, and her stools were loose. The child's fever was treated with acetaminophen. She has not been active and today has been increasingly irritable, refusing any oral intake. She has a wet cough; it has not seemed to respond to over-the-counter antitussive medicines. Both parents are concerned that the child seems "like she's losing too much fluid" and "doesn't seem like herself." They also state that "everyone is sick at day care."

PMHx: Normal birth history; no previous hospitalizations.

Meds: Tylenol as above

All: NKDA

Immun: UTD to 2 years

SHx: Lives with mother and father, and attends day care; mother is expecting second child.

FHx: Noncontributory

VS: Temp 39.2°C (102.5°F), HR 150, RR 42

PE: *Gen:* child lies quietly on mother's lap listless but without acute distress, not appearing in any acute distress. *HEENT:* mild rhinorrhea; somewhat dry oral mucosa; otherwise normal. *Neck:* supple. *Chest:* tachypneic, with decreased breath sounds at bases; no crackles or wheezes. *CV:* tachycardic; otherwise normal exam. *Abdomen:* tenderness on right side on deep palpation; otherwise normal. *Skin:* delayed cap refill of 5 seconds, slightly decreased turgor.

THOUGHT QUESTIONS

- What is in this patient's differential diagnosis?
- What diagnostic studies would you like performed?

DISCUSSION

The differential diagnosis for this patient includes gastroenteritis and other intra-abdominal processes. In addition, accompanying upper respiratory tract symptoms and rash would usually suggest a systemic viral illness. Urinary tract infections and pneumonia should be included in the differential diagnosis because of the age of the patient and the presence of systemic constitutional complaints. In infants who present with these nonspecific symptoms, a logical step-wise approach to diagnostic studies should be undertaken, based on the patient's symptoms and overall level of illness. For example, if an acute abdominal process or perforation is suspected, a KUB or other abdominal imaging might be performed. Significant respiratory distress, hypoxia or focal findings on lung exam could prompt obtaining a chest X-ray. Labs such as CBC and blood culture should be obtained when sepsis is suspected, electrolytes for severe dehydration or suspected metabolic abnormality, and liver enzymes if toxic ingestion or hepatitis is considered. A urinalysis can suggest infection and provide information on hydration status.

CASE CONTINUED

Due to her ill appearance and refusal to take oral fluids, the child was admitted for intravenous hydration and further evaluation. A CBC and blood culture were obtained, as were serum electrolytes and a urinalysis and urine culture. Results of note included a serum HCO_3 level of 14, and a WBC count of 25,000 (66% neutrophils and 19% bands). Urinalysis revealed no abnormalities. After hydration, the child appeared more alert, but had persistent cough and vomiting, and was noted to have increased respiratory distress with RR of 56 and oxygen saturation of 91% on room air. A chest x-ray revealed a consolidation of her right lower lobe with a small pleural effusion, suggesting a bacterial pneumonia. The patient was treated with the appropriate antibiotics and discharged home after an uncomplicated hospital course.

QUESTIONS

10-1. For the patient in this case, what is the most common cause of bacterial pneumonia?
A. *Mycoplasma pneumoniae*
B. Group B streptococci
C. *Chlamydia pneumoniae*
D. *Streptococcus pneumoniae*
E. *Haemophilus influenzae* type b

10-2. Which of the following conditions is associated with an increased risk of bacterial pneumonia?
A. Bronchopulmonary dysplasia
B. Cystic fibrosis
C. Gastroesophageal reflux/aspiration
D. Sickle cell disease
E. All of the above

10-3. When assessing the older child or adolescent with suspected pneumonia, which of the medications listed is useful against *Mycoplasma pneumoniae* infection?
A. Ribavirin
B. Penicillin
C. Amoxicillin
D. Amoxicillin-clavulanic acid
E. Erythromycin or other macrolides

10-4. When assessing the neonate (0–2 months) with a suspected pneumonia, which of the following organisms should be considered?
A. Group B streptococci
B. *Listeria monocytogenes*
C. *Escherichia coli*
D. *Chlamydia trachomatis*
E. All of the above

ANSWERS

10-1 D, 10-2 E, 10-3 E, 10-4 E. Pneumonia remains an important diagnosis in pediatrics. History, physical examination, and the underlying cause all usually depend on the age at presentation. Several risk factors are associated with bacterial pneumonia.

In neonates, ages 0 to 2 months, common bacterial causes of pneumonia include treatment for group B streptococci, *E. coli*, and *L. monocytogenes* (common pathogens of neonatal sepsis). *Chlamydia trachomatis* pneumonia may also present in this age group in infants born to infected mothers; it often presents in the second month of life, and can be associated with conjunctivitis.

In infants after the neonatal period, the most common causes of pneumonia remain viral (RSV, adenovirus, influenza). Viral pneumonia is generally preceded by upper respiratory tract infection symptoms, and can also be accompanied by signs and symptoms of respiratory distress. Many infants will also have nonspecific constitutional symptoms such as fever, lethargy, poor feeding, irritability, and vomiting. The physical examination may not be especially revealing. Bacterial pneumonia (predominantly *S. pneumoniae*) must also be considered.

In older infants and toddlers, the presentation may be similar to that of postneonatal infants. Symptoms of cough, tachypnea, and respiratory distress may suggest pneumonia. Chest pain and dyspnea are seen less often than in the older child. Auscultation may reveal crackles and decreased breath sounds. Lobar consolidation may often cause diaphragmatic irritation, ileus, and a clinical picture consistent with an intra-abdominal process (as was true in this case). Viral agents remain prominent, but common bacterial pathogens now include *S. pneumoniae* (most common) and *H. influenzae* type b.

In older children, fever, chills, productive cough, dyspnea, and pleuritic chest pain may all be suggestive of pneumonia. Auscultative findings include crackles, dullness to percussion, and decreased breath sounds. In otherwise healthy children, atypical pathogens such as *Mycoplasma pneumoniae* and *Chlamydia pneumoniae* are more common than *S. pneumoniae*.

Chest x-ray may help define the pattern of involvement (lobar consolidation is often suggestive of bacterial pneumonia) and denote other processes involved (i.e., pleural effusions). CBC and blood culture (nearly 20% may have associated bacteremia) may aid in diagnosis and treatment. Inpatient treatment is warranted for respiratory distress and persistent hypoxia, and often for the neonate. Viral infections are generally self-limited and require supportive care. Bacterial pathogens require appropriate antibiotic coverage. Outpatient management with amoxicillin is appropriate for most cases of suspected pneumococcal pneumonia. For inpatient therapy, where parenteral antibiotics may be required, cefuroxime or penicillin are appropriate choices for empiric therapy. For cases of suspected

H. influenzae or *S. aureus* infection, amoxicillin-clavulanic acid or a second- or third-generation cephalosporin may be required. For suspected <u>mycoplasma pneumoni</u>a cases, <u>erythromycin or another macrolide is the drug of choice</u>.

 SUGGESTED ADDITIONAL READING

Ishimine P. Fever without source in children 0 to 36 months of age. *Pediatr Clin North Am*. 2006;53(2):167–194.
Sandora TJ. Pneumonia in hospitalized children. *Pediatr Clin North Am*. 2005;52(4):1059–1081, viii.

Persistent Shortness of Breath

CC/ID: 6-year-old girl with cough for 3 weeks.

HPI: T.I. was well until 3 weeks ago, when she developed cough, rhinorrhea, sore throat, and low-grade fever. She refused to play outside at that time, stating that she "was out of breath from coughing." Her rhinorrhea, sore throat, and fever resolved, but the cough has persisted. Mother states that it is worse at night, and although she is active, "she still gets tired when she plays." She gets occasional headaches and has no current nausea, vomiting, or diarrhea. She has no rashes currently. Mother has tried several over-the-counter cough remedies without success. She states that she thinks it is a lingering "cold" and that over the past year, "they seem to take longer to clear," as they did for her at that age.

PMHx: None; normal birth history with no complications.

Meds: As above

All: NKDA

SHx: Lives with mother and father; mother smokes "outside the house"; pets: one cat.

FHx: Mother has "recurrent bronchitis attacks."

VS: Temp 37.1°C (98.8°F), BP 95/55, HR 100, RR 20

PE: *Gen:* well-appearing girl in no apparent distress, with intermittent cough during exam. *HEENT:* oropharynx slightly erythematous; TMs within normal limits; no intranasal lesions. *Lungs:* decreased breath sounds at bases bilaterally, with rhonchi throughout fields; increased expiratory phase, with wheezing in middle lung fields (medial > lateral); no crackles. *CV:* RR&R; normal S_1, S_2; no murmur. *Ext:* no clubbing; no cyanosis; no edema.

THOUGHT QUESTIONS

- What is in the differential diagnosis at this point?
- What bedside maneuvers can help in narrowing the diagnosis?
- What laboratory or imaging studies may be useful for this patient?
- What further history would you obtain?

DISCUSSION

The differential diagnosis for chronic cough is extensive and includes reactive airway disease (RAD: asthma), gastroesophageal reflux disease (GERD), aspirated foreign body, sinusitis, and allergies. Less likely in the face of an otherwise normal history and physical examination would be immune deficiency, cystic fibrosis, ciliary or parenchymal abnormalities, and psychogenic causes. In this case, a peak flow measurement was obtained and was found to be 50% of the expected value for her height, indicating an obstructive airway process. Laboratory tests were not performed, and a chest x-ray revealed hyperinflation and several areas of likely atelectasis at the bases bilaterally. Given the above findings and history (nighttime cough, cough with exercise), the clinical diagnosis of asthma was made.

A thorough history should be obtained for every patient with a suspicion of asthma. This should include a detailed history of the cough, medications, precipitating factors, ill contacts, travel, pets, environmental factors at home and school, family history, and a review of systems.

Although asthma is generally a clinical diagnosis that is reversible with bronchodilators and anti-inflammatory agents, some laboratory testing may be useful to distinguish between other causes of chronic cough. This would possibly include a CBC (eosinophilia may suggest asthma/atopy), sputum samples for Gram stain and culture, and immunologic studies. A purified protein derivative (PPD) test should be placed for suspicion of tuberculosis. Further imaging and studies should be guided by your history and physical examination (Fig. 11-1).

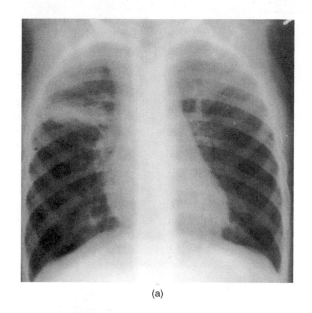

(a)

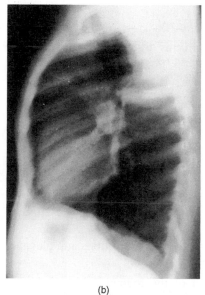

(b)

FIGURE 11-1.   These radiographs of a 3-year-old child with asthma exacerbation demonstrate severe hyperinflation, increased anteroposterior diameter of the chest, and several areas of atelectasis. (*From Marino B, Snead K,
McMillan J. Blueprints in Pediatrics. 2nd ed. Malden, MA: Blackwell Science; 2001:275, with permission.*)

CASE CONTINUED

After a nebulized β-agonist bronchodilator treatment, the patient's peak flow improved and she was sent home with an asthma action plan describing daily use of a low-dose inhaled corticosteroid, with a short-acting β-agonist for use as needed. She returned 6 weeks later to the emergency department in respiratory distress with shortness of breath, tachypnea (RR 50), audible wheezing, subcostal retractions, and supraclavicular retractions. Her pulse oximetry reading was 88% on room air. The lung examination revealed decreased breath sounds and no wheezing in all fields. Blood gas analysis revealed a pH of 7.48, a $Paco_2$ of 28, a Pao_2 of 65, and a base deficit of –2. She had not been taking her medications for several weeks because she had improved and her parents felt she did not need any further therapy.

QUESTIONS

11-1. Based on this description, which of the following would now be an appropriate course of initial therapy?
- A. Cromolyn sodium
- B. Oxygen and leukotriene receptor agonists
- C. Oxygen and inhaled bronchodilators
- D. IV fluids
- E. Oxygen, inhaled bronchodilators, and systemic corticosteroids

11-2. Which of the following is most consistent with asthma?
- A. Chest x-ray with lobar consolidation
- B. Irreversible bronchospasm
- C. Pulmonary function tests showing decreased expiratory flow rates
- D. Decreased mucus secretions and plugging
- E. Stridulous breathing

11-3. Which of the following best describes the blood gas analysis of the patient in this case?
- A. Compensatory respiratory acidosis
- B. Compensatory metabolic alkalosis
- C. Primary respiratory alkalosis
- D. Primary metabolic acidosis
- E. High anion gap acidosis

11-4. Which of the following is a predisposing factor in childhood asthma?
   A. Atopy
   B. Genetic predisposition
   C. Smoke exposure
   D. Urban households
   E. All of the above

 ANSWERS

11-1. E. The immediate therapy for a child suffering from an acute asthma attack involves relief of acute airway constriction (via bronchodilators and oxygen therapy) and control of airway inflammation (via corticosteroids). Corticosteroids generally require 4 to 6 hours for effectiveness, but are indicated for initial therapy.

11-2. C. Because asthma is an obstructive airway disease, increased lung volumes and decreased expiratory flow rates are seen in pulmonary function tests. X-ray findings usually reveal hyperinflation and peribronchial thickening. Mucus secretions and plugging are usually increased, and expiratory wheezing is usually the hallmark of the physical exam. Airway bronchospasm and obstruction is generally at least partially reversible.

11-3. C. In an acute asthma attack, a low $Paco_2$ indicates an adequate value secondary to tachypnea. (In fact, a "normal" $Paco_2$ should immediately raise concern for inadequate ventilation and the patient rapidly tiring.) This is most consistently reflected in the blood gas analysis as a primary respiratory alkalosis.

11-4. E. Previous RSV infection and poverty are also among the many risk factors for asthma.

 SUGGESTED ADDITIONAL READING

Guill MF. Asthma update: clinical aspects and management. *Pediatr Rev.* 2004;25:335–344.
Guill MF. Asthma update: epidemiology and pathophysiology. *Pediatr Rev.* 2004;25:299–305.

Wheezing and Rash

CC/ID: 5-year-old boy with wheezing and rash presents to the emergency room.

HPI: A.R. was healthy prior to this afternoon, when he and his parents were at a local park for a birthday party. He had been seen playing with some other children, when it was noticed that he had difficulty breathing and was wheezing, with swelling of his face, and redness of his face and neck. His voice sounds a "little hoarse" to his parents, and he is crying.

PMHx: Normal birth history; no previous hospitalizations or illnesses; history of mild asthma.

PSHx: None

Meds: β-Agonist inhaler taken as needed; takes multivitamin supplement.

All: NKDA

SHx: Lives with parents; no siblings; no pets because of allergies.

VS: Temp 37.2°C (99°F), BP 82/40 (systolic 80–125), HR 145 (90–110), RR 35 (18–25); pulse oximetry 88% on room air

PE: *Gen:* appears in moderate distress, with swollen face, audible wheezing, and hoarse voice. *HEENT:* erythematous swelling of eyes and face; TMs clear; oropharynx erythematous without lesions. *Chest:* visible suprasternal and intercostal retractions; wheezing in all fields with adequate air entry; no crackles. *CV:* RR&R; tachycardic; no murmur; capillary refill time <3 seconds. *Skin:* erythematous, raised, circumscribed, edematous white/evanescent plaques on face, neck, and upper extremities/trunk. *Neuro:* gross nonfocal. Rest of exam is within normal limits.

THOUGHT QUESTIONS

- What further history would you like to obtain?
- What is in your differential diagnosis at this point?
- What are your immediate concerns regarding this patient?

DISCUSSION

This child shows all of the signs and symptoms of an anaphylactic reaction. Further history from the parents reveals that the boy had been stung by a bee. The most common causes of anaphylactic reactions in children include *Hymenoptera* stings (bees and wasps); drugs such as penicillin and local anesthetics; foods such as peanuts, eggs, and seafood; and blood products, contrast media, and latex. Obtaining a history of events leading up to the episode may help determine exposure to the antigen. Also, obtaining a thorough past history indicative of underlying disorders may give clues to the cause and the clinical presentation. Previous asthma may be a risk factor for bronchospasm during anaphylactic reactions. Underlying spina bifida or urologic disorders may predispose an individual to latex allergies.

The differential diagnosis for systemic anaphylaxis includes seizures, arrhythmias, syncopal episodes, foreign body aspiration, acute poisoning, or ingestion/inhalation.

Anaphylaxis is an extreme systemic *type 1 hypersensitivity* allergic reaction and can be characterized by cutaneous, respiratory, cardiovascular, and gastrointestinal features. The physical exam should initially focus on vital signs and ABCs (airway, breathing, and circulation). In this patient, the vital signs and examination were indicative of airway swelling and bronchospasm, urticaria and angioedema, tachycardia, and borderline hypotension. With ingested allergens, diarrhea and abdominal pain may accompany presentation, likely due to angioedema within the gastrointestinal tract.

Urticaria and angioedema are common manifestations of anaphylaxis as well as other allergic reactions in children. They involve exposure to the previously mentioned allergens as well as hereditary forms. Children with known reactions to specific allergens such as bee stings should always be advised to carry injectable epinephrine to *treat any* future attacks.

CASE CONTINUED

You treat A.R. appropriately and discuss precautions to take in the future with his parents. Within a short time his symptoms have diminished and he is discharged to home.

QUESTIONS

12-1. Which of the following statements best describes the immunology of anaphylactic reactions?
   A. An IgM-mediated reaction that occurs several days after allergen exposure
   B. An IgE-mediated reaction that occurs several days after allergen exposure
   C. An IgM-mediated reaction that occurs several hours after allergen exposure
   D. An IgE- and histamine-mediated reaction that occurs *minutes to* hours after allergen exposure

12-2. Which of the following are typical characteristics of urticaria?
   A. Pruritic
   B. Generally resolves within 24 hours
   C. Blanching lesions
   D. Results from vascular dilatation and increased permeability
   E. All of the above

12-3. Which of the following best describes typical characteristics of angioedema?
   A. Confined to the lower dermis and subcutaneous areas
   B. Pruritic lesions with C1 esterase deficiency
   C. Poorly demarcated areas of swelling
   D. Generally resolves within minutes
   E. All of the above

12-4. Which of the following is indicated in the initial treatment of anaphylaxis?
   A. Airway support, oxygen, and IV fluids
   B. Subcutaneous epinephrine
   C. Diphenhydramine
   D. Corticosteroids
   E. All of the above

ANSWERS

12-1. D. Although anaphylaxis can evolve slowly or rapidly, the most common presentations occur within hours after exposure to an allergen. The reaction is primarily an IgE- and histamine-mediated reaction.

12-2. E. Urticaria typically describes blanching, edematous, red and white evanescent plaques, which appear as hives on the skin or mucous membranes. They are pruritic, may be raised, and generally resolve within 24 hours.

12-3. A. Angioedema is a similar process to urticaria, involving swelling in a well-demarcated area, usually devoid of pruritus. It is confined to the lower dermis and subcutaneous areas and also resolves within a few hours to days. Clinically, angioedema must be differentiated from cellulitis, erysipelas, lymphedema, and acute contact dermatitis. Angioedema may be accompanied by pruritus when associated with urticaria, whereas angioedema due to C1 esterase deficiency is not usually pruritic.

12-4. E. The immediate concerns for these patients include support of the ABCs (airway, breathing, and circulation). Oxygen, epinephrine, and diphenhydramine may help alleviate reactive symptoms. Intubation may be warranted in cases of severe obstruction. Intravenous fluids are also indicated for intravascular volume support. Corticosteroids are indicated to help curb the inflammatory response and treat persistent symptoms.

SUGGESTED ADDITIONAL READING

Chiu AM. Anaphylaxis: drug allergy, insect stings, and latex. *Immunol Allergy Clin North Am.* 2005;25(2):389–405, viii.

Moss MH. Pediatric allergy. *Immunol Allergy Clin North Am.* 2005;25(2):xi–xii.

Cough and Fever

CC/ID: 6-month-old girl with fever, cough, and rapid breathing.

HPI: R.B. presents to your winter evening clinic with a 4-day history of fever, rhinorrhea, and cough that has worsened. Since last night, she has had a progressively increasing rate of breathing and worsening symptoms. Her mother reports that during that time, R.B. has become more irritable and is having a harder time breathing. She had been tolerating her feeds well until today, and now is refusing her bottle. She has had no vomiting or diarrhea. She attends day care, where there are numerous ill contacts.

PMHx: None. *Birth:* SVD at term without complications.

PSHx: None

Meds: Acetaminophen as needed for fever

All: NKDA

Immun: UTD

DietHx: Just started solids last week; bottle feeding on formula.

DevHx: Sits without support; babbling; transferring objects. *ROS:* no rash; no wet diapers since this morning.

SHx: Lives with mother and grandmother at home; smokers in home.

FHx: Father with asthma.

VS: Temp 38.3°C (101°F), BP 95/55, HR 165, RR 58; Weight 6.5 kg (50%)

PE: *Gen:* alert, interactive, crying infant, grunting mildly with each breath. *HEENT:* normocephalic and atraumatic (NCAT); AFO to 1 cm; pupils equal, round, and reactive to light and accommodation

(PERRLA); copious nasal secretions, nasal flaring. Oropharynx ery-thematous; TMs with erythema/no exudates/good landmarks. *Chest:* intercostal retractions; shallow rapid breathing; wheezing audible in all fields; decreased aeration at bases; some crackles heard at bases. *CV:* RR&R; tachycardic; normal S_1, S_2; no murmur; capillary refill is 2.5 seconds; pulses normal. *Abdomen:* distended but soft; positive bowel sounds; no visceromegaly; nontender. *Neuro:* grossly nonfocal. *Skin:* no lesions.

THOUGHT QUESTIONS

- What are some initial evaluations or therapeutic meas-ures that can be taken for this patient?
- What is the differential diagnosis for this patient?
- What diagnostic tests may aid in making this diagnosis?

DISCUSSION

For the infant in respiratory distress (which is usually signified by grunting, flaring of the nostrils, and retractions/use of accessory res-piratory muscles), one must always be aware of the ABCs: airway, breathing, and circulation. Once hemodynamic stability and a patent airway with breathing are established, assessing the patient's oxygen saturation may be the next step. Oxygen is a natural bronchodilator and can help this type of patient. Fluid support may also be war-ranted. The differential diagnosis for this patient would include bron-chiolitis, pneumonia, reactive airway disease, and aspiration of foreign body. Clinical examination and history are generally suffi-cient to initially manage the patient; however, tests such as viral anti-gen assays and chest x-rays may aid in making the diagnosis.

CASE CONTINUED

Pulse oximetry on room air was 88%, which improved with oxygen therapy to 95%. The patient was admitted to the hospital, where the infant received parenteral fluids and oxygen support. A chest x-ray revealed bilateral interstitial infiltrates and hyperaeration, with mild consolidation at the bases. Bronchodilator therapy was initiated with mixed results. A rapid viral antigen test yielded positive results for RSV (respiratory syncytial virus), confirming along with the clinical and x-ray findings that the patient had bronchiolitis. The patient remained in the hospital for 48 hours, and upon time of discharge had an improved respiratory rate with no signs of respiratory distress, was tolerating oral feeds, and had an oxygen saturation of 95% on room air.

DISCUSSION

Bronchiolitis is an inflammatory process of the smaller lower airways, usually caused by RSV. Bronchiolitis can progress to respiratory failure and can potentially be fatal. RSV bronchiolitis is responsible for nearly 100,000 inpatient admissions, usually each winter and spring. Infants with congenital heart disease, chronic lung disease (usually former premature infants), or immunodeficiencies are usually at risk for more severe disease and poorer outcomes. Patients generally present with fever and upper respiratory tract infection, which is accompanied by tachypnea and wheezing. The diagnosis can be made clinically, but chest x-ray and viral antigen tests may aid in the diagnosis or in ruling out other causes. The goal of therapy is supportive care, usually achieved with oxygen and fluids; however, a significant number of patients require intensive care unit settings. Generally, the prognosis is excellent, but there may be an increased incidence of asthma subsequent to RSV infections.

QUESTIONS

13-1. Which of the following is a cause of bronchiolitis?
A. RSV
B. Adenovirus
C. *Mycoplasma pneumoniae*
D. Parainfluenzae
E. All of the above

13-2. In managing a patient with moderate or severe bronchiolitis, appropriate therapies to consider include which of the following?
A. Bronchodilator therapy
B. Oxygen
C. Corticosteroids
D. Frequent nasal suctioning
E. All of the above

13-3. Apnea is a more frequent presentation of bronchiolitis among
  A. Teenagers
  B. Infants
  C. Neonates
  D. School-aged children

13-4. Which of the following may offer passive prophylaxis against RSV?
  A. Ribavirin
  B. Palivizumab (Synagis)
  C. DTaP
  D. Air purifiers

ANSWERS

13-1. E. Although RSV is the most important cause of bronchiolitis, it should be noted that there are several other causes, including *Mycoplasma pneumoniae*. Many viral species can be identified using rapid viral antigen testing.

13-2. E. The majority of patients with bronchiolitis require no more than supportive care, as the illness is self-limited. However, those with more severe disease may require hospitalization for oxygen, fluid support and frequent nasal suctioning. Although they remain controversial, adjunctive therapies such as bronchodilators (albuterol and racemic epinephrine) and systemic corticosteroids may benefit some patients, particularly those who are more severely ill or have a history of asthma. It should be noted that although bacterial pneumonia may occur as a superinfection in patients with bronchiolitis, antibiotics are not routinely recommended.

13-3. C. In neonates, apnea may be the first presenting sign, along with poor feeding and lethargy.

13-4. B. Palivizumab (Synagis) is an intramuscular injectable monoclonal antibody that provides passive prophylaxis against RSV. An RSV polyclonal antibody called RespiGam is also available, and both may be recommended for infants at risk during the peak RSV infection months (usually from late fall to early spring).

SUGGESTED ADDITIONAL READING

American Academy of Pediatrics Committee on Infectious Diseases and Committee on Fetus and Newborn. Prevention of respiratory syncytial virus infections: indications for the use of palivizumab and update on the use of RSV-IGIV. *Pediatrics*. 1998;102(5): 1211–1216.

Coffin SE. Bronchiolitis: in-patient focus. *Pediatr Clin North Am*. 2005;52(4):1047–1057, viii.

Perlstein PH, Kotagal UR, Bolling C, et al. Evaluation of an evidence-based guideline for bronchiolitis. *Pediatrics*. 1999;104(6): 1334–1341.

Persistent Cough

CC/ID: 2-year-old boy with persistent cough.

HPI: P.D., a 2-year-old Caucasian boy, presents with a nearly 6-month history of persistent cough. The cough occurs during the day and night and is "hacking," according to the mother. He was diagnosed with asthma 4 months ago and was given bronchodilators, which help him intermittently. His coughs seem to progressively worsen with each "cold" that he gets. The cough is forceful and occasionally makes him vomit. He has had no prolonged fever, no ill contacts, and no recent travel. Mother is also concerned because he seems to be smaller than most children his age.

PMHx: Diagnosed with bronchiolitis at 12 months; repeated visits for upper respiratory infections over last few months. *Birth:* Born at home; SVD at term without complications.

PSHx: None

Meds: Albuterol PRN; over-the-counter cough medications

All: NKDA

Immun: UTD for age

DevHx: Reached milestones appropriately. *ROS:* no hemoptysis.

DietHx: History of formula intolerance ("formulas make his stools bulky and frothy").

SHx: Lives with parents and older brother; no smokers; no pets; attends day care.

FHx: Maternal uncle died in adolescence from pneumonia.

VS: Temp 36.8°C (98.4°F), BP 90/50, HR 130, RR 36; Weight 10.2 kg (<3rd percentile)

PE: *Gen:* alert, cooperative, in no acute distress; passes a bulky/frothy stool while examining. *HEENT:* normal. *Chest:* scattered wheezes audible in all fields; localized coarse crackles in middle fields; slightly increased AP diameter of chest. *CV:* RR&R; normal S_1, S_2; no murmur; capillary refill and pulses normal. *Abdomen:* mild distention; positive bowel sounds; no visceromegaly appreciated. *Skin:* no cyanosis; no edema.

THOUGHT QUESTIONS

- What is in your differential diagnosis?
- What elements of the history and physical would help in making a diagnosis?
- What diagnostic studies may help in making the diagnosis?

DISCUSSION

The differential diagnosis for chronic cough (defined as a persistent cough lasting more than 3 weeks) can include the following: asthma, gastroesophageal reflux, foreign body aspiration, laryngotracheomalacia, congenital pulmonary anomalies, cystic fibrosis, ciliary dyskinesia syndromes, recurrent viral infections, atypical pneumonia/tuberculosis, and immunodeficiencies. Because of the wide range of diseases, history and physical examination can often narrow the diagnosis. History should characterize the cough via precipitating factors, patterns, and response to therapies. Associated symptoms and past medical problems should be ascertained. A review of systems and developmental and environmental histories should be obtained. The physical examination should be comprehensive. General appearance and developmental status should be noted. The exam should note any clubbing or evidence of nasal polyps, both of which may suggest the pathologic cause. The chest exam should focus on the rate, ease of respiration, and adventitious sounds. Diagnostic studies should be driven by the history and physical exam, but may include pulse oximetry, PPD, CBC, sputum studies, chest and thoracic imaging, immune studies, and sweat chloride testing.

CASE CONTINUED

A chest x-ray was performed, which revealed large airway infiltrates, patches of mild bronchiectasis, and marked hyperinflation
(Fig. 14-1). His history of feeding intolerance and bulky/frothy
stools prompted a stool collection, which was markedly positive for
fat. Further findings on physical exam revealed mild digital clubbing. A sweat chloride test result was 90 mEq/L (>60 is abnormal),
and the diagnosis of cystic fibrosis was made. It was later learned
that the maternal uncle had cystic fibrosis too.

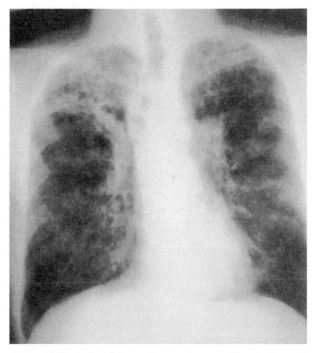

FIGURE 14-1.   Marked chronic lung disease changes (fibrosis, bronchiectasis,
and parenchymal loss) and characteristic "bleb" formation are seen in the
adolescent boy with cystic fibrosis. (*From Marino B, Snead K, McMillan J.
Blueprints in Pediatrics. 2nd ed. Malden, MA: Blackwell Science; 2001:277,
with permission.*)

DISCUSSION

Cystic fibrosis (CF) is a multisystem disease that results in disorders of the exocrine glands. Highly viscous secretions are the result of a defective chloride channel (CFTR: cystic fibrosis transmembrane receptor) and the subsequent insufficiency of water within the secretions. It is more prevalent in Caucasians, occurring in 1 in 2,500 live births. The clinical manifestations are protean and include pancreatic insufficiency, recurrent sinopulmonary disease, and failure to thrive. Through multidisciplinary therapy and new advances, life expectancy has increased (median life span is approximately 30 years).

QUESTIONS

14-1. What is the inheritance pattern for CF?
A. Autosomal dominant
B. Autosomal recessive
C. X-linked dominant
D. X-linked recessive

14-2. Which of the following is least likely to be a complication of CF?
A. Hemoptysis
B. Pneumothorax
C. Pancreatic cancer
D. Male infertility
E. Cirrhosis

14-3. Which of the following is usually clinically diagnostic of CF in the neonate?
A. Tachypnea
B. Maculopapular rash
C. Clubbing
D. Meconium ileus
E. None of the above

14-4. In managing a child with CF, which of the following is the most appropriate choice?
A. Pulmonary therapies including bronchodilators and mucolytics
B. Macrolides for suspected bacterial infections
C. Pancreatic enzyme only for those with pancreatitis
D. Avoidance of live vaccines

ANSWERS

14-1. B. Cystic fibrosis is acquired through autosomal recessive inheritance and generally involves mutations of the CFTR gene located on the long arm of chromosome 7. It should be noted that genetic testing is available for the 14 most common mutations of this gene, which account for nearly 85% of cases.

14-2. C. CF may result in multisystemic complications. Respiratory complications remain the major contributors to morbidity and mortality. Progressive hypoxia and obstructive airway disease can also lead to chronic pulmonary hypertension and right heart failure. Gastrointestinal and endocrine complications are also numerous. Impaired male fertility is virtually universal. Pancreatic cancer is generally not a complication of CF.

14-3. D. Meconium ileus is virtually pathognomonic for CF in the newborn. Nearly 20% of patients present in this fashion. Clubbing, although almost always present in the CF patient, is usually not present in the neonate.

14-4. A. Pulmonary therapies are multifaceted and may include bronchodilators, anti-inflammatory agents, and chest physiotherapy, as well as DNAse (for mucolysis). For all CF patients, pancreatic enzyme replacement along with high-calorie nutritional support and vitamin/mineral supplementation (A, D, E, K, iron) may help them to achieve near-normal growth. Bacterial infections often exacerbate disease and should be treated mainly with aminoglycosides in conjunction with other agents, since *Pseudomonas* species remain among the most important pathogens. In general, patients should receive recommended vaccine schedules without restriction, including influenza vaccine. Lung transplantation has become a viable option for those with poor pulmonary status and 1- to 2-year life expectancy.

 SUGGESTED ADDITIONAL READING

Davis PB. Cystic fibrosis. *Pediatr Rev.* 2001;22:257–264.

III

Cases in a
Newborn
Patient

Yellow Newborn

CC/ID: A 3-day-old male infant is brought in by his mother for "yellow skin."

HPI: According to his mother, C.J. has occasionally been a little "sleepy," but is otherwise acting well. There has been no fever, trouble breathing, or cyanosis. His mother's milk has just come in, and the baby seems to be feeding well. The yellow color appeared on his face on the day after birth, but has now deepened and progressed to the entire body, as well as the eyes. Mother is worried that there is something wrong with her milk.

PMHx: *Birth:* Full-term, normal spontaneous vaginal delivery (NSVD) at 39 weeks and 2 days, birth weight 3,650 g. Mother is a 28-year-old Hispanic woman, G2, P2; prenatal labs all negative; an uncomplicated pregnancy with excellent prenatal care.

Meds: None

All: NKDA

Immun: Hepatitis B at birth

THOUGHT QUESTIONS

- What is your differential diagnosis for this jaundiced infant?
- What further history or laboratory tests would you like to obtain for this newborn?

DISCUSSION

Bilirubin, a pigment derived from the degradation of heme, must be conjugated in the liver into a form that can be excreted via the intestines. Jaundice is visible when bilirubin reaches concentrations of 5 mg/dL. Many newborns develop a mild (12–15 mg/dL) and temporary unconjugated (indirect) hyperbilirubinemia termed "physiologic jaundice." This is because the newborn liver has impaired conjugation ability, and infants experience increased red cell breakdown in the first weeks of life. Breastfed infants typically experience higher and more prolonged levels of hyperbilirubinemia. The differential diagnosis for unusually prolonged or severe unconjugated hyperbilirubinemia includes factors that increase the accumulation of bilirubin, such as ABO or Rh hemolytic disease, polycythemia, or extravascular blood collection, and factors that decrease its conjugation and excretion from the body, such as dehydration or intestinal obstruction. Conjugated (direct) hyperbilirubinemia is much less common, always pathologic, and most often caused by factors that impede the passage of bile through the liver.

A thorough history of the jaundiced infant's feeding and stooling habits, weight gain, and family history for hemolytic or hepatic disease and a careful physical examination will help narrow the above differential. Since jaundice appears cephalad to caudad, severity of hyperbilirubinemia can be estimated by noting the lowest level of the yellow skin color. Laboratory tests, which may include a fractionated bilirubin level, hematocrit, and Coombs test, should be performed judiciously, based on the severity of the jaundice and the likely cause as suggested by history and physical exam.

    CASE CONTINUED

Further history reveals that C.J. breastfeeds vigorously every 3 hours for 10 minutes per side. Mom feels he empties her breast well. Occasionally he sleeps for 4 hours between feeds. He has four to five wet diapers per day, and three to four stools, which are greenish and soft. There is no known family history of liver disease, hematologic disease, or genetic disorders. No one at home is ill.

VS: Temp 37.1°C (98.8°F), HR 150, RR 55; Weight 3,530 g (70%); O_2 sat 99% on RA

PE: *Gen:* icteric male newborn, sucking vigorously on mother's breast; cries appropriately when examined. *HEENT:* icteric sclerae and mucous membranes; AFOSF; sutures normal; 4 × 6 cm soft resolving cephalohematoma on the left. Strong suck reflex. *Abdomen:* soft, nontender; normal active bowel sounds. The liver is palpable 1 cm below the costal margin; no spleen or other masses.

Neuro: normal tone; intact Moro, grasp, suck reflexes. No arching or irritability. *Skin:* jaundiced to the ankles. Capillary refill is brisk. No petechiae, rashes, or bruising.

Labs: Mother's blood type: O; baby: A. Coombs (direct and indirect) negative. Total bilirubin 20.7, direct bilirubin 0.3; Hct 52 with normal morphology, normal reticulocyte count.

THOUGHT QUESTIONS

- What is your assessment of the most likely cause of jaundice in this newborn?
- What are you most concerned about, and how would you manage this infant?

DISCUSSION

Factors such as mild dehydration from infrequent breastfeeding (newborns should feed at a minimum every 2 to 3 hours, and produce six to eight wet diapers per day), blood reabsorption from the cephalohematoma, and subclinical ABO incompatibility can exaggerate the normal physiologic hyperbilirubinemia. Because there is no evidence to suggest hemolysis, serious illness, or liver disease on history or physical examination, this is the most likely cause in this jaundiced newborn. In this case, therapy is targeted to help the infant eliminate excess bilirubin from the body until the period of physiologic jaundice has passed. Frequent feeds and adequate hydration are essential to ensure the efficient intestinal elimination of bilirubin from the body. In addition, phototherapy is typically initiated for total bilirubin levels of 20 mg/dL or higher. Phototherapy converts unconjugated bilirubin into several water-soluble stereoisomeric forms that can be excreted without conjugation.

QUESTIONS

15-1. Treating hyperbilirubinemia with phototherapy and other supportive measures is primarily performed to prevent
- A. Liver damage
- B. Hemolysis
- C. Permanent staining of the skin
- D. Kernicterus

15-2. Uncomplicated physiologic jaundice in a healthy term infant typically begins after 24 hours of life, peaks at 12 to 15 mg/dL, and resolves by
A. The first week of life
B. The second week of life
C. The first month of life
D. The sixth month of life

15-3. You are caring for a premature infant (30 weeks) whose total/direct bilirubin is 17/0.2 at 24 hours of life. Phototherapy is initiated, and the bilirubin increases to 22. The most appropriate therapeutic intervention to reduce the bilirubin level at this point is to
A. Start IV fluids
B. Start phenobarbital (to increase bile flow)
C. Perform exchange transfusion
D. Transfuse packed red blood cells

15-4. To identify potentially significant ABO incompatibility, an infant's blood type and Coombs reactivity is routinely determined in most hospitals when the mother is blood type
A. A
B. B
C. AB
D. O

ANSWERS

15-1. D. Hyperbilirubinemia is of concern to the physician for two reasons. The first is the risk for neurotoxicity (kernicterus), which occurs when unconjugated bilirubin, normally tightly bound to albumin, reaches levels high enough to exceed the binding capacity of albumin and subsequently crosses the blood–brain barrier to damage cells of the brain. In full-term newborns this can occur at levels higher than 25 to 30 mg/dL. It occurs at lower levels in premature neonates. Although truly a pathologic diagnosis, signs of kernicterus include poor feeding, hypotonia, irritability, and seizures. Phototherapy and other methods of facilitating the excretion of bilirubin are effective at preventing kernicterus. Exchange transfusion, which directly removes bilirubin from the bloodstream, is used for dangerously high bilirubin levels (usually >25 mg/dL in full-term neonates) or in patients who fail to respond to phototherapy. The second reason for concern is that elevated bilirubin levels may indicate the other processes or disorders mentioned earlier, which should be identified and treated early. The management of the jaundiced newborn should be aimed both at preventing kernicterus and at identifying and treating the cause of the jaundice.

15-2. A. Most newborns will develop a transient unconjugated hyperbilirubinemia after birth, termed "physiologic jaundice." This type of jaundice begins after 24 hours of life, peaks at a level of 12 to 15 mg/dL of indirect (unconjugated) bilirubin at around 3 days of life, and returns to normal by 1 week of age. Hyperbilirubinemia that develops in the first 24 hours, increases at a rate greater than 5 mg/dL per day, includes a direct fraction of >2 mg/dL or 15% of total bilirubin, or lasts more than 1 week should be evaluated. Risk factors for the development of more severe physiologic jaundice include prematurity, maternal diabetes, breastfeeding, and Asian or Native American ancestry.

15-3. C. Exchange transfusion is used to lower bilirubin levels in infants with significant, active hemolysis, or in those who are acutely at risk of kernicterus. In this procedure, the infant's blood is removed while simultaneously being replaced with a transfusion of O+ packed red blood cells. The procedure effectively removes bilirubin from the intravascular space while decreasing the hemolytic process that is contributing to increased bilirubin load.

15-4. D. The majority of clinically significant hemolysis from ABO incompatibility occurs when the mother is type O and the infant is type A or B. ABO hemolytic disease is caused by preformed maternal anti-A or anti-B antibodies that passively cross the placenta late in pregnancy, or during delivery, and attack A or B antigen on fetal RBCs. Due to a relatively small number of antigen sites on fetal red blood cells, the direct Coombs test (which looks for antibody-coated fetal RBCs) may be negative or weakly positive even when hemolysis is present; an indirect Coombs test (which looks for maternal anti-A or anti-B antibodies in the fetal serum) is more sensitive. Although 25% of pregnancies have the potential for ABO incompatibility, only around 10% of these develop hemolysis. Rh incompatibility is much rarer than ABO incompatibility and causes a much more severe form of hemolytic disease. All women identified as Rh negative during pregnancy should have the infant's blood tested prenatally or immediately after delivery for ABO and Rh type, hemoglobin, total bilirubin, and direct Coombs reactivity.

SUGGESTED ADDITIONAL READING

American Academy of Pediatrics Subcommittee on
   Hyperbilirubinemia. Management of hyperbilirubinemia in the
   newborn infant 35 or more weeks of gestation. *Pediatrics*.
   2004;114(1):297–316.

Tachypneic Premature Newborn

 CC/ID: 15-minute-old newborn baby boy, born prematurely at 32 weeks' GA, is brought to the intensive care nursery (ICN) with tachypnea.

HPI: Patient is a 1,430-gram baby boy born via cesarean for maternal preeclampsia and breech presentation to a 31-year-old woman, G3, P2, blood type A+, serology (–), rubella immune, and hepatitis B surface antigen (–), who has had good prenatal care. The mother presented 2 days ago to the obstetric clinic complaining of a headache and was found to have an elevated blood pressure of 190/120. She was placed on appropriate antihypertensive medication but did not respond to the therapy. Her obstetricians thus decided to deliver her fetus for maternal indications following a 48-hour course of betamethasone to enhance fetal lung maturity. Because the fetus was breech presenting, the mode of delivery was cesarean.

The infant was born blue and floppy, with poor tone and HR 60. He was resuscitated in the delivery room with 100% oxygen via face mask until pink with HR >100 and breathing spontaneously, and was then brought back to the ICN for further management. In the ICN, the face mask was briefly removed and he was noted to have a respiratory rate of 75 with moderate intercostal retractions, nasal flaring, and a blood oxygen saturation of 77% in room air (right arm).

THOUGHT QUESTIONS

- What is in this patient's differential diagnosis?
- Which test should be done to determine this baby's ability to ventilate the lungs?
- What additional blood tests should be ordered immediately?

DISCUSSION

The differential diagnosis in a premature newborn infant with respiratory distress should always include respiratory distress syndrome (RDS, or hyaline membrane disease), caused by a deficiency of surfactant in the alveoli. Additional causes in conjunction with RDS could include sepsis, pneumonia, pneumothorax, polycythemia, transient tachypnea of the newborn (from retained lung fluid), or any mass-occupying lesion or obstruction within the chest (e.g., congenital cystadenomatous malformation [CCAM], pulmonary sequestration, lobar emphysema, congenital diaphragmatic hernia, vascular ring). Mass lesions are often identified during routine prenatal fetal ultrasound examination, but many go undiagnosed until birth.

Before birth, it is helpful to determine the amniotic fluid lecithin/sphingomyelin ratio (L/S ratio) and check for the presence of phosphatidylglycerol (PG), which are measures of lung maturity. An L/S ratio greater than 2 and the presence of PG generally indicate lungs with sufficient surfactant to sustain adequate lung volumes. After birth, an arterial blood gas (ABG) should be performed on this patient to measure the serum P_{CO_2}, which assesses adequacy of ventilation. A blood gas obtained from a heel-stick or vein is also acceptable, because P_{CO_2} values are fairly close to arterial values.

Additional blood tests should include a hematocrit, CBC with differential, and blood culture.

 CASE CONTINUED

VS: Temp 36.4°C (97.5°F), BP 56/32 (MAP 40), HR 140, RR 75

PE: *Gen:* pink, tachypneic infant with nasal flaring, moderate intercostal retractions, and occasional grunting. *HEENT:* fontanel soft/flat; no cleft palate. *Lungs:* minimal air movement bilaterally; slightly "crackly." *CV:* RR&R; normal S_1, S_2; no murmur; capillary refill time 2 seconds. Remainder of exam normal for 32 weeks' GA.

Labs: ABG pH 7.20, P_{CO_2} 70, P_{O_2} 41, BE 0, Hct 51, CBC within normal limits, blood culture pending.

DISCUSSION

From the chest x-ray (Fig. 16-1) and ABG you determine that this premature infant has RDS and is not adequately ventilating his lungs (indicated by the primary respiratory acidosis with P_{CO_2} 70 on ABG). The management of RDS involves exogenous replacement of artificial surfactant, maintenance of adequate functional residual capacity (FRC) using continuous positive airway pressure (CPAP), and/or intubation and mechanical ventilation. The comprehensive management of premature infants involves providing adequate

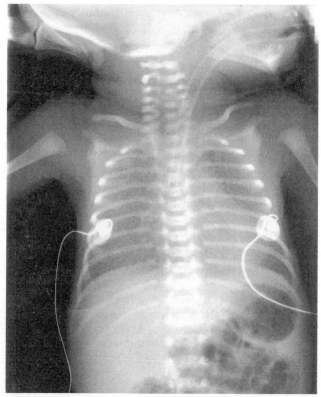

FIGURE 16-1. X-ray showing the features of respiratory distress syndrome. (*From Rudolf M, Levene M. Paediatrics and Child Health. Oxford: Blackwell Science; 1999:248, with permission.*)

nutrition, appropriate initiation of enteral feeds, maintenance of adequate blood volume, antibiotics to rule out sepsis, and monitoring for the risk of intracranial hemorrhage.

 QUESTIONS

16-1. Which of the following make up the characteristic triad of chest x-ray findings associated with RDS?
   A. Low lung volumes, small heart size, patchy infiltrates
   B. Low lung volumes, large heart size, patchy infiltrates
   C. Low lung volumes, air bronchograms, "ground-glass" appearance of lungs
   D. Large lung volumes, air bronchograms, pulmonary edema
   E. Large lung volumes, air bronchograms, patchy infiltrates

16-2. Which of the following cell types is responsible for the production of endogenous surfactant in the lung?
   A. Alveolar type I cells
   B. Alveolar type II cells
   C. Clara cells
   D. Ciliated tracheal cells
   E. Macrophages

16-3. Which of the following is a potential complication of exogenous surfactant therapy?
   A. Atelectasis
   B. Hypoglycemia
   C. Pulmonary hemorrhage
   D. Wheezing
   E. Decreased FRC

16-4. The effects of antenatal maternal steroid administration when premature delivery is anticipated include which of the following?
   A. No change in incidence of severe RDS and no change in incidence of intracranial hemorrhage
   B. Decreased incidence of severe RDS and no change in incidence of intracranial hemorrhage
   C. Decreased incidence of severe RDS and decreased incidence of intracranial hemorrhage
   D. No change in incidence of severe RDS and increased incidence of intracranial hemorrhage
   E. Increased incidence of severe RDS and increased incidence of intracranial hemorrhage

ANSWERS

16-1. C. The classic triad of radiologic findings in RDS is low lung volume, air bronchograms, and a "ground-glass" appearance of the lung parenchyma. Pulmonary edema and patchy infiltrates are *not* hallmark findings on chest x-ray of RDS. It is interesting to note that the chest x-ray can change significantly following a single dose of exogenous surfactant. In the case of an infant with respiratory distress, a very similar chest x-ray can also be the result of pneumonia caused by group B streptococcal sepsis, and therefore a rule-out sepsis workup including antibiotics must always be carried out.

16-2. B. Alveolar type II cells are responsible for the production and packaging of surfactant, which is stored in lamellar bodies within the cells prior to its release.

16-3. C. Pulmonary hemorrhage is a complication of exogenous surfactant therapy and can occur as a result of instilling fluid into the air spaces with a rapid change in lung compliance. Surfactant administration improves lung function by increasing FRC.

16-4. C. Antenatal steroids have been associated with both a decrease in severity of RDS as well as a decrease in incidence of intracranial hemorrhage.

SUGGESTED ADDITIONAL READING

Pfister RH, Soll RF. New synthetic surfactants: the next generation? *Biol Neonate.* 2005;87(4):338–344.
Soll RF, Lucey JF. Surfactant replacement therapy. *Pediatr Rev.* 1991;12(9):261–267.

CASE **17**

Cyanotic Newborn

 CC/ID: 15-minute-old full-term newborn baby boy presents to the well-baby nursery with tachypnea.

HPI: Patient is a 3,430-gram baby boy born via caesarean for failure to progress to a 31-year-old woman, G2, P2, blood type A, serology (–), rubella immune, hepatitis B surface antigen (–), who has had good prenatal care. At delivery, the infant was initially blue but had a good cry, spontaneous respirations, and improved color with Apgar scores of 9 and 9 at 1 and 5 minutes, respectively (2 for heart rate, 2 for respirations, 2 for reflexivity, 2 for tone, and 1 for color). The baby was warmed and dried and taken to the well-baby nursery for recovery. At 15 minutes of age he was noted to be cyanotic and had blood oxygen saturation values of 70% for both, right arm and right leg, and ABG values (right arm) of pH 7.44, Pco_2 35, Po_2 35, BE 0, in room air.

VS: Temp 36.6°C (97.9°F), BP 65/40 (MAP 50), HR 150, RR 100

PE: *Gen:* awake, looking around; cyanotic throughout, especially head and shoulders as compared with lower extremities. *Lungs:* good aeration bilaterally; no rales, rhonchi, or wheezing. *CV:* RR&R; prominent precordial heave; single loud S_2. No murmur. *Abdomen:* soft, nondistended; positive bowel sounds; no hepatomegaly or splenomegaly. *Ext:* equal peripheral pulses in brachial, femoral, and dorsalis pedis arteries.

THOUGHT QUESTIONS

- What is in this patient's differential diagnosis?
- What simple (nonradiologic) test can be performed to differentiate between pulmonary versus congenital heart disease?

DISCUSSION

The differential diagnosis in a term newborn with tachypnea includes transient tachypnea of the newborn (TTN, retained lung fluid), sepsis, pneumonia, pneumothorax, chest masses or obstructions (e.g., congenital cystadenomatous malformation [CCAM], pulmonary sequestration, lobar emphysema, congenital diaphragmatic hernia, vascular rings), persistent pulmonary hypertension (PPHN), and congenital heart disease. In this patient with cyanosis, PPHN or congenital heart disease or both should be considered. The congenital heart lesions that present as a cyanotic infant with tachypnea are those that lead to pulmonary overcirculation such as transposition of the great arteries (TGA), truncus arteriosus, and total anomalous pulmonary venous return (TAPVR).

The simple test to help differentiate a pulmonary versus congenital heart defect is a hyperoxia challenge. In this maneuver, the baby is placed in a 100% oxygen hood and an arterial blood gas is drawn. With pulmonary disease, the Pao_2 can be expected to rise above 150 torr, whereas in congenital heart defects it may remain less than 50 torr.

 CASE CONTINUED

You perform a hyperoxia challenge test, revealing a Pao_2 of 39 in a 100% oxygen hood, and determine that this infant most likely has congenital heart disease.

 THOUGHT QUESTIONS

- What is the next important radiologic test to perform?
- What is the significance of the cyanosis throughout?
- What is the importance of the ductus arteriosus in TGA?

 DISCUSSION

An echocardiogram is important to confirm the diagnosis of TGA and to ascertain whether an associated ventricular septal defect also exists. In cases of severe hypoxia in which the ventricular septum is intact, it may be necessary to perform an emergency atrial balloon septostomy (Rashkind procedure) to improve atrial mixing.

Cyanosis throughout this infant's upper and lower extremity reflects inadequate mixing of blood at the level of the atria and therefore inadequate delivery of oxygenated blood into the systemic circulation. This observation would necessitate a balloon septostomy as described above.

TGA is a ductal-dependent lesion, which means that patency of the ductus arteriosus is critical to survival. In these cases, it is important to start an infusion of prostaglandin PGE$_1$ to maintain ductal patency until complete surgical repair with an arterial switch can be performed (Fig. 17-1).

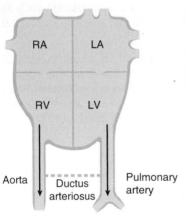

FIGURE 17-1.
Transposition of the great vessels. (*From Rudolf M, Levene M. Paediatrics and Child Health. Oxford: Blackwell Science; 1999:254, with permission.*)

 ## CASE CONTINUED

The baby was started on PGE$_1$, and a surgical arterial switch was done to correct the defect. The baby had an uncomplicated course and was discharged to home 3 weeks later on full feeds.

 ## QUESTIONS

17-1. The classic chest x-ray finding associated with TGA is
A. "Boot-shaped" heart
B. "Snowman" appearance of heart
C. "Egg on a string" appearance of heart
D. "Sail" sign

17-2. The electrocardiogram (ECG) in TGA has an electrical force axis that is
- A. Left axis deviation with left ventricular hypertrophy
- B. Right axis deviation with right ventricular hypertrophy
- C. Superior axis deviation
- D. Between 180° and 270°

17-3. Which of the following lesions comprise tetralogy of Fallot?
- A. Pulmonary stenosis, left ventricular hypertrophy, ventricular septal defect, overriding aorta
- B. Pulmonary stenosis, left ventricular hypertrophy, atrial septal defect, overriding aorta
- C. Pulmonary stenosis, right ventricular hypertrophy, ventricular septal defect, overriding aorta
- D. Aortic stenosis, right ventricular hypertrophy, ventricular septal defect, overriding aorta
- E. Tricuspid stenosis, right ventricular hypertrophy, ventricular septal defect, overriding aorta

17-4. The clinical finding of low blood pressure in the lower extremities compared with the upper extremities suggests which of the following congenital heart lesions?
- A. Tricuspid atresia
- B. Pulmonary atresia
- C. Coarctation of the aorta
- D. Tetralogy of Fallot

 ANSWERS

17-1. C. TGA is associated with the classic "egg on a string" appearance of the heart. This pathognomonic sign is caused by an oval-shaped heart due to a malpositioned pulmonary artery and the presence of a small thymus giving a narrow mediastinal shadow. The "boot-shaped" heart indicates tetralogy of Fallot, caused by an elevated and laterally displaced apex of the heart. The "snowman" appearance indicates TAPVR, caused by enlarged left and right superior vena cavae. The "sail" sign is suggestive of a pneumomediastinum resulting in a clear tracking of air separating the thymus from mediastinal structures.

17-2. B. The ECG findings in TGA are normal and can evolve into right axis deviation with right ventricular hypertrophy as the right ventricle continues to support systemic circulation. Left axis deviation occurs in conditions that lead to left ventricular hypertrophy or conduction defects with left bundle branch block. Superior axis deviation can be associated with atrioventricular canal defects or tricuspid atresia.

17-3. C. The four defining features of tetralogy of Fallot are pulmonary stenosis, right ventricular hypertrophy, ventricular septal defect, and overriding aorta. Tetralogy of Fallot is the most common cyanotic heart disease beyond the neonatal period (TGA is the most common cyanotic lesion presenting in the first week of life).

17-4. C. The hallmark of coarctation of the aorta is the finding of lower blood pressure in the lower extremities when compared with the upper extremities. This is because systemic blood flow is restricted by the stenotic aortic arch and is instead provided by right-to-left shunting of blood through a patent ductus arteriosus.

 SUGGESTED ADDITIONAL READING

Anderson RH, Weinberg PM. The clinical anatomy of transposition. *Cardiol Young.* 2005;15(suppl 1):76–87.
Tingelstad J. Consultation with the specialist: nonrespiratory cyanosis. *Pediatr Rev.* 1999;20(10):350–352.

Bilious Vomiting

CC/ID: 4-week-old baby boy presents to urgent care clinic with vomiting for past 2 days.

HPI: Patient was born prematurely at 35 weeks' gestational age by cesarean for severe variable decelerations to a 32-year-old woman, G1, P1, A +, serology (–), rubella immune, hepatitis B (–), VDRL (–), who had good prenatal care. She had a routine 20-week prenatal sonogram that revealed a normal fetus and amniotic fluid. At delivery, he was found to have a nuchal cord × 2 but was born vigorous, with Apgar scores of 6 and 9 at 1 and 5 minutes, respectively, following brief blow-by O$_2$, and a birth weight of 2,280 grams. He was discharged to home after good breastfeeding was established in 2 days. He had a normal 2-week visit, at which time his weight was noted to be 2,290 grams; his physical examination was normal. His mother states that for the past 2 days he has been vomiting up most of his formula about 30 minutes after his feeding, and over the past day has had very forceful green vomits. He has been breastfed every 3 to 4 hours, and his mother feels he has a good suck and swallow. He had a normal stooling pattern with four stools per day of mustard yellow and seedy consistency, although this morning his mother noted a single dark-brown-colored stool. He now feeds for only about 5 minutes per breast and vomits most of the quantity, which has turned green, within 10 minutes. Today his weight is 2,680 grams.

THOUGHT QUESTIONS

- What is the significance of the green vomitus?
- What is in this patient's differential diagnosis?

DISCUSSION

The green vomitus indicates that it is bilious in nature. Bilious vomiting indicates an obstructed bowel distal to the ampulla of Vater, the point where bile empties into the duodenum.

The differential diagnosis of a newborn infant with vomiting can be divided into two categories: bilious and nonbilious. Bilious vomiting generally involves conditions with partial or complete bowel obstruction, such as malrotation, volvulus, Ladd's bands, Hirschsprung disease, incarcerated hernia, torsion of Meckel's diverticulum, and intestinal atresia. Nonbilious vomiting in a newborn is largely due to gastroesophageal reflux, cow or soy milk protein intolerance, and pyloric stenosis. Although rare, nonbilious vomiting may also occur in esophageal atresia, but is usually diagnosed immediately after initiation of feeds.

 CASE CONTINUED

PMHx:/PSHx: None

Meds: None

All: NKDA

FHx: No family history of gastrointestinal disorders.

SHx: Lives at home with mother and father. At home with mother during the day.

VS: Temp 36.9°C (98.5°F), BP 57/24 (MAP 30), HR 79, RR 28

PE: *Gen:* awake, alert, and crying. *HEENT:* mucous membranes moist; throat nonerythematous. *Lungs:* clear bilaterally. *Abdomen:* soft, moderately distended; minimal bowel sounds; cries during exam, especially with palpation of abdomen; no masses or hepatosplenomegaly. *Rectum:* anus patent; no fissures noted. Stool test guaiac negative. *Skin:* slight pallor; capillary refill time 5 to 6 seconds.

THOUGHT QUESTIONS

- What aspect of the physical examination is particularly concerning?
- What radiologic test would be helpful at this time?

DISCUSSION

The compromised hemodynamic state (low blood pressure, prolonged capillary refill time of 5 to 6 seconds) is of concern because it suggests an infant who is in shock. Of primary importance will be resuscitating the infant and establishing adequate perfusion concurrent with determining the cause of the clinical symptoms.

Although an initial KUB x-ray might be a reasonable initial study to obtain, whenever a possible obstructive cause is suspected, an upper GI series with a small bowel follow-through should be performed (Fig. 18-1). If a malrotation/volvulus is suspected, an abdominal ultrasound may also help confirm the diagnosis.

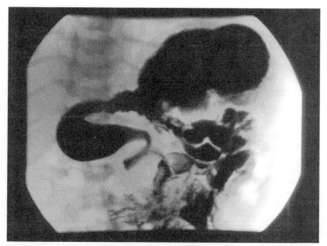

FIGURE 18-1. Malrotation with volvulus on upper GI series with small bowel follow-through. Note that the contrast in the small bowel is limited entirely to the left of midline, indicating malrotation. Also note the corkscrew appearance of the contrast, indicating volvulus within the proximal small bowel.

CASE CONTINUED

Labs: *X-rays:* KUB—gas in the stomach with paucity of air in the intestine. No free air noted. Upper GI series—contrast within stomach and extending only to the level of the ligament of Treitz, located in the right upper quadrant. *Abdominal ultrasound:* cecum located in the left lower quadrant.

You determine this baby has a malrotation with an associated volvulus.

QUESTIONS

18-1. The diagnosis of malrotation is definitive when
   A. The ligament of Treitz is abnormally located in the right quadrant, and the cecum is located in the right quadrant.
   B. The ligament of Treitz is located in the left quadrant, and the cecum is abnormally located in the left quadrant.
   C. There is a history of bilious vomiting.
   D. The ligament of Treitz is abnormally located in the right quadrant, and the cecum is abnormally located in the left quadrant.
   E. The diagnosis can only be definitive following surgical exploration.

18-2. The next step after confirming the diagnosis of malrotation with volvulus is to
   A. Consult pediatric gastroenterologists to request an emergent endoscopic procedure
   B. Consult pediatric surgeons for emergent surgical intervention
   C. Place an orogastric tube for decompression of the bowels and repeat an upper GI series in 4 to 6 hours
   D. Perform a barium enema to note the abnormal placement of the cecum in the left lower quadrant
   E. Place a red Robinson rubber catheter into the rectum to decompress the large intestine

18-3. Malrotation with associated volvulus often results in bowel ischemia or infarction due to twisting of the mesenteric blood supply, which includes the
   A. Superior gastric artery
   B. Inferior gastric artery
   C. Superior mesenteric artery
   D. Inferior mesenteric artery
   E. Gastrocolic artery

18-4. The primary metabolic derangement often associated with malrotation and volvulus is
- A. Respiratory acidosis
- B. Respiratory alkalosis
- C. Metabolic acidosis
- D. Metabolic alkalosis
- E. Metabolic alkalosis with compensating respiratory acidosis

 ANSWERS

18-1. D. The definitive diagnosis of malrotation is an abnormally placed ligament of Treitz in the right upper instead of left upper quadrant, and a cecum in the left lower instead of right lower quadrant. Retroperitoneal attachment is inadequate and the mesenteric pedicle is narrow, which can easily lead to volvulus. The symptom of bilious vomiting indicates the presence of a complete or intermittent obstruction associated with a volvulus.

18-2. B. A malrotation with associated volvulus is a surgical emergency, and a pediatric surgeon must be immediately consulted for surgical intervention. A barium enema to reconfirm abnormal placement of the cecum is unnecessary because the diagnosis is already confirmed.

18-3. C. Malrotation occurs when the small intestines abnormally rotate in utero, resulting in malposition in the abdomen and posterior fixation of the mesentery. When the intestine attaches improperly to the mesentery, it is at risk for twisting (volvulus) on its vascular supply, the superior mesenteric artery.

18-4. C. The metabolic derangement resulting from malrotation and volvulus is a severe metabolic acidosis due to bowel ischemia and infarction. This derangement should be corrected by aggressive therapy, including intubation with control of breathing and administration of fluids and alkali ($NaHCO_3$).

 SUGGESTED ADDITIONAL READING

Millar AJ, Rode H, Cywes S. Malrotation and volvulus in infancy and childhood. *Semin Pediatr Surg.* 2003;12(4):229–236.
Strouse PJ. Disorders of intestinal rotation and fixation ("malrotation"). *Pediatr Radiol.* 2004;34(11):837–851.

Rapid Heart Rate

CC/ID: 6-week-old infant brought to emergency room at midnight by parents who complain he is "breathing fast and very sleepy."

HPI: Parents report that baby was well until about 2 days ago when he started becoming increasingly "fussy" and showed decreased interest in feeding. Tonight, he has also become tachypneic but is less fussy. In fact, he seems to be sleeping more than usual and is not feeding at all. He has had no fevers or other signs of illness (no runny nose, coughing, vomiting, diarrhea, or rashes) and has not been exposed to anyone who was recently ill. There has also been no history of trauma or falls.

PMHx: *Birth:* unremarkable, with normal pregnancy and SVD at 39 weeks' GA and Apgar scores of 9 and 9 at 1 and 5 minutes, respectively. Baby was discharged home on day of life 3 and had a normal 2-week checkup as an outpatient.

Meds: None

All: NKDA

FHx: No history of metabolic or endocrine disorders in the family.

SHx: Lives at home with mother and father; no pets. Mother at home daily with infant.

VS: Temp 37.1°C (98.8°F), BP 65/45, HR 280, RR 70; 98% O_2 saturation on room air; Weight 4,405 g (birth weight 3,810 g).

PE: *Gen:* sleeping quietly; tachypneic; slightly ashen color. *HEENT:* normocephalic; anterior fontanelle soft/flat; otherwise normal. *Lungs:* clear to auscultation bilaterally; sternal and intercostal retractions. *CV:* tachycardia; regular rhythm; normal S_1, S_2; no murmurs. *Abdomen:* soft, no distention; positive bowel sounds; liver edge palpable 4 cm below costal margin; no splenomegaly; no masses. *Ext:* pulses full in upper and lower extremities. Remainder of exam normal.

THOUGHT QUESTIONS

- What is in this patient's differential diagnosis?
- What is the significance of this heart rate in an infant at rest?
- What is the most appropriate *non*hematologic test to perform?

DISCUSSION

Tachycardia often accompanies pain or agitation in an infant (sinus tachycardia), but in an infant who is resting comfortably you must consider a pathologic cause. Fever can also cause increased heart rate, but usually to a lower extent (low 200s). Sepsis should always be a strong consideration in an infant this age with poor feeding and abnormal vital signs. Other possibilities to consider include dehydration, anemia, hypovolemia (i.e., blood loss), or toxic ingestion (accidental or through breast milk). However, these factors rarely cause an increase in heart rate much above 200.

The extremely high level of tachycardia in this patient suggests that he could have a tachyarrhythmia, such as any type of supraventricular tachycardia (SVT). Whenever an abnormal heart rate is detected in an infant, special attention should be paid to assessing the patient's hemodynamic stability before proceeding with the diagnostic workup. This includes examination of pulses, skin color and perfusion, and oxygenation. Because this patient appears well compensated in these areas, you may proceed with the further investigation into the cause for his tachycardia.

This infant should have laboratory tests to evaluate for sepsis because of his young age and ill appearance. In addition, because of the suspicion of arrhythmia, the most useful supplemental diagnostic test to perform at this time would be an ECG looking for presence or absence of P waves and any signs of re-entrant phenomena.

CASE CONTINUED

Labs: CBC: WBC 15,000, no bands, 40% segs, 40% lymphs; platelets 320,000, Hct 41 g/dL. Blood culture sent. ABG (right arm): 7.22/33/95/−6 in room air. *Chest x-ray:* normal lung fields and heart size. *ECG:* shown in Figure 19-1.

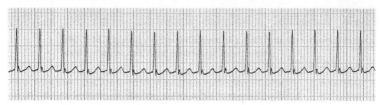

FIGURE **19-1.** Supraventricular tachycardia. Narrow QRS complex tachycardia at a rate of over 200 beats per minute. Note lack of visible P waves.

Based on the reassuring sepsis workup and the ECG results, you determine this patient has SVT, the most common type of arrhythmia in children. The base deficit of –6 on the ABG probably reflects some compromise to proper perfusion to the systemic circulation and thus warrants immediate correction of the underlying arrhythmia.

QUESTIONS

19-1. A quick review of the classification of this atrial tachyarrhythmia yields two types of SVT: automatic and re-entrant. The most common re-entry SVT is
   A. Atrioventricular re-entry tachycardia—Wolff-Parkinson-White (WPW) syndrome
   B. Atrioventricular nodal re-entry tachycardia
   C. Atrial flutter
   D. Atrial fibrillation
   E. Sinoatrial nodal re-entry tachycardia

19-2. Which of the following is *true*?
   A. P waves are always absent in SVT.
   B. A delta wave on ECG represents an initial slurred ventricular conduction delay and is called pre-excitation.
   C. SVT only occurs in infants.
   D. SVT is associated with prolonged PR interval.
   E. All SVTs are characterized as having a narrow complex.

19-3. Which of the following list of treatments may be used to treat SVT in infants?
   A. Ice bag to face, adenosine, digoxin, verapamil, synchronized DC cardioversion
   B. Adenosine, digoxin, verapamil, synchronized DC cardioversion
   C. Digoxin, verapamil, synchronized DC cardioversion
   D. Ice bag to face, adenosine, digoxin, synchronized DC cardioversion
   E. Ice bag to face, digoxin, verapamil, synchronized DC cardioversion

19-4. In patients with conduction disorders due to bypass tracts (e.g., WPW syndrome), antegrade conduction occurs through which of the following?
   A. Sinoatrial node
   B. Atrioventricular node
   C. His bundle
   D. Kent bundle
   E. Wolf bundle

 ANSWERS

19-1. B. Atrioventricular nodal re-entry tachycardia accounts for 90% of cases of SVT in children. SVT is the most common pediatric symptomatic arrhythmia and occurs with increasing risk in children with certain congenital heart defects (e.g., Ebstein's anomaly, left transposition of great artery), certain medications (e.g., caffeine, epinephrine), cardiomyopathy, myocarditis, cardiac tumors, hyperthyroidism, and fever.

19-2. B. Pre-excitation refers to the delay of ventricular conduction resulting in a "slurred" delta wave. An ECG finding of a delta wave in conjunction with a short PR interval comprises the Wolff-Parkinson-White (WPW) syndrome and indicates an abnormal retrograde conduction pathway between the ventricles and the atria. This condition is associated with an increased risk of serious arrhythmias, and can be treated with ablation of the abnormal conduction pathway.

19-3. D. Stable patients can be treated with careful application of ice bag to face, vagal maneuvers, or medications such as adenosine or digoxin; cardioversion should be administered to patients with signs of hemodynamic instability as soon as possible. Verapamil is contraindicated for use in infants with SVT because its vasodilating and negative inotropic effects may lead to hypotension and cardiac arrest in these patients.

19-4. D. In WPW syndrome, a bypass tract through a Kent bundle is present, whereby atrial conduction bypasses the atrioventricular node, entering an area of the left or right ventricle or septum directly.

 ## SUGGESTED ADDITIONAL READING

Chun TU, Van Hare GF. Advances in the approach to treatment of supraventricular tachycardia in the pediatric population. *Curr Cardiol Rep*. 2004;6(5):322–326.

Tingelstad J. Consultation with the specialist: cardiac dysrhythmias. *Pediatr Rev*. 2001;22(3):91–94.

Ambiguous Genitalia

CC/ID: Full-term newborn baby presents with ambiguous genitalia.

HPI: Patient is a 3,250-gram baby born via SVD through clear amniotic fluid to a 22-year-old woman, G1, P0, A+, antibody (–), rubella immune, hepatitis B surface antigen (–), VDRL nonreactive, group B streptococcus (–), who had good prenatal care. At birth the infant was pink and vigorous, with spontaneous respirations and a loud cry, and had Apgar scores of 9 and 9 at 1 and 5 minutes, respectively. After warming and drying the infant, a pediatrician was called to the delivery room to examine the baby's genitalia. The parents were reassured that the baby was in stable condition, but that a more thorough examination was necessary to determine the exact gender.

PMHx:/PSHx: None

Meds: None

All: NKDA

FHx: No history of ambiguous genitalia or endocrine disorders in the family.

SHx: Mother and father live together.

VS: Temp 36.1°C (97°F), BP 65/44, HR 120, RR 40

PE: *Gen:* awake, alert, pink. *HEENT:* normocephalic; anterior fontanel soft/flat; eyes PERRLA, with normal fundi; normal ears. *Lungs:* clear bilaterally. *CV:* RR&R; normal S_1, S_2; no murmur. *Abdomen:* soft, nondistended; positive bowel sounds; no masses. Normal liver edge. Kidneys of normal size palpable bilaterally. *GU:* small 1.5-cm soft tissue resembling penile tissue superior to bifid scrotum versus fused labia. *Skin:* no discolored spots or patches.

Labs: Na 122, K 3.5, Cl 100, CO_2 25, BUN 10, Cr 0.5

THOUGHT QUESTIONS

- ▪ What is in this patient's differential diagnosis?
- ▪ What is a key maneuver to perform on physical examination to help determine the cause of ambiguous genitalia?

DISCUSSION

The differential diagnosis of ambiguous genitalia is first divided into two major categories: virilized female or inadequate virilization of a male. The causes of a virilized female include congenital adrenal hyperplasia (CAH), androgenic drug exposure (e.g., progestins), true hermaphroditism (XO/XY karyotype), or maternal virilizing adrenal tumor. The causes of inadequate virilization of a male include steroid and steroid precursor deficiency, dysgenetic testes, Leydig cell hypoplasia, testicular feminization, partial androgen insensitivity, and 5α-reductase deficiency.

The key maneuver to focus upon during physical examination is to attempt to palpate gonads. Palpable gonads are nearly always testes and indicate that incomplete development of a male has occurred. Similarly, an ultrasound may be helpful to detect whether a uterus, cervix, and vagina are present.

CASE CONTINUED

Repeat examination reveals no palpable gonads, and abdominal ultrasound reveals the presence of a uterus and ovaries.

You determine that this patient must be a virilized female and obtain a genetics and urologic surgery consult to aid the family in deciding whether to rear the infant as a boy or a girl. You are aware that this decision is largely based on the prognosis of the underlying hormonal defect and the feasibility of genital reconstruction; today most patients are able to undergo hormonal replacement, have surgery, and be raised as girls.

QUESTIONS

20-1. The most common cause of CAH is a deficiency of which of the following?
- A. 17-hydroxylase
- B. 21-hydroxylase
- C. 11-hydroxylase
- D. 17-hydroxyprogesterone
- E. 18-hydroxylase

20-2. The diagnosis of CAH is made by measuring an elevation in which of the following?
- A. 17-hydroxylase
- B. 21-hydroxylase
- C. 11-hydroxylase
- D. 17-hydroxyprogesterone
- E. 18-hydroxylase

20-3. A key difference between 21-hydroxylase deficiency and 11 hydroxylase deficiency is that, unlike 21-hydroxylase deficiency, 11-hydroxylase deficiency is associated with
- A. Hypernatremia
- B. Hypotension
- C. Cortisol overproduction
- D. No ambiguity of genitalia
- E. Hyperkalemia

20-4. The treatment of 21-hydroxylase deficiency can include administration of which of the following list of therapies?
- A. Mineralocorticoid therapy, cortisol therapy, surgical treatment, testosterone
- B. Cortisol therapy, surgical treatment, testosterone
- C. Surgical treatment, testosterone, surgical treatment, mineralocorticoid therapy
- D. Mineralocorticoid therapy, cortisol therapy, surgical treatment
- E. Mineralocorticoid therapy, surgical treatment, testosterone

ANSWERS

20-1. B. 21-Hydroxylase deficiency accounts for 90% of the cases of CAH. Deficiency of this enzyme leads to decreased production of mineralocorticoids and cortisol and an overproduction of

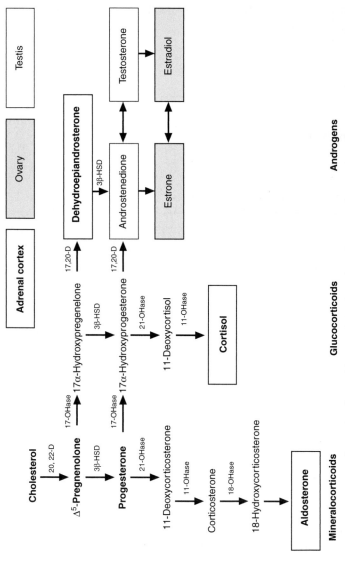

FIGURE 20-1. A schematic of steroidogenesis in the adrenal cortex. (*From Marino B, Snead K, McMillan J. Blueprints in Pediatrics. 2nd ed. Malden, MA: Blackwell Science; 2001:73, with permission.*)

androgens, causing virilization of a female (Fig. 20-1). It can also present as a salt-wasting deficiency in which symptoms of emesis, salt wasting, dehydration, and shock develop in the first 2 to 4 weeks of life. Male infants born with the defect have no genital abnormalities.

20-2. D. Measurement of elevated levels of 17-hydroxyprogesterone confirms the diagnosis of CAH. Interestingly, prenatal diagnosis in the siblings of children with 21-hydroxylase deficiency can be made by measuring elevated levels of 17-hydroxyprogesterone in amniotic fluid and HLA typing, because siblings who share the defect have the same HLA type.

20-3. A. Hypernatremia is associated with 11-hydroxylase deficiency, unlike the hyponatremic salt wasting that occurs with 21-hydroxylase deficiency (the patient in this case). 11-Hydroxylase deficiency is also associated with hypokalemia and hypertension.

20-4. D. Treatment includes cortisol, mineralocorticoids, surgical correction if necessary, and appropriate genetic counseling and recommendations for the family. Testosterone is *not* part of the therapy for 21-hydroxylase deficiency.

 SUGGESTED ADDITIONAL READING

Anhalt H, Neely EK, Hintz RL. Ambiguous genitalia. *Pediatr Rev.* 1996;17(6):213–220.

Bidarkar SS, Hutson JM. Evaluation and management of the abnormal gonad. *Semin Pediatr Surg.* 2005;14(2):118–123.

Newborn with Rash

CC/ID: Newborn girl who is small for gestational age with purpuric rash and jaundice.

HPI: Patient is a 1,950-gram baby girl born via NSVD at 39 weeks' gestational age to a 24 year-old G1, P1, blood type A+ woman who had poor prenatal care. Her prenatal labs are thus unavailable. The mother walked into the emergency department in labor and proceeded to deliver this infant within minutes after arrival. She reports that her membranes ruptured a few hours earlier and that the fluid appeared clear. She denies having any fevers during the pregnancy but does seem to recall having had a "common cold" sometime in the previous 3 months. At delivery, the baby was vigorous and was warmed and dried. Apgar scores were 9 and 9 at 1 and 5 minutes, respectively, and the baby was noted to have jaundiced skin with multiple small, round, purple-colored lesions over her trunk and extremities.

THOUGHT QUESTIONS

- What is in this patient's differential diagnosis?
- What is the significance of jaundiced skin at birth?
- What is the significance of the baby's low birth weight?

DISCUSSION

The differential diagnosis of a newborn infant with a purpuric rash includes any disorder that causes thrombocytopenia, including maternal and isoimmune ITP, maternal SLE, maternal preeclampsia, maternal medications, congenital megakaryocytic hypoplasia, giant hemangioma, sepsis, disseminated intravascular coagulation (DIC), and congenital infections (i.e., TORCH infections).

The finding of jaundiced skin at birth reflects an abnormality of bilirubin metabolism; increased bilirubin production vs decreased conjugation/excretion. Increased production is usually caused by hemolysis, which may occur in the newborn due to autoimmune processes (ABO or Rh incompatibility), red cell instability, or bleeding/bruising. Decreased conjugation and excretion of bilirubin in newborns is most commonly due to physiologically decreased bilirubin conjugation as well as increased enterohepatic circulation. Much less commonly, liver dysfunction may result in cholestasis which causes a conjugated (direct) hyperbilirubinemia.

Babies with low birth weight are referred to as small for gestational age (SGA). Low birth weight may occur after a normal intrauterine growth pattern or an abnormal one, called intrauterine growth restriction (IUGR). Another important distinction for SGA babies is whether head size and body size are proportionally small. When head size is spared in relation to body size, the infant has "asymmetric growth restriction" which is more likely to be due to placental insufficiency. Symmetric restriction of both head and body is more likely to be due to intrinsic genetic or CNS abnormalities.

 CASE CONTINUED

VS: Temp 36.7°C (98°F), BP 65/40 (MAP 50), HR 120, RR 35

PE: *Gen:* awake, eyes open, crying occasionally. *HEENT:* microcephalic (head circumference <3rd percentile); fontanelle soft, flat; eyes icteric, pupils reactive. *Lungs:* breathing room air; clear bilaterally; blood oxygen saturation 99%. *Abdomen:* soft, nondistended; positive bowel sounds; no masses; enlarged liver with edge 5 cm below costal margin. *Skin:* jaundiced; capillary refill time <3 sec; multiple 0.5-cm, round, raised, purplish lesions over trunk and extremities that do not blanch.

 THOUGHT QUESTIONS

- What is in the differential diagnosis for this infant with nonblanching purpura?
- What are appropriate laboratory tests to perform at this time?

DISCUSSION

Nonblanching purpura or petechiae usually signal thrombocytopenia. If significant liver injury also exists, the lesions may suggest centers of extramedullary hematopoiesis.

Appropriate lab tests to order are a CBC with differential, blood culture, liver function tests to assess for hepatitis, and blood titers (IgG and IgM) to detect presence of TORCH infections, including urine CMV titers.

CASE CONTINUED

Labs: *CBC:* WBC 18,000; 2% bands, 20% neut, 30% lymphocytes; Hct 45, Plt 40,000. CMV IgG and IgM positive. Urine positive for CMV.

Given the positive IgM for CMV and the presence of CMV in the urine, you determine that this infant must have congenital CMV infection.

QUESTIONS

21-1. Some of the pathogens that comprise congenital TORCH infections include which of the following?
- A. *Toxoplasma gondii,* rabies, CMV, HIV
- B. *Toxoplasma gondii,* RSV, CMV, HIV
- C. *Toxoplasma gondii,* rubella, CMV, herpes
- D. *Clostridium tetani,* rubella, CMV, herpes
- E. *Clostridium tetani,* rubella, CMV, HIV

21-2. The most common presenting clinical sign of congenital CMV infection is which of the following?
- A. Asymptomatic
- B. Jaundice
- C. Hepatosplenomegaly
- D. Purpura
- E. Microcephaly

21-3. Which of the following congenital infections presents with classical skin findings of "blueberry muffin spots"?
- A. *Toxoplasma gondii*
- B. Rubella
- C. CMV
- D. Herpes
- E. HIV

21-4. The intracranial calcifications commonly associated with congenital CMV infection are best described as
- A. Generalized (diffuse)
- B. Periventricular
- C. Cerebellar
- D. Periosteal
- E. Epidural

 ## ANSWERS

21-1. C. The organisms that make up the congenital TORCH infections are *Toxoplasma gondii*, OTHER (*Treponema pallidum*, HIV, VZV), rubella, CMV, and HSV. Rabies, RSV, and *Clostridium tetani* are *not* considered part of the TORCH infections.

21-2. A. Interestingly, the most common presentation of CMV is asymptomatic infection. CMV infection is a common infection, occurring in 1% of newborns born in the United States. Up to 10% of asymptomatic infections can manifest late sequelae that include nerve deafness and learning disabilities. Only 5% of infants with CMV manifest the syndrome of congenital CMV, which includes IUGR, purpura, jaundice, hepatosplenomegaly, microcephaly, intracerebral calcifications, and chorioretinitis.

21-3. B. Rubella syndrome presents with classic purple skin lesions known as "blueberry muffin spots." This congenital syndrome has become rare due to the success of rubella vaccine. Additional congenital anomalies that can occur secondary to infection in the first trimester include heart defects, ophthalmologic defects, auditory deficits, and neurologic malformations. Chronic infections can also lead to IUGR, radiolucent bone disease, hepatosplenomegaly, thrombocytopenia, and jaundice.

21-4. B. The intracranial calcifications commonly associated with congenital CMV are periventricular. Toxoplasmosis may be associated with intracranial calcifications that are distributed more diffusely throughout.

 ## SUGGESTED ADDITIONAL READING

Donley DK. TORCH infections in the newborn. *Semin Neurol.* 1993;13(1):106–115.
Stamos JK, Rowley AH. Timely diagnosis of congenital infections. *Pediatr Clin North Am.* 1994;41(5):1017–1033.

Jittery Newborn

CC/ID: 1-hour old newborn boy with jitteriness.

HPI: Patient is a 2,480-gram full-term (38 weeks' GA) baby boy born via elective cesarean to a 36-year-old woman, G2, P2, O +, serology (–), rubella immune, hepatitis B (–), VDRL (–), who had good prenatal care. She had a routine 20-week prenatal sonogram that revealed a normal fetus and amniotic fluid. At delivery, baby was vigorous, with Apgar scores of 9 and 9 at 1 and 5 minutes, respectively, and required only warming and drying with no additional resuscitation. At 1 hour of life he was noted to be jittery while resting in an open warmer.

THOUGHT QUESTIONS

- What is in the differential diagnosis of jitteriness in a newborn?
- What single laboratory test should be immediately performed for a jittery infant?
- What simple physical maneuver could help differentiate a true seizure from nonspecific jitteriness?

DISCUSSION

The differential diagnosis of a jittery newborn infant includes a multitude of potential causes, most simply including nonspecific neural and neurocutaneous changes associated with transition from an in utero environment. Although jitteriness due to a rapid environmental temperature fluctuation is possible, the most important pathologic causes of concern include seizures or a metabolic disturbance (i.e., glucose or electrolyte imbalance). A blood glucose level should immediately be obtained in a jittery infant to rule out hypoglycemia.

The simple maneuver of gently touching or holding the jittery extremity or extremities can be useful in determining whether the activity is due to a true seizure. Most seizure activity that manifests as jerky motion will not stop despite gently holding the extremity. Nonspecific jitteriness can often be calmed by gently wrapping the infant in a blanket.

CASE CONTINUED

VS: Temp 36.9°C (98.5°F), BP 65/40 (mean 50), HR 150, RR 35

PE: *Gen:* Awake and alert; fine shaking of limbs when started, suppressed by light pressure. *HEENT:* normocephalic; anterior fontanelle soft, flat. *Lungs:* clear bilaterally. *Heart:* RR&R; normal S_1S_2; no murmurs. *Abdomen:* soft, nondistended; positive bowel sounds; no masses or hepatosplenomegaly. *Skin:* pink, well-perfused, with capillary refill time 2 seconds.

Labs: blood glucose 20 mg/dL

THOUGHT QUESTIONS

- What is the next management step?
- What is the differential diagnosis of newborn hypoglycemia?

DISCUSSION

A newborn with low blood glucose is at high risk for developing brain injury secondary to lack of necessary nutrients for normal cellular metabolism. All hypoglycemic infants must therefore be treated immediately. Although treatment approaches may vary, blood glucose levels lower than 30 mg/dL should be treated with intravenous infusion of glucose. Usual starting doses are 2 to 3 cc/kg of D10W via peripheral IV. Higher values (>30–40 mg/dL) may sometimes be treated by initiating oral formula feedings with close follow-up of subsequent blood glucose levels.

The differential diagnosis of newborn hypoglycemia can be broadly divided into two categories: those with hyperinsulinism and those without hyperinsulinism. Babies with transient hyperinsulinism include infants of diabetic mothers and infants with RH hemolytic disease. Babies with prolonged hyperinsulinism include those with islet cell adenomas, functional hyperinsulinism, and congenital metabolic disorders (see Questions). Hypoglycemic babies without hyperinsulinism include those with intrauterine growth retardation (IUGR), birth asphyxia, polycythemia, cardiac disease, CNS disease, sepsis, maternal medications causing hypoglycemia, hypopituitarism, and defects in carbohydrate or amino acid metabolism.

 CASE CONTINUED

You admit the infant to the neonatal intensive care unit, where he remains for 2 days on an IV glucose infusion of D10W before slowly being weaned as his blood glucose stabilizes. You also complete a septic workup including CBC with differential and blood culture, and maintain the baby on IV antibiotics until sepsis is ruled out. Because his cultures are negative and his blood glucose has returned to normal, you determine the baby must have had hypoglycemia due to inadequate glycogen stores.

 QUESTIONS

22-1. Which of the following metabolic disorders is associated with hypoglycemia?
    A. Cushing syndrome
    B. Prader-Willi syndrome
    C. Hurler syndrome
    D. Hunter syndrome
    E. Beckwith-Wiedemann syndrome

22-2. Which of the following statements regarding infants of diabetic mothers is *true*?
    A. Infants may develop hypoglycemia when mothers have type 1 but not type 2 diabetes
    B. Infants may develop hypoglycemia when mothers have type 2 but not type 1 diabetes
    C. Infants may develop hypoglycemia only when mothers have type 1 or gestational diabetes
    D. Infants may develop hypoglycemia when mothers have type 1, type 2, or gestational diabetes
    E. Infants may develop hypoglycemia only when mothers have gestational diabetes

22-3. Hypoglycemia associated with panhypopituitarism is caused by a deficiency in which of the following?
  A. Growth hormone and thyroid-stimulating hormone (TSH)
  B. Growth hormone and adrenocorticotropic hormone (ACTH)
  C. Growth hormone and follicle-stimulating hormone (FSH)
  D. Oxytocin and ACTH
  E. Growth hormone and vasopressin

22-4. Which of the following blood tests is useful to obtain in a newborn patient with recurrent hypoglycemia *even when the infant is transiently euglycemic?*
  A. Serum insulin level
  B. Serum cortisol level
  C. Serum growth hormone level
  D. Serum lactate and pyruvate levels
  E. Serum amino acid levels

ANSWERS

22-1. E. Beckwith-Wiedemann syndrome should be considered in any infant with protracted hypoglycemia with hyperinsulinism. It is a congenital overgrowth syndrome associated with macrosomia, macroglossia, and abdominal wall defects in addition to hypoglycemia. There is also an associated high risk of embryonal cancers of infancy and early childhood. In a majority of infants the hypoglycemia will be only transient and resolve within the first 3 days of life. In less than 5% of infants the hypoglycemia may persist beyond the neonatal period due to hyperinsulinism. The other disorders listed do not generally present with hypoglycemia.

22-2. D. Infants of diabetic mothers can develop hypoglycemia in the neonatal period when mothers have *any* of the forms of diabetes, including type 1, type 2, or gestational diabetes. The hypoglycemia is usually transient in all three types and resolves with time, requiring only monitoring of serum glucose levels and administration of glucose via oral or IV route until levels normalize.

22-3. B. The disorders associated with panhypopituitarism that can lead to hypoglycemia include a deficiency of growth hormone and ACTH. Although there may be associated deficiencies of TSH, FSH, and/or vasopressin, these do not result in hypoglycemia.

22-4. E. Of the listed serum tests, only amino acid levels may be obtained even when infants are euglycemic. Serum insulin level, cortisol, growth hormone, and lactate and pyruvate levels should be obtained specifically when the infant is hypoglycemic.

 ## SUGGESTED ADDITIONAL READING

Fournet JC, Junien C. Genetics of congenital hyperinsulinism. *Endocr Pathol.* 2004;15(3):233–240.

Sperling MA, Menon RK. Differential diagnosis and management of neonatal hypoglycemia. *Pediatr Clin North Am.* 2004;51(3): 703–723, x.

Feeding Intolerance

CC/ID: Newborn girl with gagging or spitting up with initiation of feeds.

HPI: Patient is a 3-hour-old, full-term, 3,550-gram baby girl born via NSVD at 39 weeks' gestational age to a 24-year-old G1, P1, blood type A+ woman who had good prenatal care. Her prenatal labs were unremarkable, but pregnancy was notable for polyhydramnios on recent ultrasounds. At delivery, the baby was vigorous and was warmed and dried. Apgar scores were 9 and 9 at 1 and 5 minutes, respectively. The baby remained in the delivery room with the mother, where breastfeeding was initiated. The baby was noted to have excessive oral secretions with occasional gagging and color change, especially during feeding attempts. Sucking and swallowing mechanism appears to be intact.

THOUGHT QUESTIONS

- What is in this patient's differential diagnosis?
- What is the significance of a history of polyhydramnios?
- What would be the most appropriate initial radiologic test to perform?

DISCUSSION

The differential diagnosis of a newborn infant with difficulty on initiation of feeds can be divided into problems due to discoordinated sucking or swallowing or due to structural defects. Problems affecting sucking or swallowing include discoordination due to prematurity, weakened suck due to maternal anesthesia, hypoxia, neuromuscular disorders, sepsis, hypothyroidism, macroglossia, cleft lip or palate, cyst or tumor of mouth, micrognathia, and choanal atresia. In this

131

infant with a normal sucking and swallowing mechanism, possible structural defects of the esophagus or trachea include esophageal duplication, esophageal cyst, and tracheoesophageal fistula (TEF), either with or without esophageal atresia.

The history of polyhydramnios is suggestive of either a neuromuscular disorder or esophageal or intestinal obstruction preventing normal swallowing of amniotic fluid in utero. The simplest initial test to perform is a CXR and KUB with the placement of a feeding tube. Inability to advance a feeding tube beyond a certain point in the esophagus may strongly suggest esophageal atresia.

CASE CONTINUED

VS: Temp 36.7°C (98°F), BP 65/40 (MAP 50), HR 120, RR 35

PE: *Gen:* awake, eyes open, crying occasionally. *HEENT:* normocephalic (head circumference 50th percentile); fontanelle soft, flat; pupils reactive. Copious clear secretions noted at mouth. *Lungs:* breathing room air; mild rhonchi but good aeration throughout; blood oxygen saturation 99%. *Abdomen:* soft, mildly distended; positive bowel sounds, no masses; no hepatosplenomegaly or masses. *Skin:* well-perfused, capillary refill time <3 seconds.

Labs: CXR and KUB show equal aeration of both lung fields with a feeding tube curled upon itself at the level of the proximal esophagus. Air is noted in the stomach and throughout the intestines.

Given the clinical presentation and radiologic findings, you determine the baby has a tracheoesophageal fistula with esophageal atresia and immediately position the baby upright and place a Replogle tube to suction.

QUESTIONS

   23-1. Which of the following is the most common type of TEF?
   A. Esophageal atresia with distal TEF
   B. Esophageal atresia with no TEF
   C. H-type TEF
   D. Esophageal atresia with proximal TEF
   E. Esophageal atresia with proximal and distal TEF

23-2. Which of the following is the most specific distinguishing feature between an isolated esophageal atresia and an H-type TEF?

A. Feeding difficulty

B. Respiratory distress

C. Lack of stomach or bowel gas on KUB

D. Both have identical clinical presentations

23-3. TEF is a component of which of the following syndromes or constellation of findings?

A. Potter sequence

B. Prune belly syndrome

C. CHARGE syndrome

D. VATER or VACTERL syndrome

23-4. Which of the following best describes the oral secretions from an infant with isolated esophageal atresia?

A. Clear and projectile

B. Bilious

C. Grossly heme positive

D. Clear and copious

ANSWERS

23-1. A. The most common type of tracheoesophageal fistula is esophageal atresia with distal TEF, which comprises 85% of TEFs (Fig. 23-1). Surgical correction of esophageal atresia and distal TEF includes ligation of the fistula tract and either anastomosis of the proximal and distal esophageal ends or, in cases where the distance between esophageal ends is too great, a staged correction involving initial placement of a gastric tube and later esophageal anastomosis after adequate growth. Rarely, a colonic interpositioning surgery may be necessary, in which a large distance between esophageal ends is filled by inserting a segment resected from colon tissue.

23-2. C. Although feeding difficulty or respiratory distress or both can occur with either H-type or isolated esophageal TEF, lack of stomach or bowel gas suggests there is no connection between the oropharynx and airway with the enteric tract and is thus specific for isolated esophageal atresia.

23-3. D. TEF is part of VATER (vertebral, anal, tracheal, esophageal, radial or renal abnormalities) or VACTERL (vertebral, anal, cardiac, tracheal, esophageal, renal, and limb anomalies) syndrome. Potter sequence describes facial and limb deformities and pulmonary hypoplasia resulting from oligohydramnios (e.g., renal

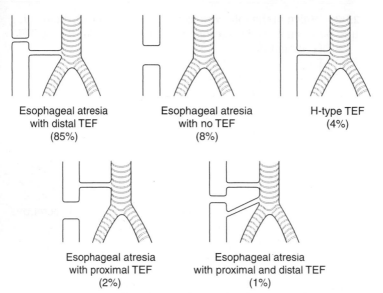

Esophageal atresia
with distal TEF
(85%)

Esophageal atresia
with no TEF
(8%)

H-type TEF
(4%)

Esophageal atresia
with proximal TEF
(2%)

Esophageal atresia
with proximal and distal TEF
(1%)

FIGURE 23-1. Types of tracheoesophageal fistulas, with relative frequencies. (*From Marino B, Snead K, McMillan J. Blueprints in Pediatrics. 3rd ed. Malden, MA: Blackwell Science; 2001:192, with permission.*)

agenesis or dysgenesis, or urinary obstruction). Prune belly syndrome describes a grossly enlarged abdomen resulting from hypoplasia of abdominal musculature due to bladder outlet obstruction or other urogenital anomalies. CHARGE syndrome includes coloboma, heart disease, atresia choanae, retarded growth and development, genital hypoplasia, and ear anomalies or deafness.

23-4. D. Oral secretions in isolated esophageal atresia are expected to be clear and copious. Projectile vomiting usually occurs with pyloric stenosis, and bilious emesis is suggestive of an obstruction distal to the ampulla of Vater. Esophageal atresia usually does not present with heme-positive secretions unless there is a history of trauma or concurrent mucosal breakdown.

 ## SUGGESTED ADDITIONAL READING

Foglia RP. Esophageal disease in the pediatric age group. *Chest Surg Clin N Am.* 1994;4(4):785–809.

Groenman F, Unger S, Post M. The molecular basis for abnormal human lung development. *Biol Neonate.* 2005;87(3):164–177.

IV

Cases Presenting with Abdominal Pain

Fever and Abdominal Pain

CC/ID: 10-year-old boy with a 2-day history of fever and abdominal pain.

HPI: A.A. has been experiencing abdominal pain for 2 days. His pain, "in the lower part of my belly, and near my belly button," is worse when he tries to sit up, and he prefers to lie still in bed. He was given acetaminophen without any resolution. He has been vomiting since last night (no blood or bile) and had initial diarrhea on the first day of his illness. This morning his parents noticed that he had a fever (measured in the axilla at 101.8°F), but that his pain is relatively improved.

PMHx: Asthma (hospitalized once for exacerbation); otherwise within normal limits.

Meds: Acetaminophen as above; herbal tea

All: NKDA

THOUGHT QUESTIONS

- What further questions would you ask as part of the history?
- What is your differential diagnosis at this point?

DISCUSSION

Abdominal pain is a very common complaint in the pediatric population. When assessing a patient, it is important to ask questions regarding the specifics of the symptom (the quality and temporal characteristics of the pain, the exacerbating and relieving factors). Other important aspects of the history include a thorough diet history, travel history, history of trauma or ingestions, stooling habits, family history, sexual behavior history, a thorough review of symptoms, and behavioral/environmental history (including ill contacts).

A particularly thorough history should be obtained because the differential diagnosis for abdominal pain is extensive. In pediatrics, common causes for acute abdominal pain account for nearly 90% of diagnoses. These include viral gastroenteritis, bacterial enterocolitis, food poisoning, dietary indiscretion, appendicitis, UTI, and group A streptococcal pharyngitis. More uncommon causes include pelvic inflammatory disease (PID), lower lobe pneumonia, insulin-dependent diabetes mellitus (IDDM), obstructive disease, intussusception, perforated bowel, trauma, and conversion reactions.

CASE CONTINUED

Further history reveals anorexia and no bowel movements over the last 24 hours, no ill contacts or new food sources, and an otherwise negative review of symptoms.

VS: Temp 38.3°C (101°F), BP 130/65, HR 100, RR 30

PE: *Gen:* supine on table; appears uncomfortable but in no acute distress. *HEENT:* dry oral mucosa; otherwise noncontributory. *Lungs:* clear to auscultation; no crackles. *CV:* RR&R, mild tachycardia; normal S_1, S_2; no murmur; otherwise normal pulses; CRT <2 seconds. *Abdomen:* nondistended; hypoactive bowel sounds in all areas; mild guarding; pain on superficial palpation in periumbilical area; tympanic abdomen; no masses. *GU:* Tanner stage 1 to 2, normal external male genitalia; no swelling or masses.

THOUGHT QUESTIONS

- Are there any other components of the physical examination that you would like to perform?
- What laboratory tests or imaging studies, if any, would you obtain?

CASE CONTINUED

A urinalysis is performed that reveals no organisms, few WBCs, and few RBCs. Based on his improving abdominal pain and clinical picture, the patient is diagnosed with an acute gastroenteritis of a likely viral origin, receives parenteral rehydration, acetaminophen for his pain and fever, and instructions on when to return to the office. He returns late that evening with persistent fever, anorexia, and worse abdominal pain. His examination now reveals pain localizing to his right lower quadrant, which increases when he is asked to move in bed. His WBC count is 19,000 with a left shift, and an abdominal CT scan reveals a perforated appendix with evidence of diffuse peritonitis.

 DISCUSSION

Appendicitis is generally a clinical diagnosis; however, laboratory values and imaging may augment clinical suspicion. In atypical cases where the diagnosis is not clear, a rectal exam may be helpful to detect tenderness or a mass. Laboratory examination may reveal a moderately increased WBC count with left shift and mild pyuria or hematuria on urinalysis. Imaging for suspected appendicitis may consist of abdominal ultrasound or CT scan. The choice of imaging is a complex and controverisal topic, resulting in wide variations in practice. Studies suggest that in centers where ultrasound is readily available it should be used to screen for appendicitis in patients at moderate risk. CT scan is more expensive and exposes the patient to radiation, but it is more sensitive and specific, and for this reason is often used preferentially in selected patients.

 QUESTIONS

24-1. The typical pediatric patient with appendicitis can present with which of the following?
   A. Fever, emesis, anorexia
   B. Periumbilical pain
   C. Right lower quadrant pain, guarding
   D. Obturator and psoas signs
   E. All of the above

24-2. Conditions that may mimic appendicitis include
   A. Lower lobe pneumonia
   B. *Yersinia* enterocolitis
   C. Urinary tract infection
   D. Diabetic ketoacidosis
   E. All of the above

24-3. For patients with suspected appendiceal perforation, which of the following apply?

- A. The appendix typically perforates 12 to 24 hours after pain begins.
- B. The incidence of perforation in young children and toddlers is low.
- C. The retrocecal appendix usually induces pain well before perforation occurs.
- D. Peritonitis, abscesses, and longer hospitalizations are rarely associated with perforation.
- E. None of the above

24-4. You are asked to review pediatric appendicitis with a group of medical students. Which of the following statements could be included in your discussion?

- A. Atypical presentation of appendicitis is quite rare in childhood.
- B. Diagnosis of appendicitis is established primarily by imaging.
- C. A high WBC count is an essential part of the diagnosis.
- D. Appendicitis is the most common indication for emergency abdominal surgery in childhood.
- E. Commonly, the majority of children with appendicitis are younger than 5 years.

ANSWERS

24-1. E. All of the symptoms mentioned are possible. Classically, fever, emesis, and periumbilical pain are followed by right lower quadrant pain (at McBurney's point), guarding, and the obturator/psoas signs. Perforation typically occurs 36 hours after pain begins, and may manifest with signs of peritoneal irritation.

24-2. E. These diagnoses make the diagnosis of appendicitis difficult, and highlight the importance of an adequate history and physical examination and a high index of suspicion for these conditions.

24-3. E. The appendix typically tends to perforate 36 to 48 hours after pain begins. This can be quite common in the younger child and toddler, who may have a longer duration of symptoms before diagnosis. The retrocecal appendix usually does not induce right lower quadrant pain until after perforation occurs. In patients with perforation of the appendix, longer hospitalization with peritonitis and abscess formation is more commonly found.

24-4. D. Appendicitis is the most common indication for emergency abdominal surgery in childhood. Atypical presentation is quite common in children, particularly with retroccal appendicitis. The diagnosis primarily clinical, although imaging is used with increasing frequency to confirm the diagnosis before surgery. Labs such as WBC count may provide additional supporting evidence for the diagnosis, but are neither sufficiently sensitive nor specific to make the diagnosis. Fewer than 10% of cases of appendicitis occur in children under age 5. It is most common between 10 and 15 years of age.

 ## SUGGESTED ADDITIONAL READING

Ashcraft KW. Consultation with the specialist: acute abdominal pain. *Pediatr Rev.* 2000;21:363–367.

McCollough M. Abdominal pain in children. *Pediatr Clin North Am.* 2006;53(1):107–137, vi.

Abdominal Pain and Vomiting

CC/ID: 6-year-old boy with vomiting and worsening abdominal pain.

HPI: M.D. presents with 2 days of vomiting and worsening abdominal pain. His vomiting is nonbloody and nonbilious, and the pain is epigastric and "near his belly button." The pain is not relieved by position or vomiting. He has no fever, cough, rhinorrhea, or diarrhea. His mother states that he has been unable to tolerate any oral intake since yesterday, but he is still urinating regularly. Some of the children at his school are ill. This morning he seems to be quite uncomfortable and very tired.

PMHx: No prior hospitalization; evaluated several times for acute gastroenteritis.

Meds: None

All: NKDA

SHx: Attends kindergarten; lives with parents; no smokers; no pets.

DietHx: "Usually eats like a horse, but never gains any weight!"

VS: Temp 37.7°C (99.8°F), BP 80/45, HR 140, RR 40

PE: *Gen:* lethargic, thin boy, breathing with difficulty; looks ill. *HEENT:* NCAT; EOMI; PERRL; mucous membranes are dry. *Neck:* supple. *Lungs:* tachypneic and labored breathing; no crackles or wheeze appreciated. *CV:* tachycardic; RR&R; normal S_1, S_2; no murmur; capillary refill time 3.5 seconds. *Abdomen:* decreased bowel sounds; periumbilical and epigastric tenderness; guarding. No visceromegaly appreciated. *Skin:* dry; no cyanosis, clubbing, or edema; decreased turgor.

THOUGHT QUESTIONS

- What further components of the history or physical examination would you like to explore?
- What signs and symptoms of dehydration are present in this patient?
- What is in your differential diagnosis at this point?
- What are some immediate measures to take in this patient?

DISCUSSION

When faced with the patient with acute abdominal pain and vomiting, obtaining a thorough history should include eliciting specifics regarding the pain, emesis, stool habits, and dietary habits and appetite. Prior surgery, a family history, travel history, and a review of symptoms will aid in the diagnosis. The physical examination findings in this patient that indicate dehydration include the vital signs—tachycardia, tachypnea, weight loss, hypotension (in decompensated or severe cases)—and poor skin turgor, dry mucous membranes, lethargy, and prolonged capillary refill time.

This patient appears to be quite ill and is facing decompensated shock. The differential diagnosis includes septic shock/meningitis, severe acute gastroenteritis, metabolic or endocrine disorders (diabetic ketoacidosis, adrenal insufficiency), toxic ingestion, GI disorders (appendicitis, perforation, pancreatitis), and trauma. Immediate measures would include assessment of the ABCs, including airway/breathing support and volume resuscitation (20 mL/kg of normal saline or lactated Ringer's solution), and appropriate monitoring of vital signs. Laboratory studies may include a CBC, blood gas measurement, serum electrolytes and glucose levels, urinalysis, and blood and/or urine for culture. Administration of empiric antibiotics should not be delayed in suspected cases of septic shock.

CASE CONTINUED

Upon assessing the ABCs, this noticeably ill-appearing child was given aggressive fluids for his apparent dehydration. An astute nurse noticed a fruity odor to his breath. His electrolyte panel yielded the following values: sodium of 155, chloride of 119, and bicarbonate of 5, with an anion gap of 31; his glucose level was 495. Arterial blood gas revealed a pH of 7.12 and P_{CO_2} of 18. His urine was positive for glucose and ketones. Based on his clinical presentation, the patient was transferred to the intensive care unit for further management of diabetic ketoacidosis. Further questioning yielded a positive family history for type 1 diabetes mellitus, and a review of symptoms revealed symptoms of polyuria, polydipsia, and polyphagia over the last several months.

DISCUSSION

Diabetes mellitus is the most common life-threatening pediatric endocrine disorder. Diabetic ketoacidosis (DKA) occurs with severe insulin deficiency, when excess ketone production (due to a lack of glucose utilization) overwhelms the blood's native buffering capacity. The result is a profound hyperglycemia, dehydration, metabolic acidosis, and lethargy. The mainstays of treatment of DKA include restoration of fluid volume, inhibition of lipolysis/return to glucose utilization, replacement of body salts, and correction of acidosis. The management of diabetes and its complications requires a multidisciplinary approach involving medical, nutritional, behavioral, and environmental interventions.

QUESTIONS

25-1. DKA presents with which of the following acid-base abnormalities?
- A. Metabolic alkalosis with compensatory respiratory acidosis
- B. Metabolic acidosis with compensatory respiratory alkalosis
- C. Respiratory acidosis with compensatory metabolic alkalosis
- D. Respiratory alkalosis with compensatory metabolic acidosis

25-2. Which of the following best describes an associated metabolic disturbance in DKA?
- A. Symptoms of hypoglycemia are due to catecholamine release and no available cellular glucose.
- B. Hypokalemia is often the result of decreased serum pH level.
- C. Ketonuria resolves when glucagon levels increase.
- D. Serum bicarbonate levels are usually normal or high.
- E. There is a normal anion gap metabolic acidosis.

25-3. You are counseling the family of the above patient with type 1 diabetes mellitus. Which of the following statements would be appropriate to include in your discussion?
- A. It becomes clinically significant after 90% of B-cell function is destroyed.
- B. Anti-islet cell antibodies may be present.
- C. It may be complicated (long term) by small and large vessel disease.
- D. It may be managed via insulin, diet and exercise therapy, and blood sugar monitoring.
- E. All of the above

25-4. Which of the following best describes type 2 diabetes mellitus?
- A. It is caused by excessive corticosteroid synthesis.
- B. Patients may commonly be thin and underweight.
- C. Patients very rarely present with skin findings.
- D. It is characterized by insulin resistance.
- E. It must be managed with insulin therapy.

ANSWERS

25-1. B. In DKA, metabolic acidosis occurs from ketone production and dehydration. The natural physiologic response to this is a compensatory respiratory alkalosis.

25-2. A. Global catecholamine release in the face of a general lack of cellular glucose availability can result in symptoms of hypoglycemia. In states of acidosis and lowered serum pH, the inability of potassium to stay in the cell results in a hyperkalemia. Increased catabolic mediators, such as glucagon, produce ketone bodies, which will manifest as ketonuria until the process is reversed. The general acidosis is reflected also by a low serum bicarbonate level. Ketone bodies account for a high anion gap metabolic acidosis.

25-3. E. Type 1 diabetes mellitus has many proposed causes; genetic, autoimmune, and environmental factors have all been implicated. The basic disorder is characterized by a lack of insulin production at the cellular level. It is only after 90% of pancreatic B-cell function has been destroyed that loss of insulin secretion becomes clinically significant. The mainstays of medical management include insulin replacement therapy, diet and exercise modification, and proper daily monitoring of blood glucose levels.

Long-term complications include microvascular disease and accelerated large vessel atherosclerosis.

25-4. D. Type 2 diabetes mellitus is becoming more of a concern because an increasing number of cases are being found in the pediatric population. The primary underlying abnormality is thought to be due to insulin resistance. Most affected patients are overweight, and acanthosis nigricans (a hyperpigmentation with a velvety texture, often found on the nape of the neck or antecubital fossa) is commonly found on physical examination. Insulin may be required for some patients, but some patients may be treated with oral medications. Nevertheless, diet and exercise remain the mainstays of any therapeutic regimen.

 SUGGESTED ADDITIONAL READING

Agus MS. Diabetic ketoacidosis in children. *Pediatr Clin North Am.* 2005;52(4):1147–1163, ix.

Haller MJ. Type 1 diabetes mellitus: etiology, presentation, and management. *Pediatr Clin North Am.* 2005;52(6):1553–1578.

Kaufman FR. Type 2 diabetes in children and youth. *Endocrinol Metab Clin North Am.* 2005;34(3):659–676, ix–x.

Scrotal Pain and Swelling

CC/ID: 16-year-old boy with scrotal swelling and pain.

HPI: T.T. presents this evening to the emergency department with several hours of worsening pain and swelling of his scrotal area. The pain began late this afternoon and is worsened by any movement. He also complains of nausea and has vomited twice in the waiting room. He has had no fever, no dysuria, and no urinary urgency. He confides that he has become sexually active, and is afraid that this is a result of recent unprotected intercourse.

PMHx: Exercise-induced asthma

PSHx: None

Meds: Albuterol inhaler as needed

All: Penicillin

FHx: Noncontributory

SHx: Lives at home with parents and older sister; 10th grade honor student; plays soccer; denies any toxic habits or exposures.

VS: Temp 37.1°C (98.8°F), BP 135/75, HR 120, RR 32

PE: *Gen:* anxious, lying on table. *HEENT:* within normal limits. *Chest:* slightly tachypneic; clear to auscultation. *CV:* tachycardic; RR&R; normal S_1, S_2; no murmur. *Abdomen:* bowel sounds; mild suprapubic tenderness; otherwise, soft, nondistended, and nontender; no masses. *Ext/Back:* no flank or side pain. *Skin:* no rashes; skin warm with no rash. *GU:* Tanner stage 5 external genitalia; swelling and redness of the right hemiscrotum; pain upon movement or palpation of the entire right testis; absent right cremasteric reflex; no relief of pain upon elevation of the scrotum. *ROS:* no weight loss; no recurrent fever; no rash; no discharge.

THOUGHT QUESTIONS

- What is your differential diagnosis at this point?
- What components of the history and physical examination help narrow this diagnosis?
- What diagnostic studies may help in the diagnosis?

DISCUSSION

For the patient who presents with scrotal swelling and pain, the differential diagnosis should include traumatic injury, torsion of the testis or appendix testis, incarcerated hernia, hydrocele, epididymitis, scrotal abscess, Henoch-Schönlein purpura, and leukemic infiltrate of the testis. Questions regarding pain (quality, location, timing/onset, radiation, and alleviating or precipitating factors) and a thorough review of systems can help narrow the diagnosis. In any adolescent, "HEADSS" questions should be asked regarding home life and family relationships; educational level, employment, eating, and exercise; activities, hobbies, and peer relationships; drug use or abuse; sexuality and sexual activity; and suicidal ideation or attempts, depression and mental health, and safety/risk. On physical examination, localization of the pain near the upper pole of the testis with a tender nodule may suggest torsion of the appendix testis, the most common cause of acute scrotal swelling and pain in the preadolescent male. An absent cremasteric reflex, associated with an exquisitely tender and slightly retracted testis, indicates a testicular torsion and is a surgical emergency. Epididymitis is associated with scrotal pain (which radiates along the spermatic cord into the flank and is relieved by lifting the scrotum), fever, and symptoms of frequency/urgency and dysuria.

In many patients, a definitive diagnosis cannot be discerned from the history and physical examination, so imaging may be necessary to depict anatomy and blood flow. High-resolution color Doppler ultrasonography can greatly aid diagnosis and is the procedure of choice in examining the acutely painful scrotum with unclear cause.

CASE CONTINUED

Based on the patient's history and positive physical findings, he was clinically diagnosed with testicular torsion. The patient was promptly referred for surgical management, and the right testis was salvaged. At his 2-week postoperative visit and in an appropriately confidential manner, you counsel him regarding safe sex practices, STDs, and pregnancy.

QUESTIONS

26-1. Testicular torsion
A. Occurs most commonly in preadolescent males (ages 9 to 12)
B. Can be associated with the "blue-dot" sign
C. Can be treated with analgesics and observation
D. May result from an absent or narrow posterior mesenteric attachment

26-2. Which of the following may cause painless scrotal swelling?
A. Varicocele
B. Hydrocele
C. Testicular tumor
D. Inguinal hernia
E. All of the above

26-3. A 15-year-old boy presents with slight testicular pain and swelling of his scrotum over 3 days. He has had fever, and last week he suffered from parotid gland swelling. What is his likely diagnosis?
A. Trauma
B. Torsion of the appendix testis
C. Mumps orchitis
D. Idiopathic scrotal edema

26-4. When counseling parents of an infant with cryptorchidism, which of the following statements should you include in your discussion?
A. It is less common in premature males than term males.
B. There is no risk for malignancy.
C. By age 1 year, most cases will have resolved.
D. Hormone therapy is more successful than surgery.

ANSWERS

26-1. D. Testicular torsion most commonly occurs in the adolescent male and is a surgical emergency. Most patients lack the posterior mesenteric attachment to the tunica vaginalis that keeps the testis from rotating around the spermatic cord. In some cases the attachment may be too narrow. The "blue-dot" sign is associated with torsion of the appendix testis (an embryonic remnant of the developing gonad) and may be observed as a tender, discolored nodule on the upper pole of the testicle. Torsion of the appendix testis can often be managed with analgesics alone.

26-2. E. Varicocele is a dilation of the venous plexus of the spermatic cord and presents classically as a palpable mass ("bag of worms" appearance) above the left testis. Hydrocele is produced by accumulation of peritoneal fluid inside a patent processus vaginalis and can be associated with hernias. Inguinal hernias can also be a cause of scrotal swelling.

26-3. C. Mumps orchitis classically presents within 1 week following parotitis, although it may occur in the absence of salivary gland involvement. Immunization history should be obtained. These patients may have fever, pain, and swelling for 4 to 10 days. Occasionally, infection can result in testicular atrophy and decreased fertility.

26-4. C. Cryptorchidism is defined by testes that have not fully descended into the scrotum and cannot be manipulated into the scrotum with gentle pressure. It occurs in 3% to 4% of term males and is more common in premature babies. Testes that remain outside the scrotum are at increased risk for traumatic injury and malignancy. The majority of cases resolve by age 1 year. Surgical repair has a much higher success rate than hormonal therapy.

 ## SUGGESTED ADDITIONAL READING

Adelman WP, Joffe A. Consultation with the specialist: testicular masses/cancer. *Pediatr Rev*. 2005;26:341–344.

Haynes JH. Inguinal and scrotal disorders. *Surg Clin North Am*. 2006;86(2):371–381.

Jayanthi VR. Adolescent urology. *Adolesc Med Clin*. 2004;15(3): 521–534.

Infant with Indigestion

CC/ID: 7-month-old with indigestion.

HPI: E.S. is a 7-month-old boy having "cramps" for the past several weeks. His parents state that they think he is experiencing pain from indigestion, because he has been "repeatedly drawing his arms and legs up to his belly" and subsequently crying during these episodes. He has been feeding well, without fever, vomiting, or diarrhea. The "cramps" seem to occur in clusters, particularly when he is about to fall asleep and occasionally after a meal. The parents feel that this may be a result of introducing solid foods to him last month. They have tried simethicone drops without any resolution.

PMHx: NSVD at term without complications

Meds: Simethicone drops

All: NKDA

Immun: UTD

FHx: Noncontributory

DevHx: Maintains head supported; unable to sit independently; not yet babbling; not yet transferring objects. *ROS:* Noncontributory.

DietHx: Age-appropriate solids introduced at 5 months; breast-feeding.

VS: Temp 37.1°C (98.8°F), BP 90/50, HR 110, RR 26

PE: *Gen:* supine on table; alert/will regard face; in no apparent distress. *HEENT:* nondysmorphic; NCAT; EOMI; PERRL; tympanic membranes within normal limits. *Lungs:* normal exam with no crackles or wheeze. *CV:* normal exam with no murmur; pulses and capillary refill time normal. *Abdomen:* bowel sounds; soft, no distention and no tenderness; no visceromegaly. *Neuro:* normal tone and reflexes; grossly nonfocal exam.

THOUGHT QUESTIONS

- What developmental milestones have not been appropriately met by this patient?
- What is in your differential diagnosis at this point?
- What further components of the physical examination or history would you explore?

DISCUSSION

The 7-month-old infant should be able to sit independently with adequate head and trunk support, to transfer grasped objects from one hand to the other, and to begin some monosyllabic babbling. The differential diagnosis for this patient may include gastrointestinal conditions such as colic, formula/food intolerance, constipation or gastroesophageal reflux as well non-abdominal episodic events such as myoclonic jerks or seizures. With the associated developmental delay noted in this child, an underlying neurologic problem manifesting as seizures should be highly considered. Further questions to ask may be related to the nature of the episodes: association with fever or feeds, relieving or exacerbating factors, relation to eating or sleeping, associated symptoms (vomiting, pallor, cyanosis, posturing), and status of the child after the episode (alert, drowsy, altered consciousness). Given the concern for a neurologic disorder, aspects of the physical exam to focus on in this patient include growth parameters, muscle strength and tone, cranial nerve function and any skin lesions suggestive of neurocutaneous disorders.

CASE CONTINUED

Height, weight, and head circumference are normal for his age. Upon further handling of the child, he exhibits a repetitive cluster of flexor contractions of the neck and trunk, with adduction and flexion of his arms and legs after which he appears sleepy and difficult to arouse for a few minutes. A subsequent electroencephalogram (EEG) reveals a characteristic hypsarrhythmia pattern. The patient is diagnosed with infantile spasms.

DISCUSSION

Infantile spasms are a form of pediatric epilepsy with a characteristic clinical presentation and EEG pattern. The term "epilepsy" describes a pattern of repeated seizures, and the cause is unknown in >50% of cases. Known causes of epilepsy include metabolic derangements, trauma, infections, neoplasms, toxins, and hereditary/genetic disorders. Conditions which can mimic seizures in children include tic disorders, reflux, breath-holding spells, syncope, movement disorders, and benign positional vertigo.

 QUESTIONS

27-1. Which of the following types of seizures are considered "generalized"?
   A. Absence
   B. Infantile spasms
   C. Tonic-clonic
   D. Atonic
   E. All of the above

27-2. Partial seizures are typically characterized by
   A. Impaired consciousness
   B. Limited initial involvement of focal area of cortical origin
   C. Classic symmetric three-per-second spike and wave pattern
   D. Initial involvement of both cerebral hemispheres
   E. Preceding febrile illness

27-3. Which of following is part of the initial management of status epilepticus?
   A. IV or rectal benzodiazepines
   B. ABC (airway, breathing, circulation) evaluation
   C. Assessment and correction of metabolic problems
   D. Assessment for underlying infection or trauma
   E. All of the above

27-4. Which drug is inappropriately matched with its seizure type and common side effects?
  A. Ethosuximide: tonic-clonic/partial; associated with tremor and weight loss
  B. Valproic acid: tonic-clonic/partial; associated with hepatotoxicity, weight gain, and nausea
  C. Phenobarbital: tonic-clonic/partial; associated with hyperactivity, ataxia, and sedation
  D. Phenytoin: tonic-clonic/partial; associated with nystagmus and gum hyperplasia
  E. Carbamazepine: tonic-clonic/partial; associated with diplopia, blood dyscrasia, and ataxia

ANSWERS

27-1. E. Generalized seizures are always associated with impaired consciousness and are indicative of bilateral hemispheric involvement. Tonic-clonic (sustained contraction followed by rhythmic contractions), absence (brief staring episodes signified by symmetric three-per-second spike-and-wave pattern on EEG), and atonic (abrupt total loss of muscle tone) are types of generalized seizure. These seizures can also be followed by a postictal phase of confusion and lethargy. Infantile spasms are a type of generalized seizure that presents between 2 to 8 months and are recurrent mixed flexor-extensor contractions that last 10 to 30 seconds each. They are frequently associated with developmental milestone loss and can also be associated with neurocutaneous disorders.

27-2. B. Partial seizures are traditionally clinically apparent, with a limited involvement of focal cortical origin in one cerebral hemisphere. Only complex partial seizures are associated with impaired consciousness. Partial seizures involve foci in one hemisphere and can occasionally progress to generalized convulsions. Generalized seizures are characterized by clinical features that indicate initial involvement of both cerebral hemispheres. The three-per-second spike-and-wave pattern is typical of absence seizures. A preceding febrile illness is not required to make this diagnosis.

27-3. E. Status epilepticus is defined as prolonged or recurrent seizure activity (usually >20–30 minutes) with no return of consciousness. The ABCs should be evaluated and maintained. Benzodiazepines can initially break the seizure and can be followed by doses of phenytoin (or fosphenytoin) or phenobarbital (used in neonates and younger children). Assessing and treating underlying causes such as metabolic derangements, underlying infection, or trauma should be included in the management.

27-4. A. Ethosuximide is generally used to treat absence seizures and is associated with rash, anorexia, and blood dyscrasias. Treatment with antiepileptic medications requires knowledge of their uses and toxicity (Table 27-1). Monitoring drug levels and noting their interactions can help in management.

TABLE 27-1   Common Indications and Side Effects of Anticonvulsants

Medication	Indications	Side Effects/Toxicity
Carbamazepine (Tegretol)	Partial, tonic-clonic	Diplopia, nausea and vomiting, ataxia, leukopenia, thrombocytopenia
Ethosuximide (Zarontin)	Absence	Rash, anorexia, leukopenia, aplastic anemia
Phenobarbital (Luminal)	Tonic-clonic, partial	Hyperactivity, sedation, nystagmus, ataxia
Phenytoin (Dilantin)	Tonic-clonic, partial	Rash, nystagmus, ataxia, drug-induced lupus, gum hyperplasia, anemia, leukopenia, polyneuropathy
Valproic acid (Depakene, Depakote)	Tonic-clonic, absence, partial	Hepatotoxicity, nausea and vomiting, abdominal pain, weight loss, weight gain, anemia, leukopenia, thrombocytopenia

From Marino B, Snead K, McMillan J. *Blueprints in Pediatrics.* 2nd ed. Malden, MA: Blackwell Science; 2001:234, with permission.

 SUGGESTED ADDITIONAL READING

Friedman MJ. Seizures in children. *Pediatr Clin North Am.* 2006;53(2):257–277.

Hill A. Neonatal seizures. *Pediatr Rev.* 2000;21:117–121.

Abdominal Pain and Bloody Diarrhea

CC/ID: 14-year-old boy with crampy abdominal pain and bloody diarrhea.

HPI: C.U. presents with abdominal pain and diarrhea that have been intermittent over the past several months. They are associated with fever, and the diarrhea is occasionally bloody. The pain is not relieved by antacids, is mildly relieved by over-the-counter pain medications, and is not generally exacerbated by eating. He has had decreased appetite and energy levels during this period, and his mother notes a nearly 10-pound weight loss over the last year. He has no cough or rhinorrhea, no headache, and no noted trauma. The patient and his family are avid campers and traveled to South America last year, but no other members are ill nor are there any known ill contacts. His pain has been particularly bad over the last 2 days, with cramping in his lower abdomen.

PMHx:/PSHx: None

Meds: As above

All: NKDA

Immun: UTD

SHx: Lives with mother, stepfather, and two younger siblings; no smokers, no pets. Not sexually active; no toxic habits; plays soccer and Sim City.

DietHx: Well-balanced diet; no particular foods seem to palliate or exacerbate symptoms; usually doesn't have "junk food."

VS: Temp 38.2°C (100.8°F), BP 100/55, HR 120, RR 24

PE: *Gen:* pale, alert, in no apparent distress. *HEENT:* NCAT; EOMI; normal exam. *Neck:* supple. *Lungs:* normal exam. *CV:*

mildly tachycardic; normal S_1, S_2; grade 1–2/6 systolic ejection murmur at left sternal border; pulses and capillary refill normal. *Abdomen:* soft, nondistended; positive for right lower quadrant fullness/mass; positive bowel sounds, somewhat hypoactive; no hepatosplenomegaly. *GU:* normal external male genitalia, Tanner stage 2.

THOUGHT QUESTIONS

■ What is in your differential diagnosis?

■ What further aspects of the physical examination or history will aid in the diagnosis?

■ What diagnostic studies may aid you in your diagnosis?

DISCUSSION

The differential diagnosis for abdominal pain and bloody diarrhea is quite extensive and can include infectious and non-infectious causes. Infectious enteritis may be caused by *E. Coli*, *Campylobacter jejuni*, *Yersinia enterocolitica*, *Clostridium difficile*, amebiasis and *Giardia*. Non-infectious causes include Henoch-Schonlein purpura, allergic olitis, lymphoma, inflammatory bowel disease, gynecologic causes, appendicitis and Meckel's diverticulum. History and physical examination should include a thorough history of present illness, medications (antibiotics, chemotherapy agents), and family, a review of growth curves, and a thorough review of systems. The physical examination should always include a rectal exam and inspection of the skin and extremities. Laboratory studies that may aid in making the diagnosis include a CBC, stool studies (for toxins, ova and parasites, and culture), protein markers, erythrocyte sedimentation rate (ESR), and imaging studies.

CASE CONTINUED

Further history reveals long-standing red and tender nodules that intermittently come and go on his shins. He has also had transient knee pain over the last several weeks. A rectal exam reveals a skin tag on his perianal region and yields positive guaiac results. The ESR is markedly elevated at 105, a CBC reveals a microcytic anemia, and albumin is low at 3. An upper GI study with small bowel follow-through shows narrowing at the terminal ileum (string sign). Contrast enema and subsequent endoscopy with biopsy confirms the diagnosis of Crohn's disease involvement of both the terminal ileum and large intestine, and management is initiated.

 DISCUSSION

Inflammatory bowel disease (IBD) refers to two clinically distinct but related disorders: Crohn's disease and ulcerative colitis (UC). In the pediatric population, they generally affect adolescents and are thought to be caused by a combination of genetic and environmental factors. Clinically, ulcerative colitis generally tends to present with symptoms affecting the large intestine, whereas Crohn's disease may affect any part of the GI tract. Both can be associated with fever, weight loss, and poor growth. Laboratory studies may show anemia and decreased serum protein markers. Contrast enema studies as well as upper GI contrast studies can aid in the diagnosis. Endoscopy and biopsy generally confirm the diagnosis. The nodules on the lower extremities in this patient were indicative of erythema nodosum, which can be associated with Crohn's disease.

 QUESTIONS

28-1. Which is least likely to be an extraintestinal manifestation of IBD?
   A. Arthritis
   B. Anterior uveitis
   C. Aphthous ulcers
   D. Acanthosis nigricans
   E. Ankylosing spondylitis

28-2. Which of the following is more common with Crohn's disease as compared with ulcerative colitis?
   A. Transmural involvement
   B. Almost always involves the rectum
   C. Restricted to large intestine
   D. Crypt abscesses
   E. Higher risk for developing cancer

28-3. Which of the following is commonly involved in IBD therapy?
- A. Corticosteroids
- B. Sulfasalazine
- C. Surgery
- D. Nutritional support
- E. All of the above

28-4. You are reviewing the clinical manifestations of IBD with a family. Which of the following statements is appropriate to include in your discussion?
- A. Crohn's patients usually do not present with an abdominal mass.
- B. Toxic megacolon is not associated with IBD.
- C. Fistula formation rarely occurs.
- D. Nutrient loss is common and can precede the diagnosis.
- E. Sexual development is unaffected and usually progresses normally.

 ANSWERS

28-1. D. A variety of extraintestinal manifestations may either precede or accompany GI symptoms. Additional findings may include pyoderma gangrenosum, hepatobiliary findings, sacroiliitis, nephrolithiasis, and thromboembolic disease. Approximately one-third of patients have at least one of these manifestations. Acanthosis nigricans is a skin finding commonly found with type 2 diabetes.

28-2. A. Crohn's disease extends transmurally, whereas ulcerative colitis is limited to the mucosal surface (Table 28-1).

TABLE 28-1   Comparison of Crohn's Disease and Ulcerative Colitis

Feature	Crohn's Disease	Ulcerative Colitis
Malaise, fever, weight loss	Common	Common
Rectal bleeding	Sometimes	Usual
Abdominal mass	Common	Rare
Abdominal pain	Common	Common
Perianal disease	Common	Rare
Ileal involvement	Common	None (backwash ileitis)
Strictures	Common	Unusual

(Continued)

TABLE 28-1   Comparison of Crohn's Disease and Ulcerative Colitis (*continued*)

Feature	Crohn's Disease	Ulcerative Colitis
Fistula	Common	Unusual
Skip lesions	Common	Not present
Transmural involvement	Usual	Not present
Crypt abscesses	Unusual	Usual
Granulomas	Common	Not present
Risk of cancer	Slightly increased	Greatly increased

Modified from Andreoli TE, Carpenter CJ, Plum F, et al. *Cecil Essentials of Medicine*. Philadelphia: WB Saunders, 1986:746, with permission.

28-3. E. Goals of therapy include control of inflammation, providing adequate nutrition and growth support, and encouraging the patient and his or her family to lead a normal life. Aminosalicylates such as sulfasalazine are indicated for colonic disease. Corticosteroids are useful for small intestinal disease, as well as in conjunction with other aminosalicylates. Surgery may be helpful and warranted in many IBD patients.

28-4. D. Many patients with Crohn's disease present insidiously and have only a right lower quadrant fullness or mass on initial examination. Delayed growth and sexual development and nutrient losses may precede the initial manifestations. When Crohn's disease affects the large intestine, it is clinically hard to distinguish from ulcerative colitis, because they both present with bloody diarrhea, abdominal pain, and urgency. Bleeding, toxic megacolon, and abscesses can be complications of ulcerative colitis. Internal and external fistula formation is the most common complication of Crohn's disease, and occurs in up to 40% of patients.

 SUGGESTED ADDITIONAL READING

Hyams JS. Inflammatory bowel disease. *Pediatr Rev*. 2005;26: 314–320.

CASE **29**

Cramps and Watery Diarrhea

 CC/ID: 4-year-old girl with watery diarrhea over the past 6 days presents to urgent care clinic with lethargy.

HPI: Patient was in her usual state of good health until 1 week ago, when she awoke twice in the middle of the night with diarrhea. She had just returned the night before from a family vacation to South America. The diarrhea was clear, watery, and with no blood. She complained of crampy abdominal pain occurring just prior to each watery stool. The diarrhea has continued throughout the week, occurring three to four times daily, and she has been afebrile. She has not been able to keep any foods or liquids down for at least the past 2 days, and her mother is concerned that she has appeared very weak since this morning. She has also not urinated since yesterday morning. Fortunately, she has not had any seizures, but her mental status has changed slightly today, accompanied by an increasingly tired appearance. Her mother was very careful about not letting her eat or drink suspicious foods during their trip, but does remember the girl adding some ice to her Coke at the airport cafeteria just before they left to return home. She has lost about 3 to 4 pounds over the past week (her last recorded weight was 30 pounds).

THOUGHT QUESTIONS

- What is in this patient's differential diagnosis?
- What is the significance of the weakness and lethargy?

DISCUSSION

The differential diagnosis of acute diarrhea includes infectious causes (e.g., viral gastroenteritis, bacterial enterocolitis, hepatitis, food poisoning, otitis media, UTI), GI causes (e.g., intussusception, appendicitis), toxic ingestions (e.g., salicylates, lead), and vasculitis (e.g., Henoch-Schönlein purpura). Watery diarrhea is often endotoxin mediated and is most commonly caused by *Escherichia coli* and *Vibrio cholerae.*

Weakness and lethargy in the face of a decreased urine output and weight loss indicate that this patient is probably suffering from dehydration. If she were also having seizures or high fevers accompanied by behavioral changes, additional explanations for lethargy could include sepsis (e.g., meningitis, encephalitis) or toxic ingestions.

CASE CONTINUED

PMHx:/PSHx: None
Meds: None
All: NKDA
FHx: No history of inflammatory bowel disorders.
SHx: Lives at home with mother and father. Attends day care five times a week.
VS: Temp 38°C (100.5°F), BP 88/62, HR 90, RR 28
PE: *Gen:* awake, alert, crying (no tears). *HEENT:* mucous membranes dry; eyes mildly sunken; throat nonerythematous. *Lungs:* clear bilaterally. *Abdomen:* soft, nondistended; minimal tenderness to touch especially over stomach, otherwise no guarding; positive bowel sounds; no masses. *Skin:* capillary refill time 3 seconds.

THOUGHT QUESTION

- In addition to physical exam and history of intake and output, what laboratory tests might be helpful in assessing the degree of dehydration in this patient?

DISCUSSION

In general, physical exam (including weight and vital signs) and history are the most useful and accurate tools for assessing degree of hydration in the pediatric patient. However, labs may provide additional information about electrolyte levels and acid-base status which are potentially relevant for treatment. A urine specific gravity can be used to estimate degree of dehydration in a patient with normal kidney function. A blood gas may show metabolic acidosis secondary to poor perfusion from dehydration. An electrolyte panel may show an elevated BUN, low HCO_3 or altered Na when dehydration is severe.

CASE CONTINUED

Labs: *Electrolytes* (mEq/L): Na 135, K 4, Cl 100, HCO_3 22, BUN 35, creatinine 0.8. *ABG:* pH 7.29, Pco_2 35, Pao_2 85, base excess –5. *Urine specific gravity:* 1.025.

QUESTIONS

29-1. Which of the following clinical manifestations of dehydration is the last to develop?
   A. Tachycardia
   B. Weight loss
   C. Decreased urine output
   D. Hypotension
   E. No tears when crying

29-2. Based on the physical exam of the patient presented in this case scenario, which of the following is an estimate of her degree of dehydration?
   A. She is not dehydrated.
   B. Mild (<5%) dehydration
   C. Moderate (5–10%) dehydration
   D. Severe (>10%) dehydration

29-3. The patient presented in this case scenario most likely has which type of dehydration?
- A. Hypotonic
- B. Hyponatremic
- C. Isotonic
- D. Hypertonic
- E. Hypernatremic

29-4. During replacement therapy for dehydration, most deficits are replaced over 24 hours, with half given over the first 8 hours and half over the next 16 hours. The exception is hypertonic dehydration, in which the deficit is replaced slowly over 48 to 72 hours to prevent
- A. Hypertension
- B. Tachycardia
- C. Brain edema
- D. Hydrocephalus
- E. Intracranial hemorrhage

ANSWERS

29-1. D. Hypotension is the last of the listed clinical manifestations of dehydration to appear. Tachycardia is often the first in children, although it is very nonspecific. Thus, the presentation of a child with tachycardia, no tears when crying, history of poor fluid intake or excessive fluid loss, weight loss, and decreased urine output should alert the clinician that cardiovascular compromise may also be imminent.

29-2. C. This patient is moderately dehydrated based on the following parameters: 5% to 10% weight loss, dry mucous membranes, altered mental status, absent tears, sunken eyes, oliguria, urine specific gravity of 1.025, elevated BUN, and pH between 7.30 and 6.92 (Table 29-1).

TABLE **29-1**   Clinical Features in Estimating the Severity of Dehydration

Clinical Feature	Mild	Moderate	Severe
Mucosa of mouth	Dry	Dry	Dry
Reported urine output	Normal (at least × 3 in 24 hours)	Reduced in last 24 hours	No urine in last 12 hours
Mental state	Normal	Lethargic or stuporous	Irritable
Pulse	Normal	Tachycardic	Tachycardic

(Continued)

TABLE 29-1   Clinical Features in Estimating the Severity of Dehydration (*continued*)

Blood pressure	Normal	Normal	Low
Capillary refilling	Normal	Slow	Very slow
Fontanelle	Normal	Sunken	Very sunken
Skin and eye turgor	Normal	Reduced	Very reduced
Percentage dehydrated	<5%	5–10%	>10%

From Rudolf M, Levene M. *Paediatrics and Child Health*. Oxford: Blackwell Science; 1999:117, with permission.

29-3. C. This patient has isotonic dehydration, given her serum sodium of 135 mEq/L. Isotonic dehydration is the most common form of dehydration and suggests that either compensation has occurred or water losses are equal to salt losses. Hypotonic dehydration in children is caused by electrolyte loss in stools; it can also occur in children supplemented with free water or dilute juices. Hypertonic dehydration is uncommon in children.

29-4. C. Brain edema due to excessive fluid shifts is a complication of rapid fluid correction in less than 48 hours for hypertonic (hypernatremic) dehydration. Brain swelling occurs as a result of rapid entry of free water into neuronal cells with high sodium concentrations. Brain edema may lead to increased intracranial pressure with mental status changes or hypoventilation and bradycardia.

The calculation of normal maintenance fluids is an important exercise and is usually based on the Holliday-Seger method: 100 mL/kg/day (for first 10 kg) + 50 mL/k/g/day (for second 10 kg) + 25 mL/kg/day (for each additional kg) = total mL/kg/day. This calculation can be simplified to determine the hourly rate as follows: 4 mL/kg/hr (first 10 kg) + 2 mL/kg/hr (second 10 kg) + 1 mL/kg/hr (each additional kg) = total mL/kg/hr.

 SUGGESTED ADDITIONAL READING

Jospe N, Forbes G. Fluids and electrolytes—clinical aspects. *Pediatr Rev.* 1996;17(11):395–403.

Lifschitz CH. Treatment of acute diarrhea in children. *Curr Opin Pediatr.* 1997;9(5):498–501.

Steiner MJ, DeWalt DA, Byerley JS. Is this child dehydrated? *JAMA.* 2004;291(22):2746–2754.

CASE 30

Abdominal Pain and Irritability

CC/ID: 2-year-old girl with abdominal pain and irritability brought in by mother.

HPI: J.O. had been generally healthy until her mother noticed increasing bouts of irritability over the past 2 months. She had previously had a vigorous appetite, but this has subsequently decreased, as has her weight. She has not had any vomiting, but over the past 3 to 4 weeks has been "pointing to her tummy" in pain. Her mother has noted some increasingly watery stools and notes that she has had some low-grade fevers, which her doctor mentioned were probably "viral" and due to being in day care. She has been noticeably more pale and seems to have less energy. She has no cough, rhinorrhea, or rashes, nor does she have any current ill contacts or any history of trauma.

PMHx: None

Meds: Acetaminophen for fever

SHx: Lives with both parents and three older siblings (all healthy); no smokers; one dog.

FHx: Maternal grandparents with hypertension; paternal uncle with epilepsy.

VS: Temp 38°C (100.4°F), HR 110, RR 28; Weight 10.25 kg (fifth percentile)

PE: *Gen:* Ill appearing, uncomfortable, pale; in no acute respiratory distress. *HEENT:* Mucous membranes are moist; TMs and oropharynx are clear. *Neck:* supple, without nuchal rigidity. *Chest:* Clear to auscultation, without wheeze or crackles. *Cardio:* Slight tachycardia; regular rhythm; soft flow murmur; pulses palpable throughout; capillary refill <2 seconds. *Abdomen:* Mild distention; hyperactive bowel sounds; firm 8- to 9-cm mass palpable in the midabdominal region; liver edge palpable 2 cm below costal margin. *GU:* Normal external female genitalia; bilateral inguinal nontender lymphadenopathy. *Skin/Extremities:* pallor; nontender bluish nodules on lower extremities.

THOUGHT QUESTIONS

- What is your differential diagnosis at this point?
- What elements of the physical exam would you further pursue?
- What further workup would you pursue?

DISCUSSION

The differential diagnosis for a patient with an abdominal mass should include hydronephrosis, splenomegaly, polycystic kidney disease, renal vein thrombosis, duodenal hematoma, polycystic ovary, and neoplastic processes such as Wilm's tumor, neuroblastoma, rhabdomyosarcoma, lymphoma, and ovarian tumors. In this patient, the history and physical are more suggestive of a chronic process, and her nonspecific symptoms (low-grade fever, irritability, weight loss), although they can be associated with a large variety of diseases, are suggestive of a neoplastic process. A full and thorough physical exam should be performed. Evaluation of an abdominal mass should start with a CBC with a differential, liver and kidney function studies, and abdominal imaging. Further analysis of urine, blood, and bone (via imaging) should be done based on clinical suspicion and/or guided by the initial evaluation.

CASE CONTINUED

Further examination reveals a hypertensive child (BP 122/80). A careful neurologic examination shows mild ataxia and an inability to observe the retina carefully due to chaotic eye movements. A CBC reveals a hemoglobin of 6.5 and a platelet count of 60,000. Further labs reveal elevated liver transaminases as well as increased BUN and creatinine levels. An abdominal CT reveals a large suprarenal mass crossing the midline, with multiple enlarged regional lymph nodes. Urine studies are positive for elevated levels of the catecholamines homovanillic acid (HVA) and vanillylmandelic acid (VMA), consistent with neuroblastoma. J.O. is admitted to the hospital for further imaging and evaluation.

 DISCUSSION

Neuroblastoma is the most common malignancy in the first year of life and the second most common solid tumor of childhood, after brain tumors outside of the central nervous system. Nearly half are diagnosed by age 2. Neuroblastomas arise from neural crest cells that form the adrenal medulla and sympathetic ganglia. Two-thirds of cases present with abdominal tumors, but presentation can also involve the thoracic cavity as well as the head and neck region. Neuroblastoma may metastasize to lymph nodes, bone and bone marrow, liver, and skin, and are commonly widespread at the time of diagnosis. Clinical manifestations can be variable depending on the origin and distribution of tumors. Abdominal neuroblastoma should be differentiated from Wilm's tumor, which arises from embryonal renal cells of the metanephros.

 QUESTIONS

30-1. Which characteristic is more suggestive of Wilm's tumor than neuroblastoma?
- A. Abdominal cavity lymphadenopathy
- B. Involvement and distortion of the renal architecture and calyces
- C. Hypertension
- D. Primarily diagnosed in children younger than 5 years
- E. Treatment with surgery and chemotherapy

30-2. Neuroblastoma of the neck region can often present with Horner's syndrome, which involves
- A. Anhidrosis
- B. Miosis
- C. Ptosis
- D. Enophthalmos
- E. All of the above

30-3. Neuroblastoma can be associated with the following risk factors:
- A. Aniridia
- B. Beckwith-Wiedemann syndrome
- C. Genitourinary abnormalities
- D. Chromosome 11 deletion
- E. None of the above

30-4. In counseling a family of a patient with neuroblastoma, you are discussing prognosis. Which of the following stages of disease carries a good prognosis?
- A. Stage I
- B. Stage II
- C. Stage III
- D. Stage IV
- E. Stage IV-S

 ANSWERS

30-1. B. Although neuroblastoma can often displace the kidney and its vasculature, it generally does not result in distortion of the calyceal system. Hypertension can be present in both disease processes, either from intrinsic renal involvement (Wilm's) or renal displacement/secretion of catecholamines (neuroblastoma) (Table 30-1).

TABLE 30-1   Comparison of Wilm's Tumor and Neuroblastoma

	Wilm's Tumor	**Neuroblastoma**
Age	Predominantly before age 5; mean age, 3 y	Predominantly before age 5; >50% before 2 y
Risk factors	Aniridia, GU abnormalities, mental retardation (WAGR syndrome); Beckwith-Wiedemann syndrome; deletion of short arm of chromosome 11	Unknown; may be associated with deletion of short arm of chromosome 1, Hirschsprung's disease, fetal hydantoin syndrome, Recklinghausen's disease
Clinical manifestations	Abdominal mass that commonly crosses midline	Abdominal mass that rarely crosses midline
	Abdominal pain	Abdominal pain
	Hypertension	Hypertension and catecholamine effects (flushing, headache, sweating, watery diarrhea)

(Continued)

TABLE 30-1   Comparison of Wilm's Tumor and Neuroblastoma (*continued*)

	Wilm's Tumor	**Neuroblastoma**
	Hematuria (microscopic/ gross)	Rare hematuria
	Associated aniridia, hemihypertrophy, GU malformations	Signs/symptoms dependent on origin/spread of tumor: mediastinal mass with respiratory distress, Horner's syndrome, bone pain and limp, periorbital infiltration; opsoclonus-myoclonus (chaotic eye movements, myoclonic jerking, truncal ataxia); palpable nontender skin nodules
Evaluation	Imaging; histological evaluation of tissue	Imaging; urine excretion of catecholamines; tissue/bone marrow biopsy
Treatment and prognosis	Surgery, chemotherapy/ radiotherapy; prognosis dependent on histology, but usually excellent	Surgery, chemotherapy/ radiotherapy; prognosis good for children <1 y and for stages I, II, and IV-S

30-2. E. Neuroblastoma with a cervical location can present with Horner's syndrome, which involves ptosis of the eyelid, miosis, enophthalmos, and anhidrosis. Of note, tumor in this location can also present with tracheal compression and respiratory distress.

30-3. E. These are all associated risk factors for Wilm's tumor. Risk factors are unknown for neuroblastoma, but may involve a chromosomal deletion (short arm of chromosome 1) and a possible association with Hirschsprung's disease and fetal hydantoin exposure.

30-4. A, B, and **E.** Stages I, II, and IV-S are all associated with a better prognosis, whereas stages III and IV have a poor prognosis. The staging is outlined as follows:

Stage I: Localized, confined to organ or structure of origin

Stage II: Extends beyond structure of origin, but not across midline

Stage III: Extends beyond midline

Stage IV: Dissemination to distant lymph nodes, bone, bone marrow, liver, or soft tissues

Stage IV-S: Age <1 year with localized tumor at stage I or II but with distant metastasis to any organ (except bone involvement)

The prognosis for Wilm's tumor is based primarily on its histology. Favorable histology and limitation of the tumor within the abdomen result in a 2-year survival rate greater than 95%. Unfavorable histology accounts for only 10% to 12% of disease, but also has a 10% to 12% survival rate.

 ## *SUGGESTED ADDITIONAL READING*

Behrman RE. Neuroblastoma. In: Behrman RE, Kliegman RM, Jenson HB, eds. *Nelson Textbook of Pediatrics*. 17th ed. Philadelphia: WB Saunders; 2004.

Chandler JC. The neonate with an abdominal mass. *Pediatr Clin North Am*. 2004;51(4):979–997, ix.

Messahel B. Clinical features of molecular pathology of solid tumours in childhood. *Lancet Oncol*. 2005;6(6):421–430.

Constipation: 2½-Year-Old

CC/ID: 2½-year-old boy with no bowel movement in 4 to 5 days.

HPI: O.T. is a 2½-year-old boy who is brought in by his mother with a history of no stool passage in 4 to 5 days. He currently has no vomiting, no cough, and no fever and is otherwise without any accompanying signs of illness. The mother states that he has seemingly had this problem since infancy, and has required various methods to prompt stooling, including rectal stimulation, suppositories, and enemas. He usually stools every 3 to 4 days. There have been no acute dietary changes, and based on his history, he has been placed on mineral oil. He occasionally "rubs his tummy" to signal discomfort, but overall appears to be at his baseline. His mother has attributed this current bout to recently starting to attend a new day-care center and recent attempts at potty training.

PMHx/
Birth Hx: Normal birth history; needed to stay an extra day "because he didn't poop until the third day." Recent UTI treated with antibiotics; negative imaging studies.

Meds: None

Immun: Needs hepatitis A no. 2.

DevHx: Beginning two-word phrases; runs well; likes to play with other children.

FHx: Maternal uncle with Crohn's disease; paternal history unknown.

SHx: Father not involved; mother's boyfriend smokes outside home; no pets, no ill contacts; daytime providers at day care and a maternal aunt; has had difficulty with toilet training: associated with temper tantrums.

ROS: As above; no rashes, no changes in behavior or activity, no urinary complaints, no weight loss, and no recent illnesses.

VS: Temp 37°C (98.6°F), HR 90, RR 26, BP 95/50; Weight 15 kg

PE: *Gen:* alert, in no acute distress; appears comfortable. *HEENT:* mucous membranes are moist; TMs and oropharynx are clear. *Neck:* supple. *Chest:* clear to auscultation bilaterally, without crackles or wheeze. *CV:* Normal pulses; capillary refill time <2 seconds; RR&R; normal S_1S_2; no murmur. *Abdomen:* mild distention; mild tenderness in left lower quadrant with palpable approximately 4 cm ×4 cm mass; normal bowel sounds; no visceromegaly appreciated. *GU:* Normal external male genitalia, Tanner stage 1. *Neuro:* Grossly nonfocal exam. *Skin/Ext:* no lesions appreciated; no signs of trauma; no clubbing or edema.

THOUGHT QUESTIONS

- What is in your differential diagnosis for this patient at this point?
- What elements of the physical exam would you further pursue?
- What further workup would you pursue to aid in the diagnosis?

DISCUSSION

Constipation occurs in over 10% of all children and is defined as abnormally reduced defecation; it may result in difficult, painful stooling, abdominal discomfort, and stool retention. Encopresis is a developmentally inappropriate release of stool and is almost always associated with severe constipation, as liquid stool leaks around a retained stool mass and is involuntarily passed.

The differential diagnosis for constipation includes functional retention, which is responsible for the majority of cases. Functional retention can be the result of traumatic events (including painful passage of hard stools, painful diarrhea, and physical or sexual abuse) or may be associated with difficult psychosocial situations or environmental changes (often associated with a sentinel event, such as inappropriate potty training methods). This may lead to further withholding of stool and increasingly painful defecation, fueling a difficult cycle. Associated symptoms of functional retention may include encopresis, abdominal pain, anorexia, and urinary tract problems (due to pelvic compression). Organic causes are responsible for less than 5% of cases, and may include Hirschsprung's disease, anatomic abnormalities of the anus or colon, medications, spinal dysraphisms, infant botulism, hypothyroidism, celiac disease, and diabetes mellitus.

 ## CASE CONTINUED

Functional retention leading to chronic constipation is suspected. The family is sent home with instructions to administer a hyperosmotic saline enema, initiate a high-fiber diet with Maltsupex extract supplement, and continue the mineral oil. The patient stools at home after the enema, and presents again 3 weeks later with similar symptoms, not having stooled for 5 days; he now has abdominal pain and distention. A rectal exam shows an empty vault, void of stool, with normal tone, and is followed by the explosive release of gas and feces. Plain films show dilated bowels with massive amounts of stool. A contrast enema reveals a transitional zone between a proximal distended segment of sigmoid colon and a normal-caliber nondistended distal segment of rectosigmoid colon. O.T. is admitted to the hospital, a surgical consultation is obtained, and a rectal suction biopsy reveals absence of ganglion cells, confirming the diagnosis of Hirschsprung's disease.

 ## DISCUSSION

Hirschsprung's disease results from the absence of intramural ganglionic cells at the submucosal plexus and myenteric plexus of the intestine, resulting in a failure of normal bowel relaxation and peristalsis. It most commonly affects the rectosigmoid colon and occurs predominantly in males (ratio of 4:1); its incidence is approximately 1 in 5,000 live births. Newborns present with delayed passage of meconium and signs and symptoms of enterocolitis. Infants and children may present with chronic constipation. Hirschsprung's disease can present at any age with signs and symptoms of intestinal obstruction. Rectal examination reveals an empty vault with normal tone. Barium enema studies usually reveal a transition zone (usually present after the first 1 to 2 weeks) between the normal distended area and the abnormally nondistended aganglionic segment. The definitive diagnosis can be made via suction biopsy, and surgical correction is necessary. Postoperative complications include stricture formation and recurrent enterocolitis.

    QUESTIONS

31-1. You suspect chronic functional constipation in a patient. Which of the following best supports this diagnosis?
    A. The patient has a history of lead poisoning.
    B. The patient has a history of botulism.
    C. The patient has a history of cystic fibrosis.
    D. The patient has a history of recurrent anal fissures.
    E. The patient has a history of vincristine use.

31-2. A family of a child with chronic functional constipation is in your office. When counseling them, which of the following statements would be best to include in your discussion?
    A. Most children can be treated through dietary changes.
    B. The majority of cases of chronic functional constipation have an organic cause.
    C. The routine use of laxatives and enemas should be encouraged.
    D. Leakage and overflow diarrhea usually occur without a retained fecal mass.
    E. The majority of cases of chronic constipation have failure to thrive.

31-3. Which of the following conditions may be associated with Hirschsprung's disease?
    A. Diabetic ketoacidosis
    B. Down syndrome
    C. Hyperthyroidism
    D. Prune belly syndrome
    E. Irritable bowel syndrome

31-4. When treating chronic constipation, which of the following therapies is best matched with its correct function?
    A. Mineral oil: bulking agent
    B. Lactulose: stool softener
    C. Docusate: hyperosmotic laxative
    D. Polyethylene glycol electrolyte solution: fiber agent
    E. Senna: peristaltic inducer

ANSWERS

31-1. D. The majority of cases of chronic constipation due to functional retention involve nonorganic causes. Recurrent anal fissures may be a result of painful defecation and passage of hard stools, fueling the cycle of voluntary withholding. The other entities listed, although causes of constipation, are generally not related to functional constipation.

31-2. A. The first steps in treatment for functional constipation should involve dietary changes. This may include increasing fluid and free water intake, decreasing the amount of simple carbohydrate-based foods, and increasing the amount of fiber and bulk in the diet through leafy vegetables and cereals. Routine use of laxatives and enemas should be discouraged. Often, poorly managed functional constipation and fecal retention can result in a retained fecal mass, and leakage of stool around the mass will result in overflow diarrhea. Although most organic causes of constipation may also be associated with failure to thrive, most children with functional chronic constipation tend to have adequate weight gain.

31-3. B. Hirschsprung's disease can be associated with Down syndrome, Waardenburg syndrome, and multiple endocrine neoplasia, among others.

31-4. E. Most therapies can be categorized as stool softeners, osmotic agents, bulking/fiber agents, and peristaltic inducers. Docusate (Colace) is a stool softener. Polyethylene glycol electrolyte solution, mineral oil, and lactulose serve mostly as osmotic agents and osmotic cathartics. Suppositories and enemas tend also to serve as hyperosmotic laxatives. Senna generally works as a stimulant of peristalsis. Psyllium and malt soup extract are traditionally used as bulking/fiber agents.

SUGGESTED ADDITIONAL READING

Abi-Hanna A, Lake AM. Constipation and encopresis in childhood. *Pediatr Rev.* 1998;19:23–31.

Biggs WS. Evaluation and treatment of constipation in infants and children. *Am Fam Physician.* 2006;73(3):469–477.

Swenson O. Hirschsprung's disease: a review. *Pediatrics.* 2002;109(5):914–918.

V

Cases Presenting with Vomiting

Vomiting and Diarrhea

CC/ID: 3-year-old girl with vomiting and diarrhea over the past 2 days presents to urgent care clinic in the afternoon.

HPI: Patient was in her usual state of good health until 2 nights ago, when she awoke twice in the middle of the night with vomiting. The vomitus was clear, nonbilious fluid with no blood. She had eaten a meal of macaroni and cheese that her 9-year-old brother had also eaten; he subsequently slept without difficulty. Her mother remembers that a friend of the little girl's from day care also had a similar vomiting bout a week earlier, which resolved on its own. She complained of crampy abdominal pain just prior to the vomiting, which improved after vomiting. By the next evening she began to have clear diarrhea (no blood) occurring three to four times throughout the day that was accompanied by a low-grade fever. Today she has not been able to keep any foods or liquids down and last urinated this morning.

THOUGHT QUESTIONS

- What is in this patient's differential diagnosis?
- What is the significance of bilious vomiting, if present?

DISCUSSION

The differential diagnosis of acute vomiting and diarrhea is extensive and includes infectious causes (e.g., viral, bacterial enterocolitis, hepatitis, food poisoning, peritonitis, pharyngitis, pneumonia, otitis media, tonsillitis, UTI), metabolic causes (e.g., diabetic ketoacidosis, adrenal crisis, renal or hepatic failure), central nervous system causes (e.g., increased intracranial pressure, meningitis, encephalitis, labyrinthitis, migraine, Reye syndrome, seizure, tumor), GI causes (e.g., appendicitis, bowel obstruction), respiratory causes (e.g., reactive airways disease), and toxic ingestions (e.g., salicylates, lead).

 ## CASE CONTINUED

The significance of bilious vomiting in any patient indicates a complete or partial obstructive process and almost always warrants corrective or exploratory surgical intervention.

PMHx/
PSHx: None

Meds: None

All: NKDA

FHx: No history of inflammatory bowel disorders.

SHx: Lives at home with mother, father, and 9-year-old brother. Attends day care twice a week.

VS: Temp 38°C (100.5°F), BP 88/62, HR 79, RR 28

PE: *Gen:* awake, alert, crying (with tears). *HEENT:* mucous membranes dry; throat nonerythematous. *Lungs:* clear bilaterally. *Abdomen:* soft, nondistended; minimal tenderness to touch, especially over stomach; otherwise no guarding; positive bowel sounds; no masses. *Skin:* well perfused; capillary refill time <2 seconds.

 ## THOUGHT QUESTIONS

- What laboratory tests, if any, are appropriate to obtain at this time?
- What is the most important aspect of the physical examination that will determine the aggressiveness of therapy?

 ## DISCUSSION

In general, labs are not necessary in the assessment or management of a child with suspected viral gastroenteritis, such as this one. If a specific infectious cause is considered, targeted testing may be performed, such as cultures of urine or stool. In the child with prolonged symptoms or severe dehydration, labs may help to establish presence of treatable conditions such as electrolyte abnormalities or acidosis.

The most important assessment of the physical examination is to determine the patient's hydration status. A moderate to severely dehydrated child may need more aggressive intervention to rehydrate.

 CASE CONTINUED

Given the low-grade fever and the history of ill contact a week prior, you determine that the most likely cause of this patient's vomiting and diarrhea is viral gastroenteritis. The child was able to tolerate small amounts of oral fluids in clinic, and she was discharged with instructions to the family about the administration of oral hydration, and assessment of dehydration.

 QUESTIONS

32-1. What is the agent most likely to cause acute gastroenteritis?
A. *Staphylococcus aureus*
B. *Clostridium perfringens*
C. Rotavirus
D. *Escherichia coli*
E. Adenovirus

32-2. What is the most appropriate treatment for a mildly dehydrated child with acute gastroenteritis?
A. Surgical laparotomy
B. Admit to hospital for IV fluids
C. Admit to hospital for IV fluids followed by inpatient oral rehydration
D. Admit to hospital for IV fluids followed by outpatient oral rehydration
E. Outpatient oral rehydration

32-3. What is the most common cause of parasitic watery diarrhea in the United States?
A. *Entamoeba histolytica*
B. *Giardia lamblia*
C. Schistosomiasis
D. *Ascaris lumbricoides*
E. *Cryptosporidium* species

32-4. What is the toxin associated with a history of antibiotic overuse?

   A. *E. coli*
   B. *Yersinia enterocolitica*
   C. *Clostridium difficile*
   D. *Clostridium perfringens*
   E. *Giardia lamblia*

ANSWERS

32-1. C. The most common agent causing acute gastroenteritis is rotavirus. *Staphylococcus aureus* and *Clostridium perfringens* are associated with food poisoning. *E. coli* frequently causes infectious diarrhea, especially watery traveler's diarrhea. Adenovirus is generally associated with respiratory illness, although extension of viral inflammation into the GI tract could also cause gastric irritation and symptoms of gastroenteritis.

32-2. E. Outpatient oral rehydration is the treatment of choice for patients with mild dehydration who are able to tolerate food or fluids orally. Inpatient IV administration of fluids is indicated only if oral rehydration is not possible.

32-3. B. *Giardia lamblia* is the most common cause of parasitic watery diarrhea in the United States. It presents with frequent, malodorous watery stools. Associated symptoms can include abdominal pain, nausea, vomiting, anorexia, and flatulence. Symptoms usually resolve in 7 to 10 days but can rarely last as long as a month.

32-4. C. *Clostridium difficile* toxin is often associated with a history of antibiotic overuse. *Salmonella*, *Shigella*, enterohemorrhagic *E. coli*, and *Yersinia enterocolitica* may be associated with blood, mucus, and fecal leukocytes.

SUGGESTED ADDITIONAL READING

Amieva MR. Important bacterial gastrointestinal pathogens in children: a pathogenesis perspective. *Pediatr Clin North Am.* 2005;52(3):749–777, vi.

Jospe N, Forbes G. Fluids and electrolytes—clinical aspects. *Pediatr Rev.* 1996;17(11):395–403.

Vomiting Infant

CC/ID: 5-week-old baby boy presents to urgent care clinic with vomiting for past 2 weeks.

HPI: Patient was born at full term (38 weeks' GA) by NSVD to a 26-year-old woman, G1, P1, A+, serology (–), rubella immune, hepatitis B (–), VDRL (–), who had good prenatal care. She had a routine 20-week prenatal sonogram that revealed a normal fetus and amniotic fluid. At delivery, baby was vigorous, with Apgar scores of 9 and 9 at 1 and 5 minutes, respectively, and a birth weight of 2,780 grams. He was discharged to home breastfeeding well 2 days after delivery and had a normal 2-week visit, at which time his weight was noted to be 2,790 grams with a normal physical examination. His mother states that for the past 2 weeks he has been having increasing spitting up, and over the last 3 days he has had very forceful vomiting described as "projectile" in nature. He has been breastfed every 3 to 4 hours, and his mother feels he has a good suck and swallow. He had a normal stooling pattern with four stools per day of mustard yellow and seedy consistency, although he has had only one such stool in the last 3 days. He now feeds for only about 5 minutes per breast and vomits most of the quantity within 10 minutes. Today his weight is still 2,790 grams.

THOUGHT QUESTIONS

- What is in this patient's differential diagnosis?
- What is the significance of today's weight?

DISCUSSION

The differential diagnosis of a newborn infant with vomiting can be divided into two categories: bilious and nonbilious. Bilious vomiting generally involves conditions with partial or complete bowel obstruction, such as malrotation, volvulus, Ladd's bands, Hirschsprung disease, incarcerated hernia, torsion of Meckel's diverticulum, and intestinal atresia. Nonbilious vomiting in a newborn is largely due to gastroesophageal reflux, cow or soy milk protein intolerance, and pyloric stenosis. Although rare, nonbilious vomiting may also occur in esophageal atresia but is usually diagnosed immediately after initiation of feeds.

The significance of today's weight is that there has been no growth since the patient's last visit nearly 3 weeks ago. In general, babies gain weight at an average of about 20 grams per day. Thus, this infant's weight should have been closer to 3,200 grams. The poor weight gain points to a definite pathologic cause associated with the vomiting history.

CASE CONTINUED

PMHx/PSHx: None

Meds: None

All: NKDA

FHx: Baby's mother reports having had a surgical procedure because of vomiting when she was an infant.

SHx: Lives at home with mother and father. At home with mother during the day.

VS: Temp 36.9°C (98.5°F), BP 88/62, HR 79, RR 28

PE: *Gen:* awake, alert, crying (no tears). *HEENT:* mucous membranes dry; eyes mildly sunken; throat nonerythematous. *Lungs:* clear bilaterally. *Abdomen:* soft, nondistended; positive bowel sounds; small 3- to 4-cm olive-sized slightly firm round mass felt just to the right of the umbilicus. *Skin:* well perfused.

THOUGHT QUESTION

■ What radiologic test would be helpful at this time?

DISCUSSION

This infant's history and physical exam are concerning for pyloric stenosis. An abdominal ultrasound can help to confirm the diagnosis of pyloric stenosis, showing a thickened ring in the region of the pylorus. Rarely, an upper GI contrast series can also be performed, but it is usually not necessary if the history, physical examination, and ultrasound are confirmatory.

 CASE CONTINUED

You determine this baby has pyloric stenosis (Fig. 33-1). The most important next step is to determine the patient's hydration status. From the physical examination, you note that he must be at least mildly to moderately dehydrated and decide to correct his fluid status before consulting the pediatric surgeons for corrective surgical repair.

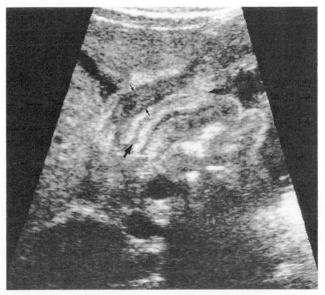

FIGURE **33-1.** Ultrasound of a baby with pyloric stenosis. Arrows indicate the elongated pyloric canal (*thick arrow*) and thickened pyloric muscle (*thin arrows*). (*From Rudolf M, Levene M. Paediatrics and Child Health. Oxford: Blackwell Science; 1999:160, with permission.*)

QUESTIONS

33-1. Additional findings associated with pyloric stenosis can often include
   A. Simian crease
   B. Visible gastric peristaltic waves
   C. A "double-bubble" sign on abdominal x-ray
   D. Bloody stools
   E. Hematemesis

33-2. What is the most common condition requiring surgery in the first 2 months of life for term newborn infants?
   A. Inguinal hernia
   B. Pyloric stenosis
   C. Cardiac atrioventricular canal defect
   D. Malrotation of the intestines
   E. Ligation of a patent ductus arteriosus

33-3. What is the surgical treatment of choice for pyloric stenosis?
   A. Nissen fundoplication
   B. Esophagomyotomy
   C. Pyloric resection
   D. Pyloromyotomy
   E. Gastrostomy tube

33-4. The metabolic derangement often associated with pyloric stenosis is
   A. Hyperkalemic metabolic acidosis
   B. Hyperkalemic metabolic alkalosis
   C. Hypokalemic metabolic acidosis
   D. Hypokalemic metabolic alkalosis
   E. Hypokalemic respiratory alkalosis

ANSWERS

33-1. B. Visible gastric peristaltic waves are often seen with pyloric stenosis. Simian crease is associated with trisomy 21 (Down syndrome), which can also have duodenal atresia and thus have the radiographic finding of a "double-bubble" sign. Bloody stools are not common in pyloric stenosis.

33-2. A. Inguinal hernia is the most common condition requiring surgical correction in term newborns. Pyloric stenosis is the second most common.

33-3. D. The surgical treatment for pyloric stenosis is pyloromyotomy, which involves making a longitudinal incision through the external pyloric musculature and suturing it in a lateral direction (at 90 degrees from the original).

33-4. D. The metabolic derangement resulting from pyloric stenosis is hypokalemic metabolic alkalosis. The loss of gastric secretions through emesis requires replacement of potassium chloride and alkali before surgical correction can be performed.

 SUGGESTED ADDITIONAL READING

Garcia VF, Randolph JG. Pyloric stenosis: diagnosis and management. *Pediatr Rev.* 1990;11(10):292–296.
Vasavada P. Ultrasound evaluation of acute abdominal emergencies in infants and children. *Radiol Clin North Am.* 2004;42(2):445–456.

Vomiting and Irritability

CC/ID: 18-month-old boy with intermittent emesis and irritability.

HPI: B.I. was well prior to 2 days ago, when mother noticed he had bouts of irritability and vomiting. Mother states that the vomiting is nonbloody and nonbilious, and "he seems to be cramping in pain." The episodes seem to be interspersed with periods of normal behavior and feeding, but she is more worried today because they have increased in frequency and he is looking more tired. He does not have any cough or runny nose, nor does he have any rash. He had just recovered from a "cold" last week and was otherwise well. He has had a slight temperature today. Mother tried giving acetaminophen without any resolution.

PMHx:/
PSHx: None

Meds: Tylenol as above

SHx: Lives with mother and father and older sibling at home; no current ill contacts. No recent travel.

FHx: None

VS: Temp 38°C (100.5°F), BP 110/65, HR 160, RR 26

PE: *Gen:* child is interactive with mother but appears tired and lethargic. Dry oral mucous membranes; decreased skin turgor. *Lungs:* clear to auscultation. *CV:* tachycardic, but with no murmur; capillary refill time is nearly 3 seconds. *Abdomen:* distended; tympanic but soft; no visceromegaly; soft palpable mass in right upper quadrant; hypoactive bowel sounds.

THOUGHT QUESTIONS

- What further history may be helpful?

- What further physical examination findings may be helpful?
- What is included in the differential diagnosis?
- What studies would be appropriate for narrowing your diagnosis?

 ## DISCUSSION

In particular, further questions regarding the bowel history are likely to contribute to the diagnosis with either positive or negative responses. These questions include frequency, quantity, concomitant symptoms, whether the patient has diarrhea, and whether the stools are bloody. The physical examination for any patient with GI complaints should include a rectal exam and a guaiac test performed to test for occult blood. The differential diagnosis for this patient includes acute gastroenteritis, intussusception intestinal obstruction, appendicitis, malrotation, Meckel's diverticula, and abdominal wall herniation. To further elucidate the diagnosis, plain films of the abdomen including a KUB and upright can provide additional information if obstruction or perforation is suspected. Ultrasound or contrast enema are the studies of choice for suspected intussusception, and an ultrasound or CT scan can be used for suspected appendicitis. If appendicitis is suspected, spiral CT is most commonly used to confirm diagnosis.

 ## CASE CONTINUED

Further questioning of the parent reveals a history of rectal bleeding at home. Rectal exam performed during the physical examination confirms this. A plan film of the abdomen reveals distended bowel loops and air-fluid levels. A subsequent air-contrast enema reveals a "coiled-spring" appearance to the small bowel and an ileocolic intussusception.

 ## DISCUSSION

Intussusception results from the telescoping of a portion of proximal bowel into adjacent distal bowel. Most commonly this is an ileocolic process. Compression of the bowel wall and obstruction of blood supply lead to ischemia and infarction. If untreated, the results can be disastrous, leading to abdominal distention, perforation, and shock. The classic triad is a history of brief, colicky, intermittent bouts of abdominal pain every 5 to 30 minutes, vomiting, and bloody stools.

QUESTIONS

34-1. Which of the following is a possible "lead point" for intussusception?
  A. Meckel's diverticulum
  B. Hypertrophied Peyer's patch
  C. Lymphoma
  D. Ingested foreign body
  E. All of the above

34-2. Abdominal exam of a patient with intussusception is most likely to reveal which of the following?
  A. Sausage-shaped mass in right side
  B. Bluish periumbilical discoloration
  C. Hepatosplenomegaly
  D. Hyperactive bowel sounds
  E. All of the above

34-3. You are counseling the family of a patient with intussusception. Which of the following statements about intussusception is appropriate to include in your discussion?
  A. It usually affects patients older than 3 years.
  B. The majority are unsuccessfully reduced via pneumatic or hydrostatic methods.
  C. Cause is unknown in the majority of cases.
  D. IV hydration and nasogastric decompression are generally not indicated.
  E. There is virtually no recurrence after reduction.

34-4. Which of the following is least likely to be included in the differential diagnosis for acute abdominal pain?
  A. Acute viral gastroenteritis
  B. Food poisoning
  C. Food allergy
  D. Bacterial enterocolitis
  E. Bowel obstruction

ANSWERS

34-1. E, 34-2. A, 34-3. C, 34-4. C. Intestinal lead points include the given answers, and more rarely Henoch-Schönlein purpura, fecaliths, traumatic hematoma, and cystic fibrosis.

The physical findings can range from peritoneal signs to a normal examination. Bowel sounds are usually hypoactive or absent. In a majority of patients (up to 80%), a sausage-shaped mass is palpable in the right side of the abdomen. Hepatosplenomegaly is generally not seen, and bluish periumbilical discoloration may be found in patients with pancreatitis.

In the overwhelming majority of patients, a cause is not found (up to 90%). The peak age of occurrence is between 3 and 18 months, and a specific lead point should be sought in older children. Pneumatic and/or hydrostatic enema can be both diagnostic and therapeutic (Fig. 34-1). These methods are successful in the majority of patients, but are also accompanied by a recurrence rate of nearly 15%. Open surgical reduction may be required. Supportive care with fluids and nasogastric decompression is the mainstay of initial management.

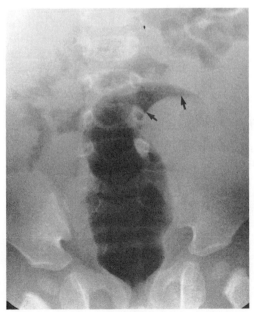

(a)

FIGURE 34-1.
Air enema of a child with intussusception. **A:** The intussusception is clearly demarcated, indenting the colonic lumen (*arrows*). **B:** Following reduction, air is now seen in the small bowel. (*From Rudolf M, Levene M. Paediatrics and Child Health. Oxford: Blackwell Science; 1999:136, with permission.*)

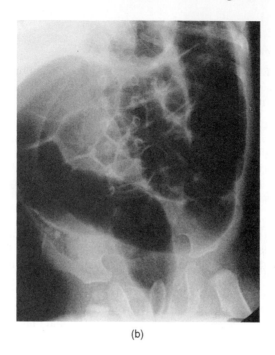

(b)

The differential diagnosis for intussusception should include those entities that are commonly associated with acute abdominal pain. This list is quite extensive, but generally does not include food allergies, which typically present with chronic abdominal symptoms.

 SUGGESTED ADDITIONAL READING

McCollough M. Abdominal surgical emergencies in infants and young children. *Emerg Med Clin North Am.* 2003;21(4):909–935.

CASE **35**

Vomiting Blood

 CC/ID: 4-year-old boy brought in by his father after he vomited blood in preschool today.

HPI: D.S. was in his usual good state of health this morning when he left for day care. Today he was playing at school when he suddenly ran to the bathroom to throw up. The teacher noticed that there were some small brownish "specks" in the vomitus, and some streaks of blood, and called his father to pick him up. D.S. has not been complaining of abdominal pain, has been eating and drinking normally, and has been stooling normally. He has not had any recent illnesses or vomiting, although he tends to have a "sensitive stomach." Currently he says he feels "fine," although he appears somewhat fearful.

PMHx: No hospitalizations; no surgeries. Has allergic rhinitis and mild eczema.

Meds: Nasal steroid spray; diphenhydramine at night

All: NKDA

Immun: UTD

FHx: Negative for hematologic disorders, peptic ulcer, or liver disease.

THOUGHT QUESTIONS

- What is your first concern with this patient?
- What are possible sources of the bleeding?

DISCUSSION

In any patient who has evidence of a GI bleed, your first concern should be the patient's hemodynamic stability. Perform a brief physical survey and check the patient's vital signs for tachycardia, an early sign of volume depletion in children. Consider a hematocrit to check for anemia. Whenever possible, try to establish whether the substance is actually blood. Gastroccult (for emesis) and Hemoccult (for stool) are rapid tests for blood. In the case of a suspected gastric or esophageal bleed, gastric lavage with warm saline can confirm the source and whether active bleeding is present.

Bleeding from the GI tract should be characterized as from either an upper or a lower GI source. An upper GI bleed, one that occurs proximal to the ligament of Treitz, presents as bright red or "coffee ground" emesis. Conversely, a lower GI bleed presents as bright red blood per rectum or in stool. Melena or heme-positive stool can signify either an upper or a lower source, so these findings require further investigation to confirm the location. In the case of D.S., the appearance of blood in vomit suggests an upper GI source. Any of the structures proximal to the ligament of Treitz (i.e., duodenal bulb, stomach, esophagus, oropharynx, and nose) could be responsible. Additional exam and history should be directed toward establishing a history of bleeding, disease, or trauma involving these structures.

CASE CONTINUED

You check the patient's vital signs, which reveal a temperature of 37°C (98.6°F), pulse of 85, respiratory rate of 21, and blood pressure of 105/70. Feeling reassured that your patient is hemodynamically stable, you perform a careful physical examination and obtain further history.

PE: *Gen:* well-appearing boy with a nasal voice. *HEENT:* right naris is crusted with blood; left appears boggy and congested. Oropharynx is normal, without bleeding or inflammation. *CV:* RR&R; no murmur; pulses and capillary refill brisk. *Abdomen:* soft, nondistended, and nontender; normoactive bowel sounds; no masses. *Skin:* pink and warm; patches of dry skin in antecubital regions; no bruising or petechiae. *Rectal:* guaiac negative for blood; normal tone.

You confirm with the family that there is no history of NSAID use or of unusual bruising or bleeding prior to this episode. D.S. denies symptoms of heartburn or gastritis, and has not been retching.

D.S's parents worry that he might be anemic, because he has nose-bleeds about once a week.

You call the teacher at the day-care center, who confirms that no sharp objects could have been ingested, and that D.S. was well prior to the episode, except that he had a nosebleed that morning that stopped after 5 minutes of direct pressure.

THOUGHT QUESTIONS

- Where is the most likely source of this patient's bleeding?
- How would you manage him?

DISCUSSION

D.S. probably vomited swallowed nasopharyngeal blood after epistaxis. The most common reason for epistaxis in children is nose pick-ing, but in this case D.S. has two additional risk factors: allergic rhinitis and the use of nasal steroids. Other causes of an upper GI bleed in a child this age include Mallory-Weiss tear, erosive gastritis, and foreign body ingestion. Management in this case would include discontinuing the nasal steroids and applying a lubricant to the nose to combat dryness. You can reassure the parents that anemia from brief, self-limited nosebleeds is very rare, and no labs are necessary.

QUESTIONS

35-1. You are examining an 8-week-old infant who was brought in because Mom has noticed some bright red, bloody streaks in her stool for 2 days. The baby has been otherwise well, feeding formula vigor-ously every 2 to 3 hours, and has been stooling soft yellow stool regu-larly. There has been no fever, vomiting, or abdominal discomfort. The vital signs and exam are within normal limits, and no fissures are noted around the anus. A guaiac test of the stool is positive for blood. In this case, the most likely cause of the blood-streaked stool is

- A. Peptic ulcer disease
- B. Volvulus
- C. Milk allergy
- D. Mallory-Weiss tear

35-2. In a patient with an active upper GI bleed, what should your *first* step be?
  A. Perform gastric lavage with warm saline solution.
  B. Assess and stabilize airway, breathing, and circulation.
  C. Send blood for CBC, type, and crossmatch.
  D. Obtain a CT scan with contrast.

35-3. What is the most common presentation for Meckel's diverticulum?
  A. Painless rectal bleeding
  B. Vomiting blood
  C. Melena and crampy abdominal pain
  D. GI obstruction

35-4. A 14-year-old boy comes to the clinic concerned that his stools are "black." He denies fever, abdominal pain, vomiting, or constipation, but has had some loose stools recently due to "stress from finals." He has been taking Pepto-Bismol with some relief. He is otherwise healthy, and vital signs and exam are within normal limits. You perform a guaiac test of his stool and a rectal exam, and both are negative for blood. What is the most likely explanation for this teen's presentation?
  A. Peptic ulcer disease
  B. Meckel's diverticulum
  C. Ingestion of large amounts of iron
  D. Use of Pepto-Bismol

ANSWERS

35-1. C. This well-appearing infant presents with evidence of lower GI bleed. Lower GI bleeds are more common than upper GI bleeds in children, and rectal bleeding is the most common presentation. The differential diagnosis of upper and lower GI bleeding depends on the age of the child. In infants, the most common causes of a lower GI bleed are rectal fissures and milk allergy. Milk allergy in infants causes a colitis that can lead to blood in the stools, as well as anemia and failure to thrive. In the perinatal period swallowed maternal blood should be considered in the differential, whereas in the adolescent patient, intestinal polyps, inflammatory bowel disease (IBD), and hemorrhoids are more likely causes. Peptic ulcer disease is an upper GI source of blood and would be more likely to present with melena or heme-positive stools, since blood is chemically changed during transit through the gut to appear dark or tarry. Rarely, however, a briskly bleeding duodenal ulcer may appear as rectal bleeding due to rapid transit time through the intestine. Volvulus may cause bright red blood in the stool, but the patient should be very ill and show evidence of obstruction. A Mallory-Weiss tear is unlikely, since the infant is not vomiting, and this is an upper GI source of blood.

35-2. B. Your *first* priority in the patient with an active upper GI bleed is to assess and stabilize the ABCs. This would include intubation if necessary, obtaining IV access, and administering volume resuscitation. Gastric lavage can help to control and identify the source of the bleeding, and should always be performed with warm saline (not ice cold, because this can cause hypothermia and inhibit clotting). A CBC, type, and cross should be sent as soon as possible to assess the severity and chronicity of the bleed and prepare for possible transfusion. Although CT scan may reveal the source of the bleeding, endoscopy is the study of choice and should be performed once the patient is stable.

35-3. C. Meckel's diverticulum, the most common anomaly of the GI tract, is usually composed of heterotopic gastric tissue. The most common presentation is painless rectal bleeding. Meckel's diverticulum is typically located in the small intestine within 2 feet of the ileocecal valve, has a peak incidence of bleeding at 2 years of age, and is present in 2% of the population (the "2-2-2" rule). The diagnosis is made by performing a special nuclear scan, called a Meckel's scan, to identify the ectopic acid-secreting cells in the diverticulum.

35-4. D. Pepto-Bismol causes black stools and can also cause a black coating on the tongue. However, the stools should be guaiac negative for blood, as in this patient. Ingestion of large amounts of iron or red meat can also cause dark stools, but these are usually positive by guaiac, due to the iron content. Dark stools can also be caused by ingestion of large amounts of blackberries, black licorice, spinach, or lead. The patient does not have physical or historical findings that suggest peptic ulcer disease, and the negative guaiac test suggests that the black stools are not caused by an upper GI bleed. With Meckel's diverticulum, the presentation is usually bright red blood per rectum.

 ## SUGGESTED ADDITIONAL READING

Leung AK, Wong AL. Lower gastrointestinal bleeding in children. *Pediatr Emerg Care.* 2002;18(4):319–323.

VI

Cases Presenting with Joint Pain

Hip Pain

CC/ID: 8-year-old girl presents to emergency room at 7 AM complaining of pain in left leg during walking.

HPI: Patient was in her usual state of good health until yesterday morning, when she noticed slight intermittent pain in her left thigh when she walked. The pain had become slightly worse throughout the day, but she was able to sleep through the night. The pain is worse this morning. She insists the leg hurts only when she walks or tries to run, and reports no history of recent trauma to her leg (especially as her mother did not allow her to play in her soccer league last week because she still had a cold). She describes the pain as being "dull" with a gradual onset and feels it mostly in her hip. It is worsened by bearing weight and improves slightly when she rests.

PMHx:/
PSHx: Normal weight gain

Meds: Tylenol PRN for pain

All: NKDA

FHx: No history of familial orthopedic, endocrine, or oncologic disorders.

SHx: Lives at home with her mother, father, and older brother, aged 12. Attends second grade and is currently in a local girls' soccer league.

VS: Temp 37°1C (98.8°F), BP 95/68, HR 74, RR 22

PE: *Gen:* awake, alert, and oriented ×3. *Ext:* left leg is well perfused. No visible bleeding, bruising, or joint swelling noted. Normal range of motion of knee and ankle, but guarding of hip on internal rotation. No pain on palpation except pain at hip while standing. Normal sensory exam and proprioception of leg. Unable to walk due to pain. Remainder of physical exam normal.

THOUGHT QUESTIONS

- What is in this patient's differential diagnosis?
- What three hematologic laboratory tests should be obtained at this time?
- What is the significance of the history of a recent cold?
- Although x-rays may also be helpful, what single procedure may yield a definitive diagnosis?

DISCUSSION

This patient's differential diagnosis mainly includes traumatic injury, infectious causes (toxic synovitis, septic arthritis or osteomyelitis), avascular necrosis of the hip (Legg-Calvé-Perthes Disease), early septic arthritis or osteomyelitis, rheumatologic disease (JRA), and, less likely, malignancy.

With this broad differential, laboratory tests should be geared toward identifying the presence of infection or inflammation, which will help to narrow the possibilities and guide further investigation. The hematologic tests to order at this time are a CBC with differential, ESR, and blood culture. The CBC and ESR lab results are elevated in septic arthritis but may be only mildly increased in toxic synovitis.

The significance of the recent cold is that it may suggest toxic synovitis, an inflammatory postinfectious arthritis that is commonly preceded by an upper respiratory viral infection.

Whenever septic arthritis is a possibility, aspiration of joint fluid is the definitive test that should be performed to confirm or eliminate this diagnosis. Septic arthritis usually yields a white blood cell count greater than 25,000 with a definitive organism. X-rays can be helpful to differentiate transient toxic synovitis or septic arthritis from osteomyelitis. In some cases of septic arthritis, there may be a notable widening of the space between the femoral head and acetabulum. Malignancies or osteomyelitis may also be detected on x-ray by irregularities or lucencies in the bone, although these findings are usually delayed by 5 or more days. Other imaging studies that are useful for examining bones and joints include MRI and bone scan. These should be considered on a case-by-case basis.

CASE CONTINUED

Labs: WBC 18,000 (60% lymphs, 25% segs, 0 bands); ESR 22 (normal up to 25). Blood culture in lab. *X-ray, left leg:* normal. No increase in joint space of left hip. No lucencies.

Based on the patient's well appearance, absence of findings on x-ray or on examination consistent with a septic joint, and reassuring laboratory studies, you determine that the patient has toxic synovitis.

QUESTIONS

36-1. Management of toxic synovitis includes which of the following therapies?
   A. Rest, anti-inflammatory medications, antibiotics
   B. Anti-inflammatory medications *only*
   C. Rest, anti-inflammatory medications, close follow-up exams
   D. Close follow-up exams *only*

36-2. If this patient had high fevers, significantly elevated WBC, ESR >25, positive finding of increased joint space on hip x-ray, and purulent fluid from joint aspiration, what would the next step be?
   A. Ask patient to return next day for repeat WBC and ESR
   B. Open joint drainage and initiation of IV antibiotics
   C. IV antibiotics only
   D. Oral antibiotics only
   E. Bone scan

36-3. What is the most common organism causing septic arthritis in a patient with sickle cell disease?
   A. *Salmonella typhi*
   B. *Haemophilus influenzae* type b
   C. *Staphylococcus aureus*
   D. *Streptococcus pneumoniae*
   E. *Neisseria gonorrhoeae*

36-4. What is the most common infectious cause of monoarthritis or polyarthritis in an adolescent?
   A. *Salmonella typhi*
   B. *Haemophilus influenzae* type b
   C. *Staphylococcus aureus*
   D. *Streptococcus pneumoniae*
   E. *Neisseria gonorrhoeae*

ANSWERS

36-1. C. Antibiotics are *not* indicated in the conservative management of toxic synovitis. Correct management includes rest, anti-inflammatory medications, and close follow-up exams to ensure that symptoms resolve by 7 to 10 days. Cases that recur or persist longer than 7 to 10 days may suggest Legg-Calvé-Perthes disease (idiopathic avascular necrosis of the femoral head).

36-2. B. The patient has septic arthritis and needs immediate surgical intervention involving open joint drainage to preserve the limb. A dose of IV antibiotics with good *S. aureus* coverage, such as nafcillin, should also be started immediately. A bone scan would not give additional information at this point because the definitive diagnosis has already been established by the purulent joint fluid.

36-3. C. Even in patients with sickle cell disease who have asplenia, the most common organism causing septic arthritis is still *S. aureus.* These patients also have increased risk of acquiring infections due to encapsulated organisms such as *Salmonella typhi.*

36-4. E. Gonococcal arthritis associated with disseminated gonococcal infection is the most common cause of polyarthritis or monoarticular arthritis in adolescents. In younger pediatric populations, the most common cause of infectious arthritis is *Staphylococcus aureus.*

 SUGGESTED ADDITIONAL READING

Blickman JG, van Die CE, de Rooy JW. Current imaging concepts in pediatric osteomyelitis. *Eur Radiol.* 2004;14(suppl 4):L55–L64.
Waters E. Toxic synovitis of the hip in children. *Nurse Pract.* 1995;20(4):44–46, 48,51.

Knee Pain

CC/ID: 11-year-old girl with fever presents to pediatric urgent care clinic with left knee pain.

HPI: Patient was in her usual state of health until 6 weeks ago, when she began to have intermittent low-grade fevers and joint swelling of her left knee. She does not remember any trauma to the leg and has not had any intercurrent viral illness. When asked about the quality of the pain, she states it is "dull," constant, limited to her knee, and hurts more at night. It is so uncomfortable that she has been limping for 2 days. Her only other symptoms include feeling tired and a slight loss of appetite. She denies any recent trips into the woods and is not sexually active.

PMHx: None

Meds: None

All: NKDA

FHx: Mother has systemic lupus erythematosus (SLE). No oncologic disorders.

SHx: Lives at home with mother and father; attends fifth grade.

VS: Temp 38°C (100.5°F), BP 105/72, HR 79, RR 28

PE: *Gen:* awake, alert, and oriented ×3. *HEENT:* normal. *Neck:* positive lymphadenopathy (bilateral anterior cervical). *Abdomen:* positive hepatosplenomegaly. *Ext, left leg:* swelling of knee joint. No erythema, but slightly warm. Decreased range of motion and minimal pain on palpation. Remainder of exam normal.

THOUGHT QUESTIONS

- What is in this patient's differential diagnosis?
- What are at least two antibody titers that are worth obtaining?

DISCUSSION

The differential diagnosis of an isolated arthritis includes juvenile rheumatoid arthritis (JRA), SLE, septic arthritis with or without osteomyelitis, toxic synovitis, Lyme disease, and residual inflammation following injury. The lymphadenopathy and hepatosplenomegaly in this case point more toward a systemic condition.

When rheumatologic disease is suspected, initial tests should include an antineutrophil antibody (ANA) and rheumatoid factor (RF), in addition to a CBC and ESR or CRP. The ANA is a sensitive but non-specific test for many autoimmune diseases, including SLE, dermatomyositis, and JRA. RF is usually negative in children with JRA, but if positive is associated with more severe prognosis and with ophthalmologic disease.

CASE CONTINUED

Labs: (+) ANA (1:640), (−) RF. WBC 15,000, Hb 11 g/dL, platelets 298,000, ESR 30 (normal up to 25). *X-ray, left knee:* no lucencies, no bony abnormalities; suggestion of slight joint soft tissue swelling.

You determine that this patient most likely has a form of pauciarticular JRA, given her history and physical exam, as well as the level of positive ANA. She does not have polyarticular JRA because she has fewer than five or more affected joints, and does not have systemic JRA because she did not exhibit temperature elevations greater than 39.4°C (103°F) for 2 weeks, has no rash, and has minimal ESR elevation (Table 37-1).

TABLE 37-1   Classification of Juvenile Rheumatoid Arthritis

	Polyarthritis	**Oligoarthritis**	**Systemic**
Total cases (%)	40–50	40–50	10–20
Number, pattern of joints involved	≥5; symmetric	≤4; may be only a single joint	Variable
Type of joints involved	Large (knees, elbows, ankles, wrists) and cervical joints	Knees and/ or ankles	Any joint
Severity of systemic involvement	Moderate	Rare	Severe[a]
Development of chronic uveitis (%)	5	20	Rare
Rheumatoid factor (+) (%)	10	Rare	Rare
ANA factor (−) (%)	50	80	10

[a]Including a high, spiking fever one to two times a day and a characteristic
rheumatoid rash (erythematous macules on trunk, extremities) lasting over 1 hour.
Modified from Cassidy JT. Connective tissue diseases and amyloidosis. In: Oski FA,
DeAngelis CD, Feigin FD, et al., eds. *Principles and Practice of Pediatrics*. 2nd ed.
Philadelphia: JB Lippincott Co, 1994:246, with permission.

 QUESTIONS

37-1. Which of the following statements supports why this patient does not have SLE?
   A. SLE does not run in families.
   B. She has a positive ANA titer.
   C. She has a negative RF titer.
   D. She does not meet at least 4 of the 11 clinical criteria to diagnose SLE.

37-2. Which of the following lists of sequelae can this patient eventually develop?
   A. Uveitis, polyarteritis nodosa, Reiter syndrome
   B. Ankylosing spondylitis, polyarteritis nodosa, Reiter syndrome
   C. Uveitis, ankylosing spondylitis, Reiter syndrome
   D. Polyarteritis nodosa only

37-3. What percentage of children with JRA will eventually "outgrow" their disease?

    A. 20%
    B. 40%
    C. 60%
    D. 80%

37-4. Which of the following statements is generally true of JRA?

    A. Morning stiffness is not a characteristic complaint.
    B. Pain symptoms are always severe.
    C. Generalized growth retardation does not occur.
    D. X-ray changes in JRA are usually mild.

 ANSWERS

37-1. D. The diagnosis of SLE is based on clinical evaluation and requires 4 of the 11 criteria for 96% certainty of disease. The 11 criteria are as follows: malar (butterfly) rash, discoid lupus rash, photosensitivity, mucocutaneous ulcers, arthritis, nephritis, encephalopathy, serositis, cytopenia, positive immunoserology, and positive ANA antibody. Furthermore, SLE is usually a familial disease.

37-2. C. Polyarteritis nodosa, a vasculitic syndrome, is *not* a sequelae of JRA. Uveitis tends to be acute, with decreased visual acuity and erythema; patients may also develop ankylosing spondylitis and features of Reiter syndrome.

37-3. D. Eighty percent of all children with JRA will "outgrow" their disease, and the prognosis is more favorable in girls with pauciarticular disease. It is, however, less favorable in the child with seropositive polyarticular disease.

37-4. D. X-ray changes in JRA are usually minimal. Morning stiffness does occur even in children and can be alleviated with early rising, warm morning baths, and heating pads and electric blankets. Pain symptoms are variable, with some children having no pain and others experiencing significant discomfort. Growth retardation occurs especially if steroids have been used to treat JRA. Some catch-up growth does occur during periods of remission.

SUGGESTED ADDITIONAL READING

Buka RL, Cunningham BB. Connective tissue disease in children. *Pediatr Ann*. 2005;34(3):225–229, 233–238.

Goldmuntz EA, White PH. Juvenile Idiopathic Arthritis: A Review for the Pediatrician. *Pediatr Rev*. 2006;27:e24–e32.

Schaller JG. Juvenile rheumatoid arthritis. *Pediatr Rev*. 1997;18(10): 337–349.

Tse SML, Laxer RM. Approach to Acute Limb Pain in Childhood. *Pediatr Rev*. 2006;27:170–180.

Shoulder Pain

CC/ID: 4-year-old boy presents to the pediatric urgent care clinic at noon complaining of pain in his right shoulder.

HPI: Patient's mother says she picked up her son from day care after she received a call that he was crying and had fallen during a game of tug-of-war (his team lost). When asked what had happened, the boy simply said he got pulled "hard" by the rope and fell forward into the sandbox. When asked where it hurt, the boy used his left hand and pointed up and down his right upper arm, keeping it still. He is not able to answer specific questions about the quality of the pain (sharp vs. dull, intermittent or constant), because he always just answers "yes." His mother reports that she has not seen him move his arm since she picked him up, and that he was in good health when he awoke this morning and has had no previous history of injuries to his right arm.

PMHx: None

Meds: None

All: NKDA

FHx: No history of familial orthopedic or connective tissue disorders.

SHx: Lives at home with his mother and father. No siblings. Attends day care 3 days a week.

VS: Temp 36.9°C (98.4°F), BP 90/60, HR 80, RR 28

PE: *Gen:* awake, alert. *Ext, right arm:* held at side, slightly flexed and pronated. No bleeding, bruising, or lacerations. No visible swelling of shoulder, elbow, or wrist joints. No pain on palpation of shoulder, elbow, or wrist joints. No pain on palpation of the humerus or bones of the arm or wrist. The boy refuses to straighten the arm or use it to reach for objects. Remainder of exam was within normal limits.

THOUGHT QUESTIONS

■ What is in this patient's differential diagnosis?

■ How does isolation of pain relate to true location of injury in limb injuries?

■ What is the significance, if any, of the position of the patient's arm?

■ What diagnostic tests, if any, would you consider at this point?

DISCUSSION

The differential diagnosis primarily includes acute traumatic conditions: fracture of the wrist, arm, or shoulder bones; dislocation of the shoulder; or subluxation of the radial head (nursemaid's elbow). Occasionally an infectious or malignant process in the bone or joint can come to the parent or child's attention after trauma, so these possibilities should be kept in mind as well. Nonaccidental trauma (child abuse) must be considered when an injury or fracture is not consistent with the history presented. Fractures in children require special attention, especially if they extend through the epiphyseal growth plate (Fig. 38-1). The mnemonic S-A-L-T-E-R may be useful in remembering the various fracture types: Slip fracture along growth plate; Above growth plate; beLow growth plate; Through growth plate; and ERasure of the growth plate.

The concept of "referred" pain in limb injuries is important to consider, because a child may perceive and thus point to an area and complain of pain even when the actual injury site is elsewhere. For this reason, careful examination of the hand, wrist, elbow, shoulder and clavicle should be performed in a case such as this one.

The slightly flexed and pronated position of the patient's arm at his side strongly suggests subluxation of the radial head (nursemaid's elbow). Additionally, lack of point tenderness on palpation is less consistent with fracture (although, rarely, some fractures may not be immediately associated with pain).

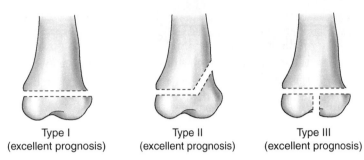

Type I
(excellent prognosis)

Type II
(excellent prognosis)

Type III
(excellent prognosis)

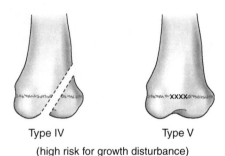

Type IV

Type V

(high risk for growth disturbance)

FIGURE 38-1.   Epiphyseal fractures: Salter-Harris classification. (*Illustration by Electronic Illustrators Group.*)

   CASE CONTINUED

Based on the typical history and physical examination, and the absence of point tenderness, you determine that this patient's injury is most likely a subluxation of the radial head (nursemaid's elbow).

   QUESTIONS

38-1. One method of reducing a nursemaid's elbow consists of applying pressure on the radial head and
   A. Applying pressure to the ulnar condyle simultaneously
   B. Fully extending the elbow while supinating the forearm
   C. Fully extending the elbow and applying sustained traction
   D. Flexing the elbow while pronating the forearm
   E. Flexing the elbow while supinating the forearm

38-2. Nursemaid's elbow should be considered in a patient without point tenderness on exam who
- A. Is unable to move the extremity
- B. Is able to pronate and supinate forearm
- C. Can only supinate forearm
- D. Is unable to flex or extend forearm
- E. Can slightly flex or extend forearm

38-3. Recurrent subluxation of the radial head should be treated
- A. Conservatively with no treatment
- B. By splinting the arm for 2 weeks
- C. By casting the arm for 2 weeks
- D. By surgical pinning of the radial head to the ulna

38-4. Which of the following statements describes the incidence of dislocated shoulder?
- A. It occurs more commonly in infants.
- B. It occurs more commonly in toddlers.
- C. It occurs more commonly in adolescents.
- D. It occurs with the same frequency throughout childhood (infants to adolescents).

 ANSWERS

38-1. D. Nursemaid's elbows are usually easily treated in the clinic setting. Pressure over the radial head as the arm is flexed and supinated will correct the subluxed radial head. There is often no need for x-ray if there is a strong history of the patient's arm being pulled and no tenderness to palpation of the bones of the wrist and arm. If there is doubt about the presence of a fracture, an x-ray should be obtained before trying to reduce the elbow in the clinic or emergency room. After reduction, there is almost immediate resolution of pain and recovery of normal range of motion.

38-2. E. Interestingly, patients are often able to lightly flex or extend at the elbow but always hold the arm in pronation until it is corrected. After reduction the arm should not be splinted, because this slows recovery; ice, ibuprofen, or acetaminophen can be recommended for pain and swelling.

38-3. A. No additional treatment beyond manual repositioning of the subluxed radial head as described is necessary. Although the problem may recur, it resolves with maturation.

38-4. C. Dislocation of the shoulder is uncommon in childhood and becomes more frequent in adolescents. The younger a child is at the time of initial dislocation, the higher the chance of developing a recurrent dislocation. Because of the high recurrence of dislocation, some orthopedic surgeons favor early reconstruction rather than conservative watchful management.

   SUGGESTED ADDITIONAL READING

Kunkler CE. Did you check your nursemaid's elbow? *Orthop Nurs.* 2000;19(4):49–52.
Sachs HC. Dislocations. *Pediatr Rev.* 2000;21(12):433–434.

Puffy Hands and Feet

CC/ID: 6-month-old African American infant presents to urgent care clinic with painful swollen hands and feet.

HPI: Patient was brought to clinic by a caretaker from his foster home when she noted that he awoke this morning and appeared to have slight swelling of his hands and feet. Over the course of the morning, he has become increasingly irritable, and the swelling has worsened. He cries immediately when his hands or feet are touched. He has been afebrile and has not had any ill contacts. His birth history is unknown because he was abandoned at birth by his mother and left in a blanket on the doorstep of an inner-city orphanage. He was in good health when he was found, has not had any illnesses to date, and has had excellent weight gain since birth. He was well until this morning, with no signs of respiratory infections; no vomiting, diarrhea, other rashes or bruising; and no reported history of trauma. He is developmentally normal.

PMHx: None

Meds: None

All: NKDA

FHx: Unknown

SHx: Lives in a foster home since age 2 months with his adoptive mother and father, both healthy. No pets. His adoptive mother stays home with him during the day.

VS: Temp 36.1°C (97°F), BP 80/65, HR 100, RR 40

PE: *Gen:* awake, alert, fussy. Cries when hands or feet are touched. *HEENT:* normocephalic, anterior fontanel soft/flat; PERRLA, normal fundi; normal ears. *Lungs:* clear bilaterally. *CV:* RR&R; normal S_1, S_2; slight flow murmur heard over entire chest. *Abdomen:* soft, nondistended; positive bowel sounds; no masses; normal liver edge. Palpable spleen tip in left upper quadrant. *Ext:* both hands and feet slightly warm to touch, with marked swelling mostly over dorsum. *Skin:* no rashes, cyanosis, bruising, or wounds.

THOUGHT QUESTIONS

- What is in this patient's differential diagnosis?
- What is the significance of a palpable spleen tip?

DISCUSSION

This patient's differential diagnosis includes sickle cell disease, trauma, osteomyelitis, juvenile rheumatoid arthritis (JRA), and tumors of bones. Because he is affected bilaterally and symmetrically in the upper and lower extremities, the most likely diagnosis is a more generalized process such as sickle cell disease.

A palpable spleen tip indicates an enlarged spleen. In sickle cell disease, splenic enlargement occurs as a result of a sequestration crisis in which the spleen suddenly becomes engorged with red blood cells, trapping a significant portion of the blood volume.

CASE CONTINUED

Labs: *CBC:* WBC 15,000, Hb 6 g/dL, Hct 20, platelets 150. No bands on differential. *X-rays, hands and feet:* marked soft tissue swelling; no fractures.

You determine that this patient has presented with dactylitis secondary to sickle cell disease and admit the child to the hospital to initiate appropriate hydration therapy and pain medication.

QUESTIONS

39-1. Which of the following lists of diagnostic tests confirms a diagnosis of sickle cell disease?
A. Newborn screening tests (in most states), hemoglobin electrophoresis, splenic ultrasound
B. Hemoglobin electrophoresis, splenic ultrasound
C. Newborn screening tests (in most states), hemoglobin electrophoresis, Sickledex preparation to demonstrate sickling of red blood cells at low O_2 tension
D. Splenic ultrasound *only*

39-2. Which of the following combinations of quantitative hemoglobin electrophoresis is characteristic of sickle cell trait?
A. 0% hemoglobin A, 2% to 3% hemoglobin A_2, 85% to 95% hemoglobin S, 5% to 15% hemoglobin F
B. 55% to 60% hemoglobin A, 2% to 3% hemoglobin A_2, 40% to 45% hemoglobin S
C. 0% hemoglobin A, 0% hemoglobin A_2, 45% to 50% hemoglobin S, 45% to 50% hemoglobin C
D. 90% to 98% hemoglobin A, 2% to 3% hemoglobin A_2, 2% to 3% hemoglobin F

39-3. The amino acid defect in sickle cell disease is a substitution in the sixth amino acid position of the β-globin chain of
A. Leucine for valine
B. Valine for glycine
C. Valine for glutamine
D. Glutamine for valine

39-4. Which of the following events in the natural course of sickle cell disease significantly increases the risk of infection by encapsulated organisms?
A. Aplastic anemia
B. Chronic hemolysis
C. Chronic penicillin prophylaxis
D. Splenic autoinfarction

ANSWERS

39-1. C. Splenic ultrasound is *not* helpful in establishing the diagnosis of sickle cell disease. It would only be useful to identify splenic enlargement—not the cause. In most states, the newborn screen includes hemoglobin electrophoresis to identify newborns with sickle cell disease. Quantitative hemoglobin electrophoresis shows 0% hemoglobin A, 85% to 95% hemoglobin S, 2% to 3% hemoglobin A_2, and up to 15% hemoglobin F.

39-2. B. Sickle cell trait is generally an asymptomatic condition in which an individual may rarely exhibit painless hematuria and/or an inability to concentrate the urine. The importance of diagnosing sickle cell trait is to provide proper genetic counseling for those individuals who wish to have children. Answer A represents homozygous sickle cell disease (the patient in this case). Answer C is hemoglobin C sickle cell disease, and answer D is for an individual without hemoglobinopathy.

39-3. C. The substitution of a valine for glutamine in the sixth position of the β-globin chain is the hallmark of sickle cell disease.

39-4. D. Splenic autoinfarction is caused by microvascular obstruction as sickled cells pass through the spleen. The associated infarction and fibrosis of splenic tissue leads to a gradual regression in splenic size, usually by age 4 years. The diminished capability of the spleen to filter encapsulated organisms places the infant and child at great risk for overwhelming sepsis, meningitis, pneumonia, arthritis, and osteomyelitis.

 SUGGESTED ADDITIONAL READING

Atweh GF, DeSimone J, Saunthararajah Y, et al. Hemoglobinopathies. *Hematology Am Soc Hematol Educ Program.* January 2003:14–39.

Wethers DL. Sickle cell disease in childhood: Part I. Laboratory diagnosis, pathophysiology and health maintenance. *Am Fam Physician.* 2000;62(5):1013–1020, 1027–1028.

Wethers DL. Sickle cell disease in childhood: Part II. Diagnosis and treatment of major complications and recent advances in treatment. *Am Fam Physician.* 2000;62(6):1309–1314.

VII

Cases
Presenting with
Refusal to Walk

CASE **40**

Limping Teen

CC/ID: 16-year-old boy presents to urgent care clinic complaining of left knee pain and a limp.

HPI: Patient was well until about 2 weeks ago, when he began to develop intermittent left knee pain mostly while walking. The pain has worsened over the past day, making it uncomfortable to walk. When asked to point to exactly where it hurts, he is vague in pointing to his left knee and says he cannot exactly pinpoint the source. He denies any history of recent trauma or previous injuries to that leg. He also denies any sports-related injuries, especially because he is currently out of sports and working on his "over-weight" problem. He has had no fevers or other intercurrent illnesses and is not sexually active.

PMHx: None

Meds: None

All: NKDA

FHx: No family history of endocrine, rheumatologic, or onco-logic disorders.

SHx: Lives at home with mother (divorced) and younger brother, age 10; healthy. Attends tenth grade.

VS: Temp 37°C (98.6°F), BP 120/81, HR 77, RR 22

PE: *Gen:* obese adolescent boy sitting in no apparent distress; awake, alert, and oriented ×3. *Ext, left leg:* Limited range of motion, with poor abduction, flexion, and internal rotation of hip. Minimal pain on manipulation but tendency toward external rotation of femur as left hip is flexed. *Left knee:* normal range of motion; no pain on palpation of joint. Normal exam of right leg and normal sensory exam of both legs. Remainder of exam normal.

THOUGHT QUESTIONS

- What is in this patient's differential diagnosis?
- What would be the appropriate radiologic study to obtain at this time? (Consider appropriate views.)
- What is the significance of the perception of knee pain in this patient?

DISCUSSION

This patient's differential diagnosis includes trauma, slipped capital femoral epiphysis (SCFE), Legg-Calvé-Perthes disease (avascular necrosis of the femoral head), and toxic synovitis of the hip. SCFE is a disorder seen early in puberty, whereas Legg-Calvé-Perthes disease generally presents between 4 and 11 years of age.

The appropriate radiologic studies to order are anterior posterior pelvic x-rays in the neutral and "frog-leg" position to properly view the femoral head.

The pain this patient perceives in his knee is known as "referred" pain. With certain injuries, the patient perceives the pain to occur at a joint other than the actual site of injury. This misperception is due to convergence of sensory pathways that conduct pain sensation to the CNS. This is especially important to keep in mind when examining children, who are often poor at localizing pain. It is therefore important to examine, and consider imaging, the entire limb even when only a single joint is reported to hurt.

CASE CONTINUED

Labs: *X-ray, left hip:* AP view—slight widening of epiphyseal physis of femoral head. "Frog-leg" view—posterior shift of femoral head, displaced 1 cm but less than two thirds the width of femoral neck. Appears as if "an ice cream scoop is falling off the cone." *X-ray, left knee and left foot:* normal.

Based on the x-ray findings, you determine that this patient has a slipped capital femoral epiphysis (Fig. 40-1).

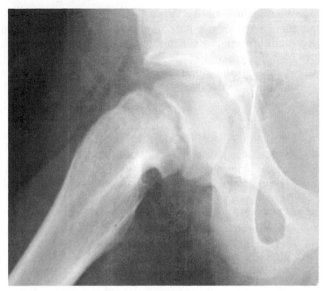

FIGURE 40-1. Lateral "frog leg" x-ray of hip. The femoral head is seen to be displaced posteriorly in relation to the femoral neck.

QUESTIONS

40-1. What should the next course of action be?
A. No medications and ask the patient to return for repeat x-rays in 1 week.
B. Prescribe Motrin and ask patient to return for repeat x-rays in 1 week.
C. Prescribe Motrin and ask patient to return for orthopedic appointment in 1 week.
D. Consult an orthopedic surgeon immediately for surgical repair.

40-2. Which of the following statements is consistent with a diagnosis of SCFE ?
A. Trauma is *not* a cause of SCFE.
B. A hormonal factor always accounts for this lesion.
C. Females are affected more commonly than males.
D. Bilateral involvement occurs in more than 50% of cases.

40-3. What is the goal of surgical repair of SCFE?
    A. Pinning the femoral head in place to prevent further slipping
    B. Pinning the femoral neck to the femoral shaft to prevent fracture
    C. Realigning and pinning of the femoral head
    D. Total joint replacement

40-4. Which of the following conditions can be a long-term complication of SCFE?
    A. Immune-mediated osteoarthritis of the femoral joint
    B. Avascular necrosis of the femoral head
    C. Loss of pain sensation in affected leg
    D. Loss of proprioception (toe-up, toe-down) in affected foot

ANSWERS

40-1. **D.** The diagnosis of SCFE in a patient should be treated by immediate surgical consultation. Casting or splinting is not effective, and prolonged disunion of the bones can lead to permanent damage.

40-2. **A.** Trauma is *not* a contributing factor to SCFE. Associated factors include obesity, male predominance, African American race, and certain endocrine disorders such as hypothyroidism.

40-3. **A.** The primary goal of treatment is prevention of further misalignment. The femoral head is thus pinned in place without realignment. If proper blood flow is maintained, and the bones remain healthy, there is no need for total joint replacement.

40-4. **B.** Avascular necrosis and late degenerative changes similar to those seen with osteoarthritis may occur as long-term consequences of SCFE.

SUGGESTED ADDITIONAL READING

Frick SL. Evaluation of the child who has hip pain. *Orthop Clin North Am*. 2006;37(2):133–140.
Loder RT. Controversies in slipped capital femoral epiphysis. *Orthop Clin North Am*. 2006;37(2):211–221.
Loder RT. Slipped capital femoral epiphysis in children. *Curr Opin Pediatr*. 1995;7(1):95–97.

Difficulty Walking

CC/ID: 8-year-old girl presents to emergency room at midnight complaining of difficulty walking.

HPI: Patient was well until 3 weeks ago, when she developed a sore throat and fever. She then traveled with her family to Washington, Oregon, Idaho, and Nevada (no camping) and returned 5 days ago with increased tiredness, back pain, neck pain, and irritability. Her mother recalls that she was "listless" and complained of a vague pain in both legs 3 days ago. When asked where it hurts, she states her legs "just feel tired." Today her mother has had to help support her while walking home from school and walking to the hospital.

PMHx: None

Meds: None

All: NKDA

FHx: No history of neurologic disorders or CNS malignancies.

SHx: Lives at home with mother, father, and two younger brothers, ages 2 and 4, both recovering from viral illness. Attends third grade.

VS: Temp 37.1°C (98.8°F), BP 99/66, HR 80, RR 25

PE: *Gen:* awake, alert, and oriented ×3; lying down, no distress. *Neck:* supple, no nuchal rigidity. *HEENT:* fundi normal; throat slightly erythematous; no exudates. *Ext, arms (bilateral):* normal sensory exam and reflexes; motor strength slightly decreased (4 out of 5) at hands, distal and proximal arms. *Ext, legs (bilateral):* Sensory exam—normal exam to pain and light-touch. Motor exam—decreased strength in feet, lower, and upper legs (2 out of 5; unable to move against gravity). Reflex exam—absent deep tendon reflex (DTR) at Achilles tendon and patellar tendon. Proprioceptive exam—normal "toe-up" and "toe-down" recognition. Babinski toe reflex—"downward" direction. Gait— unable to walk. Remainder of exam normal.

THOUGHT QUESTIONS

- What is in this patient's differential diagnosis?
- What could be the significance, if any, of whether she had gone camping?
- What are important laboratory tests to consider at this time?

DISCUSSION

This patient's examination shows symmetric bilateral ascending weakness, with intact sensation and absent reflexes. With this type of exam, her differential diagnosis includes immune-mediated demyelinating neuropathy (Guillain-Barré syndrome), tick paralysis, spinal cord compression, transverse myelitis, acute cerebellar ataxia, myasthenia gravis, poliomyelitis, botulism, diphtheric neuropathy, and porphyria.

The significance of knowing whether this patient had gone camping is that the information may help to direct the differential diagnosis toward tick-borne paralyses.

A CBC with differential, blood culture, and spinal tap for CSF are important laboratory considerations that will help distinguish between the possibilities just discussed.

CASE CONTINUED

Labs: WBC 5,400 (64% segs, 17% lymphs, 10% monos, 7% atypical lymphs); platelets 270,000. *CSF:* Gram stain negative, 1 RBC, 2 WBC, glucose 57, protein 215 g/dL (normal: 20–170 g/dL).

You repeat a physical examination and find no evidence of any ticks or tick bites. Given no history of trauma, no signs of upper motor neuron dysfunction, no acute infection, and no RBC abnormalities, you determine that this patient must have Guillain-Barré syndrome (the CSF protein levels are usually elevated after the first week of illness).

The patient is admitted to the hospital with increasing lower extremity weakness and gradually worsening upper extremity weakness and areflexia of all limbs. You have chosen to admit her to the pediatric intensive care unit primarily because you are concerned that she could develop respiratory failure requiring intubation and mechanical ventilation (12% to 20% of patients).

She remains in the hospital for 3 weeks, during which time she is treated with close monitoring, intravenous immunoglobulin (IVIG), and plasmapheresis and is finally discharged and recovers completely with normal function by another 2 weeks as an outpatient.

 QUESTIONS

41-1. Which of the following supports the idea that this patient did not have an upper motor neuron lesion?
   A. Her CSF protein level is 215 g/dL.
   B. She had a "downward" Babinski reflex.
   C. Her DTRs are absent.
   D. Her sensory exam is normal.

41-2. Although usually of unknown origins, Guillain-Barré syndrome has been associated in 20% to 40% of cases with serologic evidence of recent infection by which of the following?
   A. *Streptococcus pneumoniae*
   B. *Staphylococcus aureus*
   C. *Clostridium botulinum*
   D. *Campylobacter jejuni*

41-3. This patient's recovery of function could have been predicted to occur as
   A. Progress in the direction of onset (ascending weakness pattern followed by ascending recovery pattern)
   B. Progress in the direction opposite of onset (ascending weakness pattern followed by descending recovery pattern)
   C. Simultaneous recovery of all limbs together
   D. No particular pattern

41-4. Which of the following lists of autonomic abnormalities can be associated with Guillain-Barré syndrome?
   A. Bowel/bladder dysfunction, systemic blood pressure changes (hypotension or hypertension), abnormal sweating
   B. Bowel/bladder dysfunction, blurry vision, systemic blood pressure changes
   C. Blurry vision, systemic blood pressure changes (hypotension or hypertension)
   D. Blurry vision, abnormal sweating

ANSWERS

41-1. B. Upper motor neuron lesions are usually associated with "upward" Babinski reflex of toes. Guillain-Barré syndrome is a progressive demyelination of the peripheral nervous system (lower motor neurons) and therefore produces a pattern of ascending weakness with absent DTRs, normal Babinski reflex (downward), and intact sensation.

41-2. D. Stool cultures obtained from patients with Guillain-Barré syndrome at the onset of weakness are positive for *C. jejuni* in more than 25% of cases. Although in most cases the cause is unknown, a recent history of viral infection is often obtained from patients.

41-3. B. The onset of classic Guillain-Barré progression occurs in an ascending pattern and is followed by recovery in an opposite (descending) pattern. A variant of Guillain-Barré syndrome known as Miller-Fisher syndrome starts with acute external ophthalmoplegia and progresses in a descending pattern. Although recovery is usually complete, the primary morbidity from Guillain-Barré syndrome is respiratory failure, sometimes requiring intubation.

41-4. A. Blurry vision is *not* associated with Guillain-Barré syndrome. Miller-Fisher syndrome, a variant of Guillain-Barré, may be associated with vision abnormalities that include a slowed papillary reflex in addition to external ophthalmoplegia.

 SUGGESTED ADDITIONAL READING

Evans OB, Vedanarayanan V. Guillain-Barré syndrome. *Pediatr Rev.* 1997;18(1):10–16.
Joseph SA. Guillain-Barré syndrome. *Adolesc Med.* 2002;13(3): 487–494.

CASE **42**

Never Started Walking

CC/ID: 18-month-old boy who has not started walking.

HPI: P.L. was brought in by his mother over concern that her son was not yet walking. He recently was started in day care, where the mother noticed that he was "less advanced than the other children his age." He will cruise briefly on his own, but refuses to walk independently. Over the last several months, she has also noticed him to be more irritable and "colicky." His appetite has decreased over this time period, and his mother has noticed very little weight gain. He had been otherwise healthy, and she has not sought medical attention since his 9-month visit.

PMHx: Uncomplicated SVD at term; no chronic illness or hospitalizations.

Meds: None

All: NKDA

Immun: UTD

DietHx: "Loves to put almost anything in his mouth; not lately interested in eating much."

DevHx: Cruising and pulling to stand; not independently walking; only says "mama-dada" specifically and two to three other words; likes to play pat-a-cake; "refuses to play ball. He will not let go and throw it."

FHx: Noncontributory

VS: Temp 37.1°C (98.8°F), BP 90/45, HR 110, RR 28; Weight 9.5 kg (5%)

PE: *Gen:* alert but not very interactive; in no acute distress. *HEENT:* NCAT; nondysmorphic; EOMI; PERRL. *Lungs:* no crackles; no wheeze. *CV:* RR&R; normal S_1, S_2; no murmur. *Abdomen:* soft, nondistended/nontender; normal active bowel sounds; no masses or visceromegaly. *Skin:* no bruises or lesions noted; no clubbing, cyanosis, or edema. *Neuro:* normal tone/strength/reflexes; somewhat unsteady truncal posture; responsive to voice but not to commands. *ROS:* occasional vomiting "due likely to feeding him new foods"; no diarrhea; occasional bouts of constipation.

THOUGHT QUESTIONS

- What further components of the history or physical examination would you pursue?
- What is in your differential diagnosis at this point?
- What diagnostic evaluations may aid you in your diagnosis?

DISCUSSION

For a patient who is suspected of not meeting developmental milestones, the examiner should obtain a complete developmental history, including the areas of development affected (gross motor, fine motor, social, cognitive/language) and the pattern of development. The history should establish whether there has been a delay, arrest or regression in development, which can then guide the differential diagnosis. Additional history includes a complete review of systems and family history of other children or members with any developmentally related problems should be obtained. A social and environmental history should note the child's caretakers, stressors, and learning, playing, and living environs. It is also important to note perceptions of hearing and vision. The thorough physical examination should particularly focus on neurologic findings, growth, and developmental maturity. The broad differential diagnosis of abnormal development includes extrinsic factors (social environment, toxin exposure, nutrition) and intrinsic factors (CNS disease, muscular disease chromosomal abnormalities, metabolic derangements, sensory impairment, congenital infections, chronic systemic illness). Diagnostic testing should be based on the suspected etiology after thorough history, physical exam and formal developmental assessment, and may include imaging, sensory testing or laboratory tests (such as CBC, metabolic tests, chromosome analysis, toxin levels).

CASE CONTINUED

Further developmental history reveals that early milestones were achieved on time, through about 1 year of age. On further exam, P.L. is noted to have a clumsy pincer grasp, cannot build a tower of cubes, has no imitative behavior and does not know any body parts. The child is assessed as having arrest in development encompassing motor, social and cognitive domains. Further history reveals that 5 months ago the family had moved to a new home, built in 1928, which was undergoing partial renovation and restoration. Suspecting exposure to lead-based paint or dust, you perform a serum lead test. A level of 80 is found, and the child is diagnosed with lead poisoning.

DISCUSSION

Abnormal development is an important symptom in childhood, as it may be a sign of a correctable environmental or social condition or a treatable medical illness. For this reason, developmental screening is an essential part of health maintenance for children of all ages. Abnormal development may be limited to one area, or may affect more than one area ("global" delay). Although there are many causes of abnormal development, the cause is unknown in a significant number of patients, especially for those with delay in an isolated domain. In this case, this patient's pattern of initially normal development followed by arrest suggested a new insult of some type.

QUESTIONS

42-1. Which of the following is most likely to be associated with significant lead poisoning?
  A. Macrocytic anemia
  B. Increased cognitive ability
  C. Normal coordination
  D. Absence of GI symptoms
  E. Pica

42-2. Which of the following is the best indicator for future intellectual achievement?
  A. Fine motor development
  B. Gross motor development
  C. Language development
  D. Social development

42-3. You are counseling the family of an infant who is suspected of having cerebral palsy. Which of the following statements regarding this condition could you include in your discussion?
   A. It always involves motor areas of the brain.
   B. It always is associated with mental retardation.
   C. One percent to 2% of cases are idiopathic.
   D. Motor problems are generally progressive rather than static.
   E. A multidisciplinary approach is rarely helpful.

42-4. List the likely sequence for sexual development in males.
   A. Development of pubic hair
   B. Penile enlargement
   C. Testicular enlargement
   D. Height growth spurt

ANSWERS

42-1. A. Lead poisoning is a major preventive health issue in primary care pediatrics. Exposure to lead-based paint is the main cause, and a blood lead level above 20 defines lead poisoning. Developmental delay can be one of the associated findings, which may include cognitive and neurologic impairment. Pica refers to a propensity to put nonedible objects in the mouth, and is commonly associated with the intake of flaking lead paint. Anorexia, nausea, vomiting, abdominal pain, and constipation can occur. For severe cases, seizures, encephalopathy, and coma may result. Lead poisoning (along with iron deficiency and thalassemia) commonly is associated with a microcytic anemia. The CDC recommends universal screening for lead poisoning at 12 months and 2 years of age.

42-2. C. Of the four domains of development (Table 42-1), language is the best indicator for future intellectual achievement.

42-3. A. Cerebral palsy is a disorder of motor movements and posture resulting from an insult to the motor area of the brain. Injuries may occur before, during, or after birth. Although most patients have perinatal complications resulting in cerebral palsy, many cases have no known cause. Abnormal posture, visual/oral function, tone, and primitive/muscle-stretch reflexes are usually present and are static rather than progressive in nature. Regressing motor skills usually suggests a different subset of diagnoses. Mental retardation and intellectual impairment may be present in nearly half of cases, but are not always present. A multidisciplinary approach to care best serves these patients and their families.

TABLE 42-1 Normal Developmental Milestones

Age	Gross Motor	Visual/Fine Motor	Language	Social
1 month	Raises head slightly from prone; makes crawling movements	Tight grasp; visually fixes/follows to midline	Alerts to sound	Regards face
2 months	Head held in midline; lifts chest off table *3 months:* Holds head steadily; supports on forearms in prone	Follows past midline; fist no longer clenched *3 months:* Hands open at rest; responds to visual threat	Social smile *3 months:* Coos	Parent recognition *3 months:* Reaches for familiar objects/people
4 months	Rolls front to back; supports on wrists *5 months:* Rolls back to front; sits with support	Brings hands to midline; reaches with arms in unison; grabs rattle	Laughs; orients to voice; needs expressed through differential cry *5 months:* Orients to bell (localizes laterally)	Enjoys looking around environment
6 months	Sits unsupported; puts feet in mouth when supine *7 months:* Creeps	Reaches with either hand; object transfer; uses raking grasp	Babbles; imitates sound *7 months:* Orients to bell (localized indirectly)	Recognizes strangers; expresses displeasure when toy or parent removed
8 months	Comes to sit *9 months:* Crawls; pulls to stand	Object inspection *9 months:* Pincer grasp; holds bottle; probes with forefinger	"Dada" (indiscriminate) *9 months:* Waves bye-bye; "Mama" (indiscriminate); understands "no"	Fingerfeeding *9 months:* Explores environment; plays pat-a-cake

(Continued)

233

TABLE 42-1 Normal Developmental Milestones (continued)

Age	Gross Motor	Visual/Fine Motor	Language	Social
10 months	Cruises; walks when led with both hands 11 months: Walks when led with one hand	—	"Dada/Mama" (discriminate); orients to bell (directly) 11 months: Follows one-step command with gesture	—
12 months	Walks alone	Mature pincer grasp; marks paper with pencil; voluntary release	2 words other than "Dada/Mama", immature jargon 13 months: Uses 3 words 14 months: Follows one-step command without gesture	Imitates actions; comes when called; cooperates with dressing
15 months	Creeps up stairs; walks backward	Scribbles with crayons (imitation), stacks 2 blocks (imitation); uses spoon and cup	Uses 4 to 6 words 17 months: 7 to 20 words; points to 5 body parts; mature jargon	Give/takes toys; tests limits and rules; plays games with parents
18 months	Runs; throws toy from standing	Spontaneous scribble; feeds self; turns 2–3 pages at a time; stacks 3 blocks	2-word combinations 19 months: Knows 8 body parts	Copies parent in tasks; likes to play with other children
21 months	Squats in play; goes up steps	Stacks 5 blocks	2-word sentences; uses 50 words	Asks to have food, go to toilet
24 months	Up/down steps without help; throws ball overhand	Stacks 7 blocks; turns pages one at a time; imitates pencil stroke; removes pants and shoes	Uses pronouns inappropriately; follows 2-step commands	Listens to short stories; parallel play

234

30 months	Jumps with both feet off floor	Holds pencil in adult fashion; horizontal and vertical strokes; unbuttons	Uses pronouns appropriately; concept of "1"; repeats 2-digit forward	Tells first and last name; gets self drink without help
3 years	Rides tricycle; goes up steps with alternate feet; kicks ball	Copies circle; undresses completely; dresses partially; stacks 8 blocks	Uses 250 words; 3-word sentences; understands concept of "2," plural/past tense; speech 75% intelligible	Group play; takes turns; knows full name/age/sex; shares toys
4 years	Hops; alternates feet going down stairs	Copies cross; buttons clothing; dresses completely; catches ball 4.5 years: Copies square	Asks questions; knows colors, song, or poem from memory	Tells "tall tales"; cooperative play with a group of children
5 years	Skips alternating feet; balances on one foot	Copies triangle; ties shoes; spreads with knife	Prints first name; asks word meanings; tells simple story	Competitive games; helps in household tasks; abides by rules

TABLE 42-2   Tanner Staging of Secondary Sex Characteristics

Breast Development

Stage 1	Preadolescent; elevation of papilla only
Stage 2	Breast bud; elevation of breast and papilla as small mound; enlargement of areolar diameter (11.15 ± 1.10)
Stage 3	Further enlargement and elevation of breast and areola; no separation of their contours (12.15 ± 1.09)
Stage 4[a]	Projection of areola and papilla to form secondary mound above level of breast (13.11 ± 1.15)
Stage 5[a]	Mature stage; projection of papilla only due to recession of areola to general contour of breast (15.33 ± 1.74)

Genital Development (Male)

Stage 1	Preadolescent; testes, scrotum, and penis about same size and proportion as in early childhood
Stage 2	Enlargement of scrotum and testes; skin of scrotum reddens and changes in texture; little or no enlargement of penis (11.64 ± 1.07)
Stage 3	Enlargement of penis, first mainly in length; further growth of testes and scrotum (12.85 ± 1.04)
Stage 4	Increased size of penis with growth in breadth and development of glans; further enlargement of testes and scrotum and increased darkening of scrotal skin (13.77 ± 1.02)
Stage 5	Genitalia adult in size and shape (14.92 ± 1.10)

Pubic Hair (Male and Female)

Stage 1	Preadolescent; vellus over pubes no further developed than that over abdominal wall (i.e., no pubic hair)
Stage 2	Sparse growth of long, slightly pigmented downy hair, straight or only slightly curled, chiefly at base of penis or along labia (male: 13.44 ± 1.09; female: 11.69 ± 1.21)
Stage 3	Considerably darker, coarser, and more curled; hair spreads sparsely over junction of pubes (male: 13.9 ± 1.04; female: 12.36 ± 1.10)
Stage 4	Hair resembles adult in type; distribution still considerably smaller than in adult; no spread to medial surface of thighs (male: 14.36 ± 1.08; female: 12.95 ± 1.0)
Stage 5	Adult in quantity and type, with distribution of the horizontal pattern (male: 15.18 ± 1.07; female: 14.41 ± 1.12)
Stage 6	Spread up linea alba: "male escutcheon"

[a]Stages 4 and 5 of breast development may not be distinct in some patients.
From Marino B, Snead K, McMillan J. *Blueprints in Pediatrics*. 2nd ed. Malden, MA: Blackwell Science; 2001:52, with permission.

42-4. C, B, D, A. The sequence for sexual development in females is thelarche (breast buds), height growth spurt, pubic hair, and menarche. The events of puberty in both sexes occur in predictable sequences but may vary in their timing and velocity for each individual (Table 42-2).

  SUGGESTED ADDITIONAL READING

Colson ER, Dworkin PH. Toddler development. *Pediatr Rev.* 1997;18:255–259.

Johnson CP, Blasco PA. Infant growth and development. *Pediatr Rev.* 1997;18:224–242.

Laraque D, Trasande L. Lead poisoning: successes and 21st century challenges. *Pediatr Rev.* 2005;26:435–443.

Sore Foot and Dark Urine

CC/ID: 6-year-old boy brought in by his parents for limping.

HPI: D.J. has been limping and complaining of a blister on his left heel for two weeks, but was otherwise in good health until yesterday, when he began to feel tired and his mother thought he looked "puffy." He has been drinking well, but has only urinated a very small amount of "brownish" urine once today. D.J. complains of a mild headache, but has not had fever, rash, abdominal pain, joint pain, dysuria, diarrhea, or vomiting. There is no history of trauma, and he has never had dark urine before. His parents are concerned that the blister has not healed and now appears infected.

PMHx: No illnesses or hospitalizations.

Meds: None

All: NKDA

Immun: UTD

VS: Temp 36.8°C (98.2°F), BP 130/80, HR 90, RR 22; Weight 22 kg (65%)

PE: *Gen:* a tired-appearing but nontoxic boy. *HEENT:* mild periorbital edema bilaterally. Oropharynx is moist, without erythema or exudate. No lymphadenopathy. *CV:* no murmur; pulses and capillary refill brisk. *Lungs:* clear. *Abdomen:* no abdominal or flank tenderness or bruising; no organomegaly. *Ext:* slight ankle edema; joint and muscle exam are normal. A 3-mm superficial honey-crusted erosion is visible on the left heel; it is tender, with 2 cm of surrounding erythema. Remainder of exam is within normal limits.

THOUGHT QUESTIONS

■ What organ system seems to be predominantly affected in this child?

■ What is your differential diagnosis and how will you further evaluate him?

DISCUSSION

D.J.'s symptoms—dark urine, reduced urine output (oliguria), edema, and hypertension—suggest renal pathology. Dark urine often signifies hematuria or myoglobinuria (blood or myoglobin in the urine), which has a broad differential. Causes of hematuria or myoglobinuria in children include infection, trauma, stones, rhabdomyolysis, hematologic disorders, benign or familial hematuria, and menses. In this case, the dark urine in the presence of symptoms such as edema, oliguria, and hypertension suggests a functional problem at the glomerular level.

Renal dysfunction can often be categorized into nephrotic and nephritic syndromes. Nephrotic syndrome, a noninflammatory and usually idiopathic condition, is characterized by large proteinuria, hypoalbuminemia, edema, and hyperlipidemia. Edema is usually the presenting complaint; hypertension and hematuria are less common. Glomerulonephritis (GN) is the most common type of nephritis. It occurs from noninfectious inflammation of the glomerular basement membrane (GBM) and is usually immune-complex mediated. Hematuria is the hallmark of this disease, and proteinuria may be present but is much less severe than in nephrotic syndrome. Urinalysis is a valuable tool in differentiating nephrotic syndrome from GN. Additional studies in this case should be directed toward evaluating the patient's electrolyte and fluid status, and further characterization of the source of his renal disease. The foot lesion has the characteristic appearance of impetigo, a superficial skin infection caused by *Staphylococcus* or *Streptococcus* species, and would be a good place to culture to document streptococcal infection.

CASE CONTINUED

You ascertain from the boy's mother that there is no family history of rheumatologic disease, renal disease, diabetes, or deafness. Meanwhile, you send a urine sample to the laboratory for urinalysis and culture. The urinalysis shows numerous red blood cells and casts, a few white cell casts, no bacteria, and small protein. You culture the foot blister, and the Gram stain shows gram-positive cocci. You also draw a CBC, electrolytes, and an albumin level, which are all within normal limits except for slightly elevated BUN and creatinine levels of 25 and 1.0, respectively. Based on these results, you suspect glomerulonephritis and send a C3 complement level, which comes back low, confirming the presence of glomerular inflammation with consumption of complement. Two days later the wound culture grows group A streptococci.

THOUGHT QUESTION

- What is the most likely cause of this patient's glomerulonephritis?

DISCUSSION

The most common cause of acute GN in children is poststreptococcal glomerulonephritis (PSGN). Other less common causes of GN in children include IgA nephropathy, systemic disease such as lupus, and Alport syndrome (a hereditary progressive form of the disease often accompanied by deafness). This patient's clinical picture and recent streptococcal skin infection suggested the diagnosis of PSGN. His laboratory results confirm the diagnosis, with urinary red cell casts and a decreased C3 level.

QUESTIONS

43-1. With supportive care alone, most cases of PSGN will
- A. Resolve completely
- B. Progress to renal failure
- C. Result in mild systemic hypertension
- D. Require lifelong steroids to prevent recurrence

43-2. This patient's edema is most likely caused by which of the following?
- A. Low albumin level
- B. Early cardiac failure
- C. Salt and water retention
- D. Decreased activity level

43-3. What is the most common cause of nephrotic syndrome in children?
  A. Minimal change disease
  B. Membranous glomerulonephritis
  C. Chronic use of NSAIDs
  D. Systemic lupus erythematosus

43-4. Renal biopsy of this patient would most likely reveal
  A. Infiltration of the GBM by IgA
  B. Effacement of GBM epithelial cell foot processes
  C. Collections of IgG and C3 below the GBM
  D. Thinning of the GBM

ANSWERS

43-1. A. The management of acute PSGN is mainly supportive, because it is usually a self-limited disorder. Over 98% of children with PSGN make a full recovery, although the symptoms may take months to resolve. Complications such as hypertension and edema are treated with vasodilators, diuretics, and fluid restriction. If the patient has a positive streptococcal culture of skin or throat at the time of diagnosis, appropriate antibiotic therapy should be initiated. Steroids and other immunosuppressants have not been shown to affect course or outcome. The prognosis for other types of glomerulonephritis is much less favorable. For example, most boys and 20% of girls with Alport syndrome will progress to end-stage renal disease (ESRD) by mid-adulthood; those with rapidly progressive glomerulonephritis (a rare and devastating form of GN) usually become dialysis dependent within a few years.

43-2. C. Edema in cases of PSGN is usually caused by salt and water retention due to a decrease in glomerular function. Hypoalbuminemia is much less common than in nephrotic syndrome, and is not present in this patient.

43-3. A. Minimal change disease (MCD) is the most common cause of nephrotic syndrome in children, accounting for 75% of cases, followed by focal glomerular sclerosis (Table 43-1). Membranous GN is the most common cause in adults, but is much less common in children. Management of uncomplicated nephrotic syndrome in children includes steroids and salt restriction. Long-term prognosis for MCD is excellent, although the majority (80%) of patients will relapse at least once. Bacterial infections are the most common complication, and spontaneous bacterial peritonitis is the

TABLE 43-1 Nephrotic Syndrome and Glomerulonephritis

	Nephrotic Syndrome	Glomerulonephritis
Definition/ Pathophysiology	Noninflammatory increase in permeability of glomerular capillary wall (possibly due to loss of negatively charged proteins). Results in proteinuria, primarily albumin.	Noninfectious inflammatory process of the glomerular capillaries, usually caused by trapped antigen-antibody complexes. Results in hematuria, inflammatory cells in urine.
Histology	**MCD:** Effacement of foot processes	**PSGN:** Collections of IgG and C3 below GBM; proliferation of mesangial and capillary cells; inflammatory cell infiltration. **IgA nephritis:** IgA deposits in GBM.
Diagnosis	**Criteria:** (1) Generalized edema; (2) hypoproteinemia (<2 g/dL); (3) urine protein/creatinine ratio >2 in morning void *or* 24-hr urine protein >50 mg/kg body weight; (4) hypercholesterolemia (>200 mg/dL). Hematuria is *rare* (10%–20%).	**UA:** Gross or microscopic hematuria is the hallmark. Also may have RBC casts, proteinuria, leukocytes. **Clinical:** may have hypertension, edema (10%–20%).
Most common pediatric causes	Minimal change disease (75% in children <12).	(1) Poststreptococcal; (2) IgA nephropathy; (3) systemic disease.
Treatment	Supportive care and systemic corticosteroids; 85% to 90% response to initial treatment; 80% relapse at least once.	Supportive care and treatment of underlying disease.
Mortality (causes)	2% (peritonitis, thrombus).	Mortality is rare (cerebral hemorrhage, hyperkalemia).

most common infection. Hypercoagulability can occur due to urinary loss of coagulation factors such as antithrombin III and protein C. Interestingly, bleeding can also occur due to loss of factors IX, XI, and XII. End-stage renal disease is rare in patients with MCD, but is more common in patients with other causes of nephrotic syndrome.

43-4. C. Renal biopsy is *not* routinely indicated in cases of PSGN. However, if performed, histology reveals collections of IgG and C3 below the GBM, proliferation of mesangial and capillary cells, and inflammatory cell infiltration. Infiltration of the GBM by IgA is found in IgA nephropathy and Henoch-Schönlein purpura (HSP). Effacement of foot processes is seen in minimal change disease, the most common cause of nephrotic syndrome in children. Thinning of the GBM is seen in benign familial hematuria.

 SUGGESTED ADDITIONAL READING

Bergstein J, Leiser J, Andreoli S. The clinical significance of asymptomatic gross and microscopic hematuria in children. *Arch Pediatr Adolesc Med.* 2005;159(4):353–355.

Febrile Toddler

CC/ID: 15-month-old girl who has been refusing to walk for the last 4 days.

HPI: P.T. is a previously active child, who seems well and happy when she is sitting or lying down, but will not walk to her parents or to get toys. She has been walking since age 11 months, but now cries when placed on her feet. She has also had a low-grade fever (100°F–101°F) once or twice a day for a week, which her parents were told was due to a "virus." P.T. has had a good appetite, but recently has seemed more tired. She has not had runny nose, cough, rash, joint swelling, vomiting, or diarrhea. Her parents say they have not seen her fall, although she is such an active child that she often gets away from them.

PMHx: No hospitalizations or surgeries

Meds: Acetaminophen for fever

All: NKDA

Immun: UTD

SHx: Noncontributory

THOUGHT QUESTION

- What will you look for on physical examination?

DISCUSSION

In this toddler who seems to be refusing to walk due to pain, the source of her discomfort may be anywhere from the lumbar spine to the bottom of the feet. The physical examination should include a careful assessment of this entire region to characterize any tenderness, weakness, swelling, or deformity in the back or lower extremities. Observation is a crucial part of this examination; note the child's position of comfort, and any spontaneous use of the limbs. The remainder of the examination should assess the child's general health and stability, as well as look for stigmata of systemic disease or trauma such as rash, bruising, organomegaly, and lymphadenopathy.

CASE CONTINUED

VS: Temp 38.8°C (101.8°F), HR 120, RR 25; Weight 11 kg (75%)

PE: *Gen:* a playful, healthy-appearing child, sitting in mother's lab. She cries when pulled to a stand and holds her right leg off the ground. *HEENT:* no lymphadenopathy; normocephalic; oropharynx normal. *CV:* RR&R; no murmur. *Lungs:* clear. *Skin:* warm and pink; no bruising or rashes. *Ext:* no redness, swelling warmth, or limitation in movement of hips, knees, or ankles. The spine is palpated without discomfort. There is no redness, swelling, or deformity of the legs or feet. Careful examination of the lower right leg reveals pain on palpation of the proximal tibia.

THOUGHT QUESTIONS

■ What is your differential diagnosis at this point?
■ What further studies would you obtain?

DISCUSSION

The exam and history suggests a process in the bone of the lower leg. Possibilities include trauma (e.g., fracture, bruise), infection (e.g., osteomyelitis, septic arthritis), or malignancy (e.g., leukemia, metastatic neuroblastoma). A plain film of the leg is a good diagnostic test to start with. It may reveal fracture, a lytic lesion in the bone, or some of the early signs of bone infection such as periosteal reaction and tissue plane elevation (Fig. 44-1). Based on the plain film results, a CBC, blood culture, and ESR and/or CRP may be indicated to evaluate for infection, inflammation, and possible bone marrow involvement. More sophisticated imaging, such as nuclear bone scan or MRI, may be indicated to identify more subtle bony changes of early infection or malignancy, or to further distinguish between infectious and destructive processes.

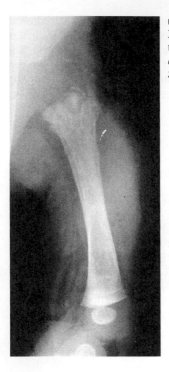

FIGURE 44-1.
X-ray of femur showing periosteal elevation. (*From Rudolf M, Levene M. Paediatrics and Child Health. Oxford: Blackwell
Science; 1999:223, with permission.*)

CASE CONTINUED

A plain film of the right leg shows elevation of soft tissue planes
around the tibial metaphysis, indicating an inflammatory process
in the bone. A CBC shows an elevated WBC count of 18,000, with
87% neutrophils. The ESR and CRP are elevated at 102 and 65
respectively. A blood culture is drawn, and because of concern for
osteomyelitis, an orthopedic consult is obtained. MRI confirms the
diagnosis, and the child is taken to the operating room for needle
aspiration of the bone for culture. She is admitted to the hospital
for parenteral therapy with nafcillin and ceftriaxone. The blood and
bone cultures subsequently grow methicillin-sensitive *Staphylococcus
aureus*, and her antibiotics are changed to nafcillin alone. P.T. is
afebrile on the second hospital day, and after 1 week of parenteral
therapy, her ESR is decreasing and her CRP has decreased to normal
(<2). The patient is discharged home on oral cephalexin to complete a
minimum of 3 weeks of antibiotic therapy, with close follow-up.

QUESTIONS

44-1. What is the most common bacterial cause of osteomyelitis in children?
- A. Salmonella in all age groups, including neonates
- B. *S. aureus* in neonates; salmonella in older infants and children
- C. *S. aureus* in all age groups, including neonates
- D. Group B streptococci in neonates; *S. aureus* in older infants and children

44-2. A medical student with whom you are working wants to know at what age children are at greatest risk for osteomyelitis. What is the best answer?
- A. Postpubertal teenagers are at the greatest risk of osteomyelitis.
- B. Toddlers (ages 2–4) are the highest-risk age group.
- C. The highest incidence occurs from thet neonatal period through toddlerhood.
- D. Incidence is bimodal, peaking in the neonatal period and again at ages 9 to 11.

44-3. What are the most common locations for osteomyelitis in children?
- A. Femur and tibia
- B. Skull and vertebrae
- C. Sternum and ribs
- D. Bones of the feet and hands

44-4. You are examining a 7-month-old infant who cries when she is placed on her feet. Her parents say she has been like this all day. She is afebrile, but her exam is otherwise similar to the child in this case, with pain on palpation of the lower leg. You obtain a plain film, which shows a minimally displaced spiral fracture of the tibia. This child's fracture is most likely a result of
- A. Osteomyelitis
- B. Osteosarcoma
- C. Accidental fall
- D. Nonaccidental trauma (child abuse)

ANSWERS

44-1. C. Most cases of osteomyelitis in infants and children are hematogenous in origin, and *S. aureus* is the most common pathogen. Immature blood vessels in the metaphysis make children's bones more vulnerable to invasion by bacteria. In the neonate, group B streptococci and *Escherichia coli* are other important pathogens. Salmonella should be considered in children with immunodeficiency, and is particularly associated with osteomyelitis in children with sickle cell disease. Children with sickle cell disease are especially vulnerable to osteomyelitis not only because they have impaired host defenses from splenic dysfunction, but also because they suffer bony damage from repeated episodes of vascular compromise.

Because of the prevalence of *S. aureus* in most cases of pediatric osteomyelitis, empiric therapy with an antistaphylococcal antibiotic (usually nafcillin) with or without a third-generation cephalosporin is usually initiated. If there is suspicion for MRSA, clindamycin or vancomycin should be used as empiric therapy. The duration of hospitalization and IV antibiotics depends on the patient's response to treatment. With good response (afebrile, CRP/ESR decreasing to normal, pain significantly improved), the patient may be discharged on an appropriate oral antibiotic to complete a minimum of 3 weeks of antibiotic therapy.

44-2. D. The incidence of osteomyelitis in children is bimodal, with peaks in the neonatal period and again at ages 9 to 11. In the older age groups, osteomyelitis is about twice as common in boys as in girls. Other risk factors include trauma or surgery involving the bone, which predisposes to bacterial invasion by rupturing small blood vessels and creating a favorable environment for bacterial growth. A history of trauma is found in approximately one third of cases of osteomyelitis. Children with impaired immune function are especially vulnerable to skeletal infection.

44-3. A. Most cases of osteomyelitis in children involve the long bones. The femur and tibia together account for about half of all cases. In neonates, more than one bone is involved in almost half of the cases. This is in contrast to older children, in whom involvement of multiple bones is rare.

44-4. D. The most likely cause of a spiral fracture of the tibia in a preambulatory infant is child abuse. This type of fracture occurs with a twisting force on the lower leg. A tibial spiral fracture in an older child is sometimes called a "toddler's fracture," because the injury is known to occur after an accidental forward fall, such as a toddler might experience while trying to walk or run. Although a 7-month-old preambulatory infant *could* be accidentally injured in such a way as to cause a twisting force on the lower leg (catching a foot in a crib, for example), this type of fracture is very unusual in preambulatory infants and is considered nonaccidental until proven otherwise. A condition such as osteogenesis imperfecta should also be considered as a predisposing factor, but its presence does *not* rule out child abuse. In this case, a careful history should be taken to elicit any history of trauma, frequent fractures, or caretaker negligence. Follow-up should include a skeletal survey to look for other fractures, and a referral to Child Protective Services (CPS) for further investigation.

 SUGGESTED ADDITIONAL READING

Gutierrez K. Bone and joint infections in children. *Pediatr Clin North Am*. 2005;52(3):779–794.

Kim MK, Karpas A. The limping child. *Clin Pediatr Emerg Med*. 2002;3(2):129–137.

VIII

Cases
Presenting with
Altered Mental
Status

Seizure

CC/ID: 2-year-old boy brought to emergency room at 3 AM by parents following 5 minutes of generalized seizure.

HPI: Parents state that their toddler was well until last evening, when they noted a runny nose, watery eyes, and increased irritability with refusal to eat dinner. At 2:30 AM they heard him cry and suddenly become silent. When they reached his room, they found him with his eyes rolled back, and he had rhythmic jerking of both his arms and legs that lasted at least 2 minutes. He did not stop breathing but turned slightly pale. Before they could dial 911, the episode stopped and he fell asleep, so they rushed him into the emergency room, where he is sleepy, but will intermittently wake and cry. When asked if he had a fever at home, the mother said that he had felt warm to the touch. He had been otherwise healthy, with no coughing, vomiting, diarrhea, or rashes, and has not had any known ill contacts.

PMHx: Birth history unremarkable: full term, SVD, Apgar scores of 9 and 9 at 1 and 5 minutes, respectively; discharged home on second day of life.

PSHx: None

Meds: None

All: NKDA

Immun: UTD

FHx: No family history of seizures or metabolic disorders.

SHx: Lives at home with healthy mother and father, no siblings. Attends day care during the week.

VS: Temp 38.9°C (102.1°F), BP 90/60, HR 105, RR 40

PE: *Gen:* sleeping quietly, awakens and cries when examined, but is consolable by mother. *HEENT:* normocephalic; no bumps, bruises. Eyes watery, no crusting; PERRLA, fundi normal. Clear rhinorrhea from nose. *Neck:* supple. *Lungs:* CTA(B). *Abdomen:* soft, nondistended/nontender; no masses. *Neuro:* normal motor, sensory, and reflex exam. *Ext:* initially too sleepy to assess gait, but after 30 minutes able to walk at baseline per mother.

THOUGHT QUESTIONS

- What is in this patient's differential diagnosis?
- What further workup would you pursue at this point?

DISCUSSION

The term "febrile seizure" refers to a relatively common and benign condition in children, accounting for 80% of first-time pediatric seizures. The etiology of febrile seizures is unknown, but they are often familial, and are suspected to occur as a result of elevated cytokine levels associated with certain febrile illnesses. Most febrile seizures are categorized as "simple"—defined as a seizure that is brief, generalized and non-recurring. A post-ictal state is often present after a febrile seizure, but should not be prolonged. Febrile seizures must be distinguished from other causes of seizure in a febrile child, such as neurologic disease or CNS infection. Therefore, absence of localizing signs or symptoms of these conditions is essential to the diagnosis. The differential for nonfebrile seizures includes metabolic derangements, cerebrovascular events, malignancy, trauma or epilepsy.

CASE CONTINUED

Given the history and presence of a fever, you are aware that the causes for this child's convulsions that carry the highest risk are meningitis or other CNS infection. Because you elicit no meningeal or encephalopathic signs on examination, and the child does not appear ill, and because he has returned to his neurologic baseline, you determine that he has had a febrile seizure. The history and physical findings are consistent with a nonspecific viral syndrome, and no further workup is necessary.

THOUGHT QUESTION

■ What are the most important points to discuss with the patient's parents regarding fever management and risk of further seizures?

DISCUSSION

The most important intervention at this time is to provide parental education about febrile seizures. Fever control with acetaminophen or ibuprofen is recommended for the child's comfort, but has not been shown to prevent recurrence of febrile seizures. Aspirin should be avoided secondary to a risk of developing Reye syndrome. Children with simple febrile seizures require no further evaluation beyond determination of the source of the fever, but febrile seizures can have up to a 50% recurrence rate with subsequent febrile illnesses. A simple febrile seizure lasts <10 minutes, is generalized, and does not recur within 24 hours. Suspected febrile seizures which do not meet these criteria are called "complex febrile seizures." Children with complex febrile seizures may undergo additional workup and close follow-up, because there is more like to be an underlying condition or illness which is the cause of the seizure.

QUESTIONS

45-1. Which of the following is true about febrile seizures?
A. Febrile seizures usually develop into epilepsy at a later age.
B. Febrile scizures are not associated with long-term cognitive problems.
C. There is generally no genetic predisposition to developing febrile seizures.
D. Febrile seizures are mostly associated with only bacterial infections that result in high fever.

45-2. Febrile seizures most commonly occur in children aged
A. Birth through 1 month
B. 1 month through 6 months
C. 6 months through 5 years
D. 5 years through 10 years

45-3. What will an EEG obtained from a child who has just had a febrile seizure most likely show?
- A. Normal
- B. A characteristic three-spikes-per-second waveform
- C. Generalized slowing
- D. Generalized slowing with occasional sharp waves

45-4. During the early months of life, the excitability of the newborn cortex
- A. Decreases gradually
- B. Increases continually into and beyond adulthood
- C. Increases initially and then decreases in the second decade of life
- D. Does not change

ANSWERS

45-1. B. Children who have febrile seizures do not have long-term cognitive, developmental or behavioral problems. Febrile seizures *may* be focal, without loss of consciousness, although this is less typical and should prompt evaluation for another etiology of the seizure. Although the etiology of febrile seizures is unknown, there appears to be a genetic component, as there is often a family history of similar seizures in first-degree relatives. Febrile seizures may be associated with any type of febrile illness, and viruses are the most common causes of febrile illness in the pediatric age group.

45-2. C. Febrile seizures are most likely to occur in children aged 6 months to 5 years, with a peak onset at 14 to 28 months of age.

45-3. A. Normal EEGs are expected in patients after a simple febrile seizure, and further imaging such as head CT or MRI will not be helpful. The characteristic three-spikes-per-second EEG waveform is associated with petit mal (absence) seizures. Generalized slowing with or without sharp spikes on EEG may occur as a consequence of global cerebral insult, such as following a hypoxic or ischemic CNS event.

45-4. C. The developing cortex of the newborn gradually becomes increasingly excitable (and thus more prone to seizures) before "maturing" and becoming less excitable in the second decade of life. Seizures are thus increasingly common during the early years and are then outgrown as the child grows older.

SUGGESTED ADDITIONAL READING

Sabo-Graham T, Seay AR. Management of status epilepticus in children. *Pediatr Rev.* 1998;19(9):306–309.

Warden CR. Evaluation and management of febrile seizures in the out-of-hospital and emergency department settings. *Ann Emerg Med.* 2003;41(2):215–222.

Shock

CC/ID: 1-month-old baby boy presents to emergency room at midnight appearing pale and gray.

HPI: Patient's mother reports that her 1-month-old infant was in his usual state of good health until about 24 hours ago, when he began to feed poorly. He normally breastfeeds about 20 minutes per breast at least every 3 to 4 hours, but over the past 24 hours he has refused to feed for more than 5 minutes per breast, and no more frequently than every 8 hours. She does not report any fevers, but the baby's father is just recovering from a cold during the past week. She has also noted that his last wet diaper was nearly 18 hours ago. He normally has a wet diaper at least every 3 to 4 hours. This evening, he became increasingly fussy and refused to feed altogether. Within a couple of hours his color suddenly became pale and gray, and he was unresponsive with shallow breathing. His parents called 911, and a paramedic team noted very poor skin perfusion, prompting intubation, starting an IV, and rushing him to the hospital emergency room. He had no vomiting or diarrhea, no obvious signs of any blood loss, and no history of trauma or toxic ingestions. He had a history of normal vaginal delivery following an uncomplicated pregnancy with good prenatal care.

PMHx: None

Meds: None

All: NKDA

FHx: No family history of congenital heart diseases or metabolic diseases.

SHx: Lives at home with mother and father, no siblings; at home with mother during day.

THOUGHT QUESTIONS

■ What is in this patient's differential diagnosis?
■ What are the three fundamental steps during a proper resuscitation?

DISCUSSION

This patient's differential diagnosis includes conditions that present as shock. Shock is classified into four major categories: hypovolemic, cardiogenic, distributive, and septic. Hypovolemic shock occurs from water and electrolyte losses such as vomiting and diarrhea or hemorrhage. Cardiogenic shock results from congenital heart diseases, ischemic heart diseases with cardiomyopathies, or arrhythmias. Distributive shock occurs from anaphylaxis, neurologic injury, or drug toxicity. Septic shock results from the common pathogens that cause infection within particular age groups.

The first three steps during any resuscitative procedure are A, B, and C: airway, breathing, and circulation. Performed in this order, these are the necessary steps in initiating any resuscitation. Establishing an airway in an obtunded individual usually requires intubation via endotracheal tube. Breathing refers to ensuring that once an airway is established, the patient is able to either breathe spontaneously or to breathe with the assistance of mechanical ventilation. Circulation involves assessment of the adequacy of proper perfusion to the vital organs and establishing IV access, or rarely, intraosseous access (in children younger than 6 years) to deliver fluids and medication.

CASE CONTINUED

VS: Temp 36.1°C (97°F), BP 50/30, HR 180, RR 70

PE: *Gen:* sleepy; unresponsive to gentle touch; withdraws appropriately to pain. *HEENT:* intubated; mucous membranes dry; eyes mildly sunken; throat nonerythematous. *Lungs:* crackles at bases bilaterally; good air entry. *CV:* tachycardia; RR&R; normal S_1, S_2; ventricular S_3 gallop. No murmur. *Abdomen:* soft, nondistended; minimal bowel sounds; no masses. Liver edge down 4 to 5 cm below costal margin. No palpable spleen tip. *Skin:* sweaty, cool extremities; capillary refill time 5 to 6 seconds.

THOUGHT QUESTION

- What is the significance of the sweating, ventricular S_3 gallop, and low liver edge?

DISCUSSION

Taken together, this constellation of clinical findings suggests a patient with congestive heart failure. It would be helpful to obtain a chest x-ray, electrocardiogram (ECG), and an echocardiogram to detect pulmonary edema, measure relative forces, and assess heart function, respectively.

CASE CONTINUED

Labs: *Chest x-ray:* pulmonary edema; enlarged heart size. *ECG:* ST segment depression; T wave inversion. *Echocardiogram:* decreased contractility of left ventricle and moderately decreased ejection fraction.

After no improvement in condition despite adequate volume resuscitation, a normal CBC, and negative blood culture, you determine that this patient most likely has congestive heart failure and shock due to cardiomyopathy (e.g., myocarditis). The patient was probably exposed to the same viral infection that had affected her father earlier, and ST segment depression indicates that the heart has sustained ischemic changes.

QUESTIONS

46-1. What is the most common cause of myocarditis in North American children?
- A. Adenovirus
- B. Coxsackie A virus
- C. Coxsackie B virus
- D. Respiratory syncytial virus
- E. Rhinovirus

46-2. Which of the following vascular beds are considered vital end organs?

    A. Coronary, cerebral, renal

    B. Coronary, hepatic, cerebral

    C. Hepatic, cerebral

    D. Renal, hepatic

46-3. Which of the following represents the most sensitive measure of low intravascular fluid status?

    A. Tachypnea

    B. Tachycardia

    C. Decreased urine output

    D. Loss of consciousness

46-4. Which of the following medications is *not* part of the initial management of acute septic shock?

    A. Glucose infusion

    B. Antibiotics

    C. Normal saline

    D. Lactated Ringer's solution

 ANSWERS

46-1. **C.** Coxsackie B virus and echovirus are enteroviruses and are the most common causes of myocarditis in North American children. Coxsackie A virus is responsible for the more common hand-foot-and-mouth disease. Adenovirus and RSV are more commonly associated with respiratory tract infections.

46-2. **A.** The coronary, cerebral, and renal vascular beds constitute the vital end organs. The hepatic vascular bed is *not* considered a vital end organ. Similarly, the skin, pancreas, and splanchnic vascular beds are also not considered vital end organs. During shock, autonomic mechanisms preferentially preserve blood flow to the brain and heart at the expense of the other organs.

46-3. **B.** Tachycardia is considered the most sensitive measure of intravascular fluid status and is thus the first presenting sign of a low fluid volume. Decreased urine output can also gradually present with hypovolemia, and a loss of consciousness can occur with prolonged hypovolemia. Tachypnea is usually not a sensitive measure of decreased fluid volume.

46-4. **A.** Glucose infusion is *not* considered a resuscitation medication for septic shock. It is important to treat septic shock with aggressive fluid boluses and the initiation of antibiotics. Soon after hemodynamic stability has been established, appropriate glucose infusions should be administered.

     SUGGESTED ADDITIONAL READING

Leonard EG. Viral myocarditis. *Pediatr Infect Dis J.* 2004;23(7): 665–666.

McKiernan CA, Lieberman SA. Circulatory Shock in Children: An Overview. *Pediatr Rev.* 2005;26:451–460.

Irritability

CC/ID: 14-month-old girl with 1-day history of irritability.

HPI: R.T. was brought in to the emergency department by her mother after she was noted this morning to be increasingly irritable. She refuses to eat or drink, and when not crying, "she is very tired, and not interacting with me as much as she normally does." She had been cruising (walking) for the last 2 to 3 weeks, but now cries when she is left to stand. She has had no fever and no other symptoms of illness. The mother was concerned about the irritability and her inability to console the infant. She tried giving the baby acetaminophen this morning, without any relief. She has brought her in for visits in the past regarding irritability and a "strange rash on her back and legs." A careful review of systems reveals no other symptoms. The mother reveals that her husband, from whom she is separated, took care of the child this past weekend until this morning. He usually takes care of the infant every weekend. By phone, he describes her as being playful this past weekend, but that she "may have climbed onto the sofa and fallen down this morning." He does not know of any rashes.

PMHx: Born at 28 weeks' gestational age; neonate intensive care unit stay for 2 months; asthma.

Meds: Albuterol as needed; inhaled corticosteroids; acetaminophen as above

All: NKDA

Immun: UTD; received RSV prophylaxis last winter

DevHx: Global mild developmental delay (babbles/coos, starting to cruise).

VS: Temp 37.1°C (98.8°F), BP 115/60, HR 150, RR 30

PE: *Gen:* alert, but uncomfortable; crying and difficult to examine; appears small for age. *HEENT:* NCAT; EOMI; tympanic membranes within normal limits; oropharynx clear. *Skin/Ext:*

refuses to move right leg or bear weight; cries upon palpation of right middle thigh, which appears swollen; multiple linear (1 cm) paired scars on buttocks and lower extremities of varying age; circular bluish discolorations on back.

THOUGHT QUESTIONS

- What currently lies in your differential diagnosis?
- What laboratory studies or evaluations and treatment are indicated for this child?

DISCUSSION

Changes in behavior warrant suspicion of any infectious causes, including meningoencephalitis. Also, seizure activity and CNS disturbances, trauma, ingestions or toxic exposures, GI disturbances (such as intussusception), and metabolic disturbances should be included. In this case, nonaccidental trauma should be strongly suspected in this child, because the clinical examination and history do not match appropriately. To evaluate this possibility, a detailed physical examination and skeletal survey (generally x-rays of the long bones, skull, spine, thorax, pelvis, and extremities) should be performed.

CASE CONTINUED

The skeletal survey reveals a spiral fracture of the right humerus and multiple old symmetric fractures of the posterior ribs. On closer examination, the infant's "rash" is suspiciously consistent with burn marks from contact with a cigarette lighter. You are further suspicious when you recall that the child is developmentally incapable of climbing onto an elevated surface and that fractures occurring before true ambulation are usually inflicted. You conclude that this child has been subjected to nonaccidental trauma and notify Child Protective Services. The infant is admitted to the hospital for further management, which includes a CT scan of the head and ophthalmologic exam (for suspicion of sequelae of shaken baby syndrome).

THOUGHT QUESTIONS

- What are the risk factors for nonaccidental trauma?
- What is your legal responsibility as a physician?

DISCUSSION

Physical abuse is unfortunately a common causes of mortality and morbidity in infants and children. Almost half of children brought in for medical attention as a result of physical abuse are younger than 1 year. Parents, male paramours, and step-parents are the most common perpetrators. Other types of abuse include sexual abuse, emotional abuse, and neglect (which actually results in more deaths than sexual and physical abuse combined). Risk factors include chronic disease or prematurity, age younger than 3 years, perception of the child as "difficult" or "abnormal," single parents, and history of abuse in the parent or caregiver.

A history which is inconsistent with injury or exam findings, delay in seeking treatment, or a pattern of unusual or unexplained injuries all warrant suspicion of physical abuse. Physical findings of burns, bruises or other injuries in specific patterns (shape of a hand or object) or locations (non-bony prominences such as buttocks, back or ears) may be suggestive of abuse. Certain types of fractures are considered suggestive of abuse as well, such as metaphyseal chip fractures of the extremities, spiral fractures of non-weight-bearing extremities, and posterior rib fractures. When sexual abuse is suspected, a thorough examination and collection of appropriate specimens is recommended, including evaluation for sexually transmitted infections (STI's). Health care workers are considered "mandated reporters," which means that they are legally required to report any reasonable suspicion of child abuse or neglect to the appropriate child protective agencies. The health care worker should also document and treat any injuries, and should order labs when indicated to rule out a medical explanation for suspicious injuries.

QUESTIONS

47-1. Which of the following conditions can be confused with nonaccidental trauma?
  A. Osteogenesis imperfecta
  B. Coagulopathies
  C. Mongolian spots
  D. Folk remedies causing bruising
  E. All of the above

47-2. Which of the following is a risk factor for a child to be abused?
  A. Age <3 years old
  B. Chronic illness or disease
  C. Foster children
  D. Low socioeconomic status
  E. All of the above

47-3. Which of the following is consistent with findings of shaken baby syndrome?
  A. Subdural hematomas
  B. Metaphyseal chip fractures
  C. Retinal hemorrhages
  D. Usually little or no evidence of external injury
  E. All of the above

47-4. You are reviewing the causes and effects of abuse with your clinical team. Which of the following statements should be included in your discussion?
  A. Failure to thrive and developmental delay can result from child abuse.
  B. Nonaccidental burns are usually superficial and in a splash-and-droplet pattern.
  C. Common bruises from childhood play usually are not on bony protuberances.
  D. Crying and toilet training are uncommon triggers for abuse.
  E. All of the above

ANSWERS

47-1. E. It is important to understand the various conditions and situations that can mimic physical abuse. Also included are insect bites, impetigo (which can mimic cigarette burns), vasculitic lesions/nevi, and conditions that can mimic or predispose to fracture (e.g., rickets, leukemia, Caffey disease).

47-2. E. All of the answers are associated with a higher risk for abuse. It should also be noted that abuse is more common in infants and toddlers, but it can occur at *any* age.

47-3. E. In children younger than 2 years, 80% of head injury deaths result from abuse. Because of the large relative size of the infant head, the pliable skull, lax ligaments, weak cervical spine, and increased plasticity of brain parenchyma, the head is more susceptible to injury from being shaken. Infants may present with profound lethargy, variable tone, posturing, shock, and irritability. Metaphyseal chip fractures result from shearing forces on the corners of long bones.

47-4. A. Failure to thrive and developmental delay can be the result of all forms of abuse. Accidental burns generally present with a splash-and-droplet pattern and are usually superficial in nature. Play usually results in bruising on bony protuberances such as the elbows and knees. Crying and toilet training are among the most common triggers for an abusive incident.

   SUGGESTED ADDITIONAL READING

Gushurst CA. Child abuse: behavioral aspects and other associated problems. *Pediatr Clin North Am.* 2003;50(4):919–938.
Johnson CF. Sexual abuse in children. *Pediatr Rev.* 2006;27:17–27.
Sirotnak AP, Grigsby T, Krugman RD. Physical abuse of children. *Pediatr Rev.* 2004;25:264–277.

CASE **48**

Confusion After a Fall

CC/ID: 14-year-old boy with confusion and vomiting.

HPI: E.H. is brought in by his parents and a friend for increasing confusion and episode of vomiting after a skateboarding accident in which he fell and hit his head. He was not wearing a helmet at the time, and remembers falling backward off a staircase railing and hitting the left side of his head. The friend claims that he was briefly unconscious, but awoke seconds later. In the hour following the accident, he has been more "confused," according to his parents, has vomited once, and complains of a "major headache."

PMHx: History of asthma and eczema.

Meds: None

All: None

FHx: Maternal grandfather with stroke. Paternal grandmother with Alzheimer disease.

THOUGHT QUESTIONS

- What further history would you elicit at this point?
- What is your differential diagnosis?

DISCUSSION

The history given by the parents and patient in this case seem consistent, but ideally the source of injury should be described by the child and caretaker separately (inconsistencies should raise suspicions of abuse). An accurate account of the mechanism of injury and the immediate events following are important. Loss of consciousness should be elucidated, as well as amnesia, seizures, and visual impairment. Any changes in mental status (including confusion, inappropriate words, and changes in orientation) should be noted. Vomiting, headache, and changes in mental status suggest increased intracranial pressure. As with any painful symptom, the specific components of the headache should be further described.

The differential diagnosis for confused states and vomiting should include trauma and abuse, causes of encephalopathy and encephalitis, meningitis, toxic ingestion, and vascular anomalies leading to hemorrhage. Intracranial masses should be associated with insidious progress of symptoms. In most cases, a thorough history will narrow this list to the appropriate diagnosis and course of action. Evaluation of the child with suspected head trauma starts with the ABCs (airway, breathing, circulation), a brief but thorough history, and subsequent physical examination and secondary survey.

 ## CASE CONTINUED

Upon further questioning, the patient and parents deny any seizure activity and claim that the headache is mostly concentrated at the site of the injury. His family has no history of epilepsy or neurologic problems. He has been otherwise well and without any complaints, except some pain at his left wrist. He denies any toxic exposures or habits.

VS: Temp 37.2°C (99°F), BP 110/70, HR 80, RR 24

PE: *Gen:* supine; sleepy but responsive; alert and oriented to name and place. *HEENT:* laceration behind left ear lobe; tenderness on occiput and left mastoid, with posterior auricular bruising on left side. No CSF rhinorrhea or otorrhea. PERRL/EOMI. *Neck:* supple; full range of motion. *Abdomen:* soft, nondistended/nontender; no visceromegaly; positive bowel sounds. *Back:* spine straight; no bruises. *Skin/Ext:* palpable pain at left wrist; decreased ability to extend wrist; anatomical snuffbox tenderness. *Neuro:* CN 2–12 grossly intact. He has mild bilateral lateral visual field deficits; deep tendon reflex and strength response are normal; he seems confused as to what time of day it is, and asks "whether or not you've seen my chicken." He becomes more combative during your exam and cannot recall his parents' names or do any complex functions (serial 7s). His gait is unsteady, and he seems to veer left.

THOUGHT QUESTION

- What further laboratory studies or evaluations and treatment would you perform on this patient at this point?

CASE CONTINUED

Because of this patient's confusion and clinical exam, a CT scan of his head and cervical spine is performed, which reveals a left basilar skull fracture and an epidural hematoma. Neurosurgical assistance is sought immediately. Incidentally, he also suffered a left navicular bone fracture in his wrist, further highlighting the importance of a full-body examination and secondary survey.

DISCUSSION

Hemorrhage occurring after trauma is usually epidural or subdural rather than intraparenchymal. Physical signs and clinical evidence can suggest the diagnosis, but a CT scan of the head is the imaging choice for an expeditious therapeutic course. Intracranial pressure (ICP) reduction and monitoring may often be required for the patient with cerebral edema. A concussion is defined as a brief loss of consciousness after head injury, associated with anterograde or retrograde amnesia, without apparent brain injury. Minor head trauma is a common complaint in children, and does not always require imaging. Imaging or observation should be considered in the very young child and those with prolonged loss of consciousness or abnormal neurologic findings.

QUESTIONS

48-1. The primary determinant of neurologic outcome in head trauma is
- A. Size of the hematoma
- B. Associated seizure activity
- C. Length of associated unconsciousness
- D. Mechanical force of the injury
- E. Location of initial impact

48-2. You are reviewing the evaluation and initial management of a 6 year-old patient with an intracranial bleed sustained in an automobile accident with your clinical team. Which of the following statements is appropriate to include in your discussion?
  A. Cranial nerve function rarely helps to localize the injury.
  B. Vomiting, headache, and mental status changes are suggestive of increased ICP.
  C. Cerebral edema is a rare complication.
  D. Cervical collar application is usually unnecessary.
  E. Children with head trauma have a poor prognosis in comparison with adults.

48-3. Which of the following is characteristic of a *subdural* bleed?
  A. Appears as a biconcave lesion on CT scan
  B. Associated with rupture of middle meningeal artery
  C. Presence of a hematoma between the dura and arachnoid layers
  D. Can be classically associated with a "lucid interval"
  E. CSF rhinorrhea is the hallmark finding.

48-4. Which of the following is an acceptable method to manage a patient with increased ICP from traumatic brain injury?
  A. Sustained hyperventilation
  B. Corticosteroids
  C. Mannitol
  D. Fluid restriction to keep blood pressure low
  E. Glucose infusion

ANSWERS

48-1. C. The primary determinant of neurologic outcome is the length of unconsciousness.

48-2. B. Because of the uncertainty of possible cervical spine injuries, upon initial evaluation in the field a cervical stabilization collar should *always* be placed. Cranial nerve abnormalities, particularly papillary findings and extraocular movements, can help localize injury and suggest elevated ICP or herniation. Appropriate clinical monitoring for seizures and cerebral edema can help alert the clinician of these relatively common sequelae of head trauma. Children with head trauma tend to have better outcomes than adults.

48-3. C. Subdural bleeds usually appear as crescentic bleeds on CT scan (Fig. 48-1; Table 48-1). Subdural bleeds are usually associated

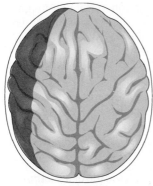 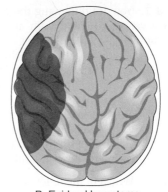

A. Subdural hematoma   B. Epidural hematoma

FIGURE 48-1. Imaging findings for subdural and epidural bleeds. **A:** Subdural hematoma. **B:** Epidural hematoma. Note the crescentic mass associated with subdural bleed versus the biconcave-shaped mass associated with epidural bleed. (*Illustration by Electronic Illustrators Group.*)

TABLE 48-1 Differentiating Acute Subdural and Epidural Bleeds

	Subdural	Epidural
Location	Between the dura and arachnoid layers	Between the skull and the dura
Symmetry	Usually bilateral	Usually unilateral
Etiology	Rupture of bridging cortical veins	Rupture of middle meningeal artery or dural veins
Typical injury	Direct trauma or shaking	Direct trauma in the temporal area
Consciousness	Intact but altered	Impaired–lucid–impaired
Common associated findings	Seizures, retinal hemorrhages	Ipsilateral pupillary dilatation, papilledema, contralateral hemiparesis
Appearance on CT with contrast	Crescentic	Biconcave
Prognosis	High morbidity; low mortality	High mortality; low morbidity
Complications	Herniation	Skull fracture; uncal herniation

From Marino B, Snead K, McMillan J. *Blueprints in Pediatrics.* 2nd ed. Malden, MA: Blackwell Science; 2001:235, with permission.

with rupture of bridging cortical veins. Epidural bleeds generally occur between the skull and dura. CSF rhinorrhea is not the hallmark of subdural hematomas. Subdural bleeds generally are associated with intact but altered mental status. (Note: association of impaired mental status followed by a lucid interval and subsequent impairment is not as common in pediatrics as in the adult population.)

48-4. C. The only acceptable method of those listed is mannitol. Hyperventilation can be used for acute herniation, but should not be sustained. Corticosteroids are not indicated in managing intracranial pressure from traumatic brain injury. Hypotension is associated with poor outcomes, so fluids should not be restricted below the rate required to maintain adequate blood pressure. In fact, higher than normal blood pressures may be necessary in order to ensure adequate cerebral perfusion pressure in patients with high ICP. Glucose administration is contraindicated, as it is associated with poor outcomes.

 SUGGESTED ADDITIONAL READING

Coombs JB, Davis RL. A synopsis of the American Academy of Pediatrics' practice parameter on the management of minor closed head injury in children. *Pediatr Rev.* 2000;21:413–415.

Dias MS. Traumatic brain and spinal cord injury. *Pediatr Clin North Am.* 2004;51(2):271–303.

Gedeit R. Head injury. *Pediatr Rev.* 2001;22:118–124.

Thiessen ML. Pediatric minor closed head injury. *Pediatr Clin North Am.* 2006;53(1):1–26, v.

Erratic Behavior

CC/ID: 12-year-old girl with erratic behavior.

HPI: T.I. is brought into the emergency department by her mother this evening after erratic behavior over the last 2 to 3 days. Her mother states that she has been intermittently tearful, angry, and occasionally confused, muttering to herself repeatedly. Yesterday, she had vomiting (nonbloody and nonbilious), malaise, and no appetite, which all seem to have improved somewhat. There has been no fever, no diarrhea, no ill contacts, and no recent travel or new foods. Her mother says that she has been silent all evening and becomes excessively angry when approached.

PMHx: Noncontributory

PSHx: None

Meds: None

All: NKDA

VS: Temp 37.1°C (98.8°F), BP 110/65, HR 90, RR 22

PE: *Gen:* quiet, reluctant, but alert and oriented ×3. *HEENT:* NCAT; EOMI; PERRL. *Neck:* supple. *Lungs:* normal exam. *CV:* normal exam. *Abdomen:* soft; right upper quadrant and epigastric tenderness, with liver edge palpable 3 cm below costal margin; positive bowel sounds; no other masses. *Rectal:* exam normal. *Back/Ext:* mild back pain; otherwise normal. *ROS:* no dysuria; no headache; no weight loss.

THOUGHT QUESTIONS

- What is in your differential diagnosis?
- What elements of the history are helpful toward making a diagnosis?
- What diagnostic tests may aid in your diagnosis?

DISCUSSION

The differential diagnosis for this patient includes food poisoning, gastroenteritis, gallstone disease, hepatitis, Epstein-Barr infection, gastritis and peptic ulcer disease, and toxic ingestions. For the patient with erratic behavior or with altered mental status, a thorough history should include an attempt to identify any substance ingested and the specific nature of the ingestion (when? how much? types of substances?) and the subsequent behaviors. This can often be a challenge in the unwitnessed event for a toddler, or in the case of an adolescent. It is helpful to obtain a detailed social history, including details of the home environment, school, stressors and sexual activity, and toxic exposures as well as history of any trauma. In the patient with altered mental status or behavioral changes, initial screening evaluation may include an fingerstick glucose pulse oximetry, ECG, serum electrolytes and osmolarity, and determination of serum pH. Toxicology screens can also be helpful. In patients such as the one in this case, other directed laboratory tests that may be helpful are a CBC, urine pregnancy test, urinalysis, liver function tests, and pancreatic enzyme tests.

 CASE CONTINUED

Upon further questioning, her mother says her menarche was nearly 2 years ago and she has normal cycles. In the emergency department, you order a CBC and urinalysis, which are normal, and a pregnancy test, which is negative. Her liver enzymes are greatly elevated (ALT 2,100), and her prothrombin time (PT) is mildly elevated at 13.9. A urine toxicology screen for opiates, amphetamines, LSD, and marijuana is negative. Serum levels for aspirin and acetaminophen are undetected. A CT scan of the abdomen is done and is normal. She is still quite angry and tearful and now becomes combative. As you try to calm her down, she reveals that she is scared for herself for "what she did" but that her mother "deserves it!" Further questioning reveals that her parents have decided to file for divorce, and the patient subsequently admits to ingesting 15 extra-strength acetaminophen tablets nearly 2.5 days ago. She is admitted, treated, and evaluated by psychiatry for follow-up.

DISCUSSION

Acute ingestions are challenging, but should be suspected in any patient with altered mental status, acute behavioral changes, seizures, arrhythmias, and coma. Most cases occur in children <5, but fatalities are rare in this age group. Adolescents account for the majority of fatalities, mostly from intentional ingestion in attempted suicide. It is important to note that multiple substances may be involved. Acetaminophen is a commonly ingested substance, and generally affects the liver via toxic by-products during metabolism via the cytochrome P450 system, resulting in necrosis and damage. Acetaminophen toxicity initially clinically manifests with vomiting/nausea, anorexia, and pallor. This may progress over days to abdominal pain and back pain, and subsequently to signs and symptoms of liver dysfunction. Acetaminophen levels in plasma, particularly noted within 24 hours of a known single-dose ingestion, can be used to extrapolate hepatic toxicity. In many cases, levels may be undetected due to the length of time elapsed since the ingestion. In most cases, prognosis is excellent with the appropriate treatment.

QUESTIONS

49-1. Which of the following reflects a metabolic disturbance seen with salicylate ingestion?
- A. Normal anion gap metabolic acidosis with respiratory acidosis
- B. Normal anion gap metabolic acidosis with respiratory acidosis
- C. High anion gap metabolic acidosis with respiratory acidosis
- D. High anion gap metabolic acidosis with respiratory alkalosis
- E. Normal anion gap metabolic alkalosis with respiratory alkalosis

49-2. Which substance is properly matched with its antidote?
- A. Acetaminophen: calcium gluconate
- B. Opiates: flumazenil
- C. Iron: activated charcoal
- D. Diazepam: naloxone
- E. Carbon monoxide: hyperbaric oxygen

49-3. Which of the following is most likely to be effective in managing an acute ingestion of iron?
   A. Syrup of ipecac after waiting 1 hour
   B. Rumack nomogram analysis
   C. Gastric lavage
   D. Activated charcoal
   E. Pyridoxine

49-4. You are counseling a family on the preventive and clinical aspects of poisoning. Which of the following statements is appropriate to include in your discussion?
   A. Aspirated hydrocarbons pose little threat to lung tissue.
   B. Moist mucous membranes, increased sweating, and bradycardia are found in anticholinergic ingestion.
   C. Mydriasis, tachycardia, and elevated blood pressure are found in sympathomimetic ingestion.
   D. Activated charcoal can be used for alcohol ingestions.
   E. Mydriasis, tachycardia, and elevated blood pressure are found in cholinergic ingestion.

 ANSWERS

49-1. D. Salicylates remain an important cause of pediatric poisoning and can cause a high anion gap metabolic acidosis with a compensatory respiratory alkalosis. A common mnemonic used to remember the causes of a metabolic acidosis with anion gap is MUDPILES (Methanol, Uremia, DKA, Paraldehyde, INH/iron, Lactic acidosis, Ethanol and ethylene glycol, Salicylate).

49-2. D. Commonly ingested substances have specific antidotes that may aid in the treatment. Diazepam and other benzodiazepines can be treated with flumazenil. Acetaminophen poisoning may be treated with N-acetylcysteine. Opiate poisoning can be treated with naloxone. Iron ingestions and poisoning may be treated with deferoxamine. Carbon monoxide poisoning is traditionally treated with hyperbaric oxygen.

49-3. C. For acute ingestions, assessment of ABCs and hemodynamic stability should occur first. Although ABCs should always be assessed first, the next sequence of treatments is generally determined by the nature and timing of the poisoning. Activated charcoal is an excellent way to bind toxins and minimize their absorption. Its use is ineffective, however, in ingestions of heavy metals (iron, lead, lithium) and is contraindicated in caustic or hydrocarbon ingestion.

TABLE 49-1 Signs, Symptoms, and Treatment of Specific Pediatric Poisonings

Substance	Clinical Manifestations	Antidote/Treatment
Acetaminophen	Nausea/vomiting, anorexia, pallor, diaphoresis; may progress over days to jaundice, abdominal pain, liver failure	**A:** N-acetylcysteine **T:** Gastric emptying if <2 hours since ingestion; activated charcoal if <4 hours since ingestion. Draw blood level at 4 hours and use available nomogram to assess risk of hepatotoxicity. If toxic, start oral N-acetylcysteine and continue for 72 hours.
Anticholinergics (atropine, tricyclic antidepressants, antihistamines, phenothiazides)	Fever, mydriasis, flushing, dry skin, tachycardia, hypertension, cardiac arrhythmias, delirium, psychosis, convulsion, coma	**A:** Physostigmine for atropine and antihistamines **T:** $NaCO_2$, $MgSO_4$ for tricyclic antidepressants
Cholinergics (organophosphates and other pesticides)	Nausea/vomiting, sweating, meiosis, salivation, lacrimation, bronchorrhea, urination, defecation, weakness, muscle fasciculation, paralysis, confusion, coma	**A:** Pralidoxime chloride **T:** Gastric lavage, activated charcoal; prophylactic atropine
Opiates	Pinpoint pupils, bradypnea, hypotension, hypothermia, stupor, coma	**A:** Naloxone **T:** Evaluate and secure airway as needed; gastrointestinal decontamination if appropriate; naloxone
Sedatives/hypnotics	Nystagmus, meiosis or mydriasis, hypothermia, hypotension, bradypnea, confusion, ataxia, coma	**A:** Flumazenil for benzodiazepines **T:** Evaluate and secure airway if needed; maintain hemodynamic stability; activated charcoal with cathartic; supportive care

Modified from Marino B, Snead K, McMillan J. *Blueprints in Pediatrics*. 2nd ed. Malden, MA: Blackwell Science; 2001:7, with permission.

Induction of emesis with ipecac syrup is no longer recommended routinely. Gastric lavage can be used in cases of acute ingestion, may help to remove and dilute stomach contents, and can be effective especially if used within the first hour of ingestion. Pyridoxine is a helpful antidote in isoniazid poisoning, and Rumack nomogram analysis is helpful in acetaminophen poisoning to predict hepatic toxicity. Poison Control hotlines are an extremely valuable resource and should be rapidly accessed by caregivers and health care providers in these situations.

49-4. C. Mydriasis, tachycardia, and hypertension are usually characteristics of sympathomimetic substances. Cholinergic substances generally are associated with other symptoms, such as meiosis, salivation, and lacrimation. Anticholinergic ingestions are characterized by dry mucous membranes, decreased sweating, dilated pupils, and tachycardia (Table 49-1). Hydrocarbons in the lung trigger a profound inflammatory reaction and can result in a chemical pneumonitis. Preventing aspiration is the primary goal in hydrocarbon ingestion. Oral activated charcoal is a safe and effective treatment for most pediatric ingestions; exceptions include alcohol, hydrocarbons, heavy metals and lithium.

 SUGGESTED ADDITIONAL READING

Bryant S. Management of toxic exposure in children. Emerg Med Clin North Am. 2003;21(1):101–119.
McGuigan ME. Poisoning potpourri. *Pediatr Rev.* 2001;22:295–302.

CASE **50**

Refusing to Go to School

CC/ID: 10-year-old boy who refuses to go to school.

HPI: A.J. has just started fifth grade and says he "hates school." His parents are concerned because he has already failed two tests this year. A.J.'s teacher recently had a meeting with his parents to discuss his poor performance and "behavior issues," which include temper tantrums in the classroom and refusal to participate in class. She even mentioned that he might benefit from medication to "help him concentrate." A.J.'s dad made the appointment because he wants to make sure "everything is OK, medically." A.J. had previously done well in school, and his parents are getting worried because he seems more withdrawn and now is angry about going to school.

PMHx: No significant illnesses or hospitalizations.

SHx: Lives with parents and 6-year-old sister. Dad is an accountant; Mom is an attorney.

FHx: No illnesses in the family.

Meds: None

All: None known

Immun: UTD

THOUGHT QUESTIONS

- What are some possible causes of school failure in a child this age?
- What additional information would you like to gather to help guide your evaluation?

DISCUSSION

School is an important stage for the performance and evaluation of the developmental tasks of late childhood. One way to organize causes of school failure is to divide them into those that are intrinsic or extrinsic to the patient. Intrinsic causes include learning disabilities, attention deficit hyperactivity disorder (ADHD), mental retardation, sensory impairment (hearing and vision), seizure disorders, emotional illness, chronic illness, and temperamental dysfunction. Extrinsic causes include family dysfunction, stress and social problems (including drug use), cultural or family expectations, and ineffective schooling.

Further history should be targeted toward further characterizing the nature of the school disfunction and ruling out treatable medical causes. Medical illnesses that can affect learning include chronic disease, seizures, lead poisoning, anemia, and sensory impairment. Additional history should include patterns of development and behavior, areas of school difficulty, and the child's perspective on what is going on. The physical exam should be complete enough to identify or exclude medical conditions that may explain poor school performance, and should include hearing and vision screening.

 ## CASE CONTINUED

A.J.'s father reports that there were no significant delays in A.J.'s early motor, cognitive, or social development. On further questioning, he notes that A.J.'s grades over the last year have shown a steady decline in performance. However, he is proud to point out that A.J. still gets A's in math, "just like Dad." At home he has not been acting out the way his teacher was describing in the classroom. In fact, he spends most of his time in his room, working on his homework or playing math games on the computer. You speak with A.J. alone and he denies symptoms of depression, feeling ill, use of drugs, or difficulty seeing or hearing. He is frustrated by his bad grades, and often gets angry in class when the teacher singles him out to read out loud. "She makes me feel dumb," he says. "And I feel like my parents are disappointed in me."

Hearing/
vision screen: Normal for age.

VS: Temp 36.7°C (98°F), HR 106, RR 24; Weight 32 kg (25%), height 138 cm (50%)

PE: *Gen:* healthy-appearing, slender young man in no apparent distress. *HEENT:* moist mucous membranes; normal oropharynx; supple neck; no lymphadenopathy; TMs normal bilaterally. *GU:* Tanner 0 (prepubertal) with normal external genitalia. *Neuro:* strength 5/5 upper and lower extremities; CN 2–12 intact; sensation equal to your exam; DTRs in upper and lower extremities 2+. *Skin:* no rashes or pigmented lesions.

THOUGHT QUESTIONS

- What intrinsic and/or extrinsic factors do you think are contributing to A.J.'s recent trouble in school?
- What would you recommend to his family at this point?

DISCUSSION

A.J. may have several factors contributing to his school failure. Since his performance is math is relatively unaffected, his difficulties seem to be isolated to subjects requiring reading. This is classic for children with dyslexia, a learning disability specific to reading and recognizing the written word. Also consistent with dyslexia is A.J.'s need to spend a long time on homework assignments, and the fact that his cognitive development and function is otherwise normal. Dyslexia often first becomes apparent in later elementary school, when reading and writing become an important factor in most school activities. Although A.J. denies feeling depressed, his behavior indicates that he is being emotionally affected by his trouble in school. At home, he is withdrawn and quiet, whereas at school his frustration manifests as anger and disruptive behavior. Other social factors include pressure to meet his parents' expectations, and a disruptive relationship with his teacher.

At this point, A.J. would most likely benefit from a learning assessment by his school. Schools are required to perform a learning assessment at a parent's request, and to provide the necessary services to address a student's learning needs. Children with dyslexia may benefit from learning reading skills and being given more time to complete assignments and tests.

QUESTIONS

50-1. A.J.'s father wants to know if A.J. has ADHD, which he has heard about from friends. In order to meet the current diagnostic criteria for this disorder, A.J would need to meet each of the following criteria: (1) at least six clinically significant symptoms of inattention *or* of hyperactivity/impulsivity for 6 months, (2) significant impairment in social, academic, or occupational functioning, and (3) some of these symptoms being present before age 7, as well as which of the following?

    A. A family history of ADHD
    B. Impaired functioning in two or more social settings
    C. Self-injury from impulsive behavior
    D. Response to stimulant medication

50-2. After further investigation, A.J. is diagnosed with dyslexia. His father wants to know if this could have anything to do with his own reading difficulty as a child. You can answer him that

    A. Dyslexia is a spontaneous disorder, without familial heredity.
    B. Dyslexia is usually related to early perinatal brain damage, and is therefore not heritable.
    C. Dyslexia is heritable, but only 5% to 10% of patients have a family history of reading difficulty.
    D. Dyslexia is heritable, with about 50% of patients having a family history of reading difficulty.

50-3. A.J.'s mother wants to know how to fix this problem so that her son can live up to his potential. You can answer her that

    A. Medications such as those used to treat ADHD can also be effective in children with dyslexia.
    B. Dyslexia tends to get worse over time, and A.J. will likely develop other learning difficulties in the future.
    C. Children with dyslexia can be taught ways to compensate for their impairment, but the condition is usually persistent.
    D. Dyslexia tends to resolve over time, and most patients outgrow it by early adulthood.

50-4. What is the most common cause of school failure in the pediatric population?

    A. Seizure disorder
    B. Neurodevelopmental disorder (learning disability or ADHD)
    C. Mental retardation
    D. Hearing impairment

ANSWERS

50-1. B. The current guidelines for diagnosis for ADHD include the following criteria: (1) at least six symptoms of inattention *or* six symptoms of hyperactivity/impulsivity are present and have been persistent for 6 months, (2) some of the symptoms were present before 7 years of age, (3) impairment from the symptoms is present in more than one setting, and (4) impairment is clinically significant in social, academic, or occupational functioning.

Attention deficit hyperactivity disorder is one of the most commonly diagnosed neurobehavioral disorders of childhood. The estimated prevalence of ADHD in school-aged children is 3% to 9%, and the disorder is diagnosed about three times as often in boys as in girls. Among school-aged children with ADHD, girls are more likely to have the predominantly inattentive subtype. The main focus of treatment of ADHD is to maximize function. First-line treatment includes stimulant medications (methylphenidate or dextroamphetamine), which have been shown to have short-term efficacy in improving symptoms and behaviors in most children. Behavior therapy may be helpful for some children.

50-2. D. Family history is one of the most important risk factors for dyslexia. There is an approximately 50% chance of dyslexia in the parent, child, or sibling of a patient with dyslexia. Dyslexia is the most common learning disability in children, occurring in about 80% of children diagnosed with a learning disability. Although initially thought to be more common in males, more recent studies report similar prevalence in males and females. The etiology of dyslexia is unclear; however, functional brain imaging in dyslexic readers shows decreased activity in the posterior left hemisphere and increased activity in frontal regions in comparison with nondyslexic subjects.

50-3. C. Dyslexia is generally a persistent, chronic condition, with most dyslexic individuals experiencing lifelong difficulty with reading. Typically students are able to function well in school with the use of accommodation strategies, such as longer times to complete assignments or tests. There is no good evidence that early intervention or treatment can "cure" the problem. However, new intensive approaches that provide systematic instruction in phonemic awareness, phonics, fluency, vocabulary, and comprehension strategies have shown promise for some children.

50-4. B. Neurodevelopmental dysfunction is the most common cause of school failure in children. The two most common neurodevelopmental disorders of childhood are learning disabilities and ADHD. Learning disabilities are the most common cause of school failure in the general population, with an estimated prevalence of 7% to 10%. Emotional disturbance and ADHD are the two next most common causes. The estimated prevalences of some intrinsic causes of school failure in the general population are as follows: learning disabilities, 7% to 10%; emotional disturbance, 5% to 10%; ADHD, 3% to 9%; chronic illness, 5%; and mental retardation, 2% to 3%.

 ## SUGGESTED ADDITIONAL READING

Byrd RS. School failure: assessment, intervention, and prevention in primary pediatric care. *Pediatr Rev.* 2005;26(7):227–237.

Committee on Quality Improvement and Subcommittee on Attention-Deficit/Hyperactivity Disorder. Clinical practice guideline: diagnosis and evaluation of the child with attention-deficit/hyperactivity disorder. *Pediatrics.* 2000;105:1158–1170.

Phillips DM, Longlett SK, Mulrine C, et al. School problems and the family physician. *Am Fam Physician.* 1999;59(10):2816–2824.

IX

Cases Presenting with Abnormal Growth

CASE **51**

Teen with Poor Appetite

CC/ID: J.D. is a 15-year-old girl brought in by her mother for "looking thin."

HPI: J.D. says everything's fine, and she feels great, but her mother thinks she is wasting away: "A few months ago she was a beautiful girl, now look at her," she says. Mom states that the patient hardly eats anything, and seems "depressed." She is worried that she may be on drugs or have cancer. The patient replies that she just isn't hungry for dinner when she gets home from track practice, and that mom's cooking is "greasy," so "I eat with my friends." She denies fevers, abdominal pain, diarrhea, vomiting, or headache, but has been mildly constipated. She weighed 110 lb (50 kg) at her last doctor's visit 9 months ago.

PMHx: No hospitalizations or surgeries.

Meds: None

All: NKDA

Immun: UTD for age

SHx: Sophomore in high school; straight-A student. Runs cross-country for the track team. Parents are lawyers, recently divorced; 10-year-old brother is healthy, but having school trouble.

VS: Temp 36.0°C (96.8°F), BP 105/70, HR 52 (normal 60–80), RR 14; Weight 42.5 kg (7%), height 165 cm (70%)

PE: *Gen:* a polite, cooperative, and very thin young lady wearing baggy sweats. *HEENT:* no lymphadenopathy; oropharynx normal. Hair is thin and brittle. Mucous membranes slightly pale. *CV:* bradycardia; regular rhythm; no murmurs. *Lungs:* clear. *Abdomen:* soft, flat, with normal bowel sounds; no masses. *Skin:* cool and dry; no rashes or bruising. Fine, downy hair noted on abdomen. *GU:* Tanner 4 female, normal external genitalia.

THOUGHT QUESTIONS

- ■ What types of illnesses are you concerned about in this patient?
- ■ What further history would you like to obtain?

DISCUSSION

Causes of weight loss in teenagers can be considered in two broad categories: organic and nonorganic. Organic causes include chronic infection (e.g., TB, HIV, EBV), malignancy (e.g., leukemia, lymphoma, CNS, and bone tumors), endocrine disturbance (e.g., hyperthyroidism, diabetes mellitus, adrenal or pituitary insufficiency), and GI disease (e.g., inflammatory bowel disease, malabsorption). Nonorganic causes include drug use, depression, and eating disorders such as anorexia nervosa and bulimia nervosa.

Although organic causes must be considered, the patient does not have evidence of chronic illness or infection on initial history or physical exam. The next step would be to interview her confidentially to confirm the history and obtain information on dieting behavior, sexual activity, drug use, and any social stressors that may be contributing to her weight loss.

CASE CONTINUED

You ask J.D.'s mom to step out of the room and ask J.D. what she thinks about her mom's concerns. She agrees she may have "lost a little weight," but says "I'm just getting healthy." She tells you that she became a vegetarian and stopped eating fat several months ago because her friends were doing the same thing. She feels like "the biggest girl on the track team" and still needs to lose some weight, but it has become much harder now. She admits that she feels exhausted and cold all the time, and is having trouble sleeping. She blacked out in the shower last week, and didn't tell her mother. J.D. denies sexual activity or drug use, and has not been using vomiting or laxatives to control her weight. Her last normal period was over 5 months ago.

THOUGHT QUESTION

- What is the most likely diagnosis, and how will you manage this patient?

DISCUSSION

Based on the history and physical findings, you can make a likely diagnosis of anorexia nervosa (AN), the third most common chronic condition of childhood after asthma and obesity. AN is a psychiatric disorder characterized by an intense fear of becoming obese, disturbance in perception of one's body shape or size, the absence of at least three consecutive menstrual cycles in postmenarchal females, and refusal to maintain body weight above the 15th percentile for age and height. Other common findings include excessive physical activity, preoccupation with food, and sleep and mood disturbances. Mortality is approximately 5% to 10%.

Treatment is aimed at restoring nutritional balance to achieve weight gain and restore menstruation, correcting physiologic abnormalities, and addressing the underlying psychiatric disturbance. The most important determinants of short- and intermediate-term outcome are medical and nutritional stabilization; individual and family therapy are crucial for good long-term prognosis. Psychotropic medications have a limited role in the pediatric population, but may be helpful for some patients. Criteria for admission include electrolyte imbalance, abnormal vital signs (hypothermia, hypotension), or cardiac rhythm disturbances. Most treatment programs combine behavior modification and psychotherapy with medical and nutritional support. Success of treatment is moderate, estimated at 50% to 70%.

QUESTIONS

51-1. What is the most common cause of death from anorexia nervosa?
- A. Cardiac arrest
- B. Electrolyte imbalance
- C. Infection
- D. Suicide

51-2. By diagnostic criteria, anorexia nervosa can be differentiated from bulimia nervosa by the presence of
    A. Extreme weight loss or refusal to maintain minimum body weight
    B. Excessive exercise in order to control weight
    C. Episodes of binge eating
    D. Distortion of body image

51-3. An attending physician asks you if this patient exhibits the characteristics of the female athlete triad, which refers to typical findings in female athletes with eating disorders. This triad is composed of
    A. Anorexia, amenorrhea, and osteoporosis
    B. Anorexia, sport-related injuries, and low self-esteem
    C. Anorexia, hair loss, and vomiting to control weight
    D. Anorexia, decreased muscle mass, and use of laxatives

51-4. A friend with a teenage daughter asks you about her daughter's risk of developing bulimia or anorexia. What is the best answer regarding the prevalence of these two eating disorders in the population?
    A. They are equally prevalent, but anorexia is more common in women.
    B. Anorexia is five times as common as bulimia.
    C. Bulimia is five times as common as anorexia.
    D. They are equally prevalent, but bulimia is more common in women.

 ANSWERS

51-1. D. The most common cause of death from anorexia nervosa is suicide, followed by death from the cardiac complications of starvation, refeeding, or electrolyte imbalance.

51-2. A. One of the most helpful criteria to differentiate anorexia nervosa from bulimia nervosa is the presence of extreme weight loss or refusal to obtain or maintain minimum body weight (Table 51-1). Weight loss is *not* part of the diagnostic criteria for bulimia nervosa. Intense fear of gaining weight and amenorrhea are other criteria for anorexia nervosa that are not characteristic of bulimia nervosa. Both disorders are characterized by body image distortion, and extreme exercise is common in both as well. Although binge eating and purging behavior are part of the criteria for bulimia nervosa, they may also be present in patients with the binge/purge type of anorexia nervosa.

TABLE 51-1   Diagnostic Criteria for Eating Disorders

Anorexia Nervosa	Bulimia Nervosa
1. Intense fear of becoming fat or gaining weight, even though underweight.	1. Recurrent episodes of binge eating, characterized by:
2. Refusal to maintain body weight at or above a minimally normal weight for age and height (i.e., weight loss leading to maintenance of body weight <85% of expected, or failure to make expected weight gain during period of growth, leading to body weight <85% of that expected).	a. Eating a substantially larger amount of food in a discrete period of time than would be eaten by most people in similar circumstances during that same time period.
	b. A sense of lack of control over eating during the binge.
	2. Recurrent inappropriate compensatory behavior to prevent weight gain (i.e., self-induced vomiting, use of laxatives, diuretics, fasting, or hyperexercising).
3. Disturbed body image, undue influence of shape or weight on self-evaluation, or denial of the seriousness of the current low body weight.	3. Binges or inappropriate compensatory behaviors occurring, on average, at least twice weekly for at least 3 months.
	4. Self-evaluation unduly influenced by body shape or weight.
4. Amenorrhea, or absence of at least three consecutive menstrual cycles.	5. The disturbance does not occur exclusively during episodes of anorexia nervosa.
Types	**Types**
Restricting: no regular bingeing or purging (self-induced vomiting or use of laxatives and diuretics).	*Purging:* regularly engages in self-induced vomiting or use of laxatives or diuretics.
Binge eating/purging: regular bingeing and purging in a patient who also meets the above criteria for anorexia nervosa.	*Nonpurging:* uses other inappropriate compensatory behaviors (i.e., fasting or hyperexercising), without regular use of vomiting or medications to purge.

From American Psychiatric Association. *Diagnostic and Statistical Manual of Mental Disorders.* 4th ed. Washington, DC: American Psychiatric Association; 1994, with permission.

51-3. A. The female athlete triad comprises anorexia, amenorrhea, and osteoporosis. Amenorrhea is thought to be due to a combination of weight loss and hypothalamic-pituitary disturbances. The average weight at which menstruation is restored is at 90% of ideal body weight, but amenorrhea persists in 25% of patients after restoration of healthy weight. Bone density studies are recommended in all anorexic females because of the high likelihood of osteoporosis. Osteoporosis is usually reversible with nutrition. Although sports-related injuries, hair loss, and decreased muscle mass are common in malnourished female athletes, they are not part of the female athlete triad. Vomiting and use of laxatives may be present in patients with the binge/purge type of anorexia, but these findings are more common in patients with bulimia.

51-4. C. Bulimia nervosa is approximately five times as common as anorexia nervosa, which occurs in about 1% of females aged 14 to 18 years. Both disorders are more common in females, with males representing 5% to 10% of those affected. The incidence of eating disorders has been steadily increasing in the last 20 years, and is greatest among high-risk groups such as college students, gymnasts and other athletes, and those with a history of sexual abuse. Although previously reported primarily in the middle and upper socioeconomic groups, anorexia is now recognized to occur in all socioeconomic and racial/ethnic groups.

 SUGGESTED ADDITIONAL READING

American Academy of Pediatrics, Committee on Adolescence. Identifying and treating eating disorders. *Pediatrics*. 2003;111: 204–211.

Fisher M. Treatment of eating disorders in children, adolescents, and young adults. *Pediatrics Rev*. 2006;27:5–16.

Misra M, et al. Effects of anorexia nervosa on clinical, hematologic, biochemical, and bone density parameters in community-dwelling adolescent girls. *Pediatrics*. 2004;114(6):1574–1583.

Weight Loss and Pallor

CC/ID: $3^1/_2$-year-old boy is brought in by his mother for poor appetite and pallor.

HPI: G.G. had been healthy until 3 to 4 weeks ago, when he developed a fever, cough, and fatigue. At that time, his mother was told by the doctor that he had a virus, but she now reports that he has "never really recovered." The cough has resolved, but he has continued to have low-grade fevers, is sleeping more than usual, and "hardly eats at all." His mother thinks he looks thin and pale, and she has noticed dark circles under his eyes. He has not had vomiting, diarrhea, abdominal pain, or runny nose. He does not have any rashes, but Mom thinks he has "tons of bruises." His weight at his last visit 3 weeks ago was 35 lb (16 kg).

PMHx: None

Meds: None

SHx: Parents are divorced; patient lives with mother. Two older brothers are healthy.

VS: Temp 38.1°C (100.5°F), BP 95/72, HR 105, RR 22; Weight 13.5 kg (25%)

PE: *Gen:* thin, tired-appearing, pale boy sitting in mother's lap. *HEENT:* mucous membranes are pale but moist, with pinpoint purple macules scattered on the buccal mucosa. TMs and oropharynx clear; no nuchal rigidity. Nontender anterior and posterior lymphadenopathy is noted bilaterally, and nodes are also palpable in the supraclavicular, occipital, and inguinal areas. *CV:* tachycardia with a soft flow murmur. *Abdomen:* soft and nontender. Spleen tip palpable but nontender; liver edge 2 cm below the costal margin. *Skin:* pale, but warm and well perfused. Several large bruises of various colors are noted over both shins and on the elbows; three nonblanching, pinpoint macules noted on abdomen. Remainder of exam within normal limits.

THOUGHT QUESTIONS

- What is your differential diagnosis at this point?
- What further workup would you pursue?

DISCUSSION

G.G.'s weight loss and ill appearance suggest a chronic rather than an acute process. He has a constellation of nonspecific symptoms of inflammation and hematologic dysfunction (fever, lymphadenopathy, hepatosplenomegaly, and pallor) that can be attributed to a large variety of diseases. In broad categories, these include infection (e.g., viral infections such as EBV or HIV, and subacute or chronic bacterial infections), rheumatologic disease (e.g., lupus and JRA often present with nonspecific systemic findings in children), and malignancy. Malignancy is of particular concern in this child, because his pallor, mucosal petechiae, bruising, and fever suggest bone marrow dysfunction.

With this broad differential diagnosis, the most useful first screening lab test would be a CBC with differential. The CBC is a good indicator of infection or inflammation, as well as bone marrow function, and the results may guide further testing. Other blood tests to consider as indicated by examination and history in cases like this include an ESR or CRP, an ANA, blood cultures, and specific viral serologies. When malignancy is suspected, a bone marrow aspirate should be performed prior to significant intervention, especially treatment with steroids.

CASE CONTINUED

You draw blood for a CBC, which reveals a WBC count of 3,000, hematocrit of 23, and platelets of 57. The automated differential shows 86% lymphocytes and 10% neutrophils. Shortly thereafter, the laboratory calls because the manual differential reveals 5% blasts. The findings on physical examination, along with the presence of pancytopenia on CBC and blasts on peripheral smear, suggest acute lymphocytic leukemia (ALL), the most common malignancy in children. You consult the oncology service and obtain additional labs and a bone marrow biopsy, which confirms the diagnosis of ALL with 35% lymphoblasts present on bone marrow examination. G.G. is admitted for further evaluation and for the initiation of chemotherapy. The oncologist informs you that his age, initial lymphocyte count, and lymphoid cell lineage place him in a favorable prognostic category, and he is felt to have an excellent chance of full recovery.

 ## DISCUSSION

Leukemias are the most common childhood malignancies, representing 25% to 30% of the malignancies diagnosed each year. CNS tumors, lymphoma, and neuroblastoma follow in frequency. About 97% of all childhood leukemias are acute, and 80% of these are lymphocytic. Presenting features include signs of bone marrow infiltration and dysfunction (pallor, bruising, petechiae, fever or prolonged infection), bone or joint pain (caused by leukemic expansion of bone marrow cavity), lymphadenopathy, and weight loss. The diagnosis is suggested by the presence of blasts and evidence of bone marrow failure on peripheral blood counts, and confirmed by bone marrow examination.

 ## QUESTIONS

52-1. G.G.'s parents have been reading about leukemia on the Internet and ask you whether a bone marrow transplant will be needed to cure their child. What is the best answer regarding the usual course of therapy for ALL in children such as G.G.?

  A. The overall cure rate for ALL in children is 99% after one round of chemotherapy.
  B. The overall cure rate for ALL in children is around 80%, and bone marrow transplant is only indicated in those who do not respond to standard chemotherapy.
  C. The overall cure rate for ALL in children is around 80%, with bone marrow transplant as part of the routine treatment regimen.
  D. Bone marrow transplant is not used to treat ALL in children.

52-2. Your senior resident mentions that G.G. should be monitored carefully for tumor lysis syndrome upon initiation of chemotherapy. Findings of tumor lysis syndrome include

  A. Hyperuricemia, hyperkalemia, and hyperphosphatemia
  B. Hypernatremia, hypermagnesemia, and alkalosis
  C. Anemia, thrombocytopenia, and fever
  D. Leukocytosis, fever, and petechiae

52-3. During chemotherapy, G.G. develops severe neutropenia, with a total WBC count of 250 and an absolute neutrophil count of 100. On the seventh hospital day, he develops a fever of 39.5°C (103°F) and shaking chills. On examination, he has severely ulcerated, painful oral mucosa, and is pale with diffuse bruising and petechiae. After you ensure that the patient's airway, breathing, and circulation are adequately supported, what should the next step in management be?

    A. Treat the fever with acetaminophen and observe the child for further fevers.

    B. Start an antifungal agent for likely fungal mucositis.

    C. Obtain cultures of blood and urine and start broad-spectrum antibiotics.

    D. Check tumor lysis labs and initiate alkalinization.

52-4. You are taking care of a 6-month-old white girl with ALL. Her initial presenting labs included a WBC count of 4,000 and a platelet count of 200,000. Her surface markers indicate that she has a non-T, non-B cell type of ALL. Regarding her prognosis for a good outcome, the factor that is the most *unfavorable* (high risk) is her

    A. Age

    B. Female gender

    C. Low WBC count

    D. Type of ALL

ANSWERS

52-1. B. The overall cure rate for childhood ALL is 80%. Bone marrow transplant is indicated only for patients who do not respond to standard treatment. Treatment of leukemia, which is initiated in the hospital, includes treating the complications from the disease at presentation (transfusing blood products, stabilizing electrolytes, restoring nutrition, and treating infection), treating the leukemia itself (specific regimens vary by institution, but include chemotherapeutic phases of induction, consolidation, and maintenance therapy), and managing the complications of therapy.

52-2. A. Tumor lysis syndrome is due to a rapid release of intracellular contents such as potassium, phosphate, and purines during lysis of tumor cells from rapid growth or chemotherapy. It is rare in solid tumors, and is most often seen in malignancies with a high growth rate, such as T-cell ALL and Burkitt's lymphoma. It is most likely to occur during the first 5 days of chemotherapy. The resulting hypocalcemia, hyperphosphatemia, hyperkalemia, and hyper-uricemia can cause hypocalcemic tetany, arrhythmias, and renal failure from precipitation of uric acid. Management includes vigorous hydration and alkalinization, removal of uric acid, and correction of electrolyte disturbances. Other complications commonly seen during initiation of chemotherapy include neutropenia, anemia, thrombocytopenia, and mucositis.

52-3. C. Fever and neutropenia is considered an oncologic emergency. Patients with severe neutropenia are at risk for serious, invasive infections from a variety of organisms, including bacteria and fungus. Your first priority is to stabilize the patient's ABCs; then obtain cultures of blood and urine and start broad-spectrum antibiotics as soon as possible. Mucositis is common in children with severe neutropenia and does not necessarily imply fungal infection. Patients with severe neutropenia *are* at risk for fungal infection, but antifungals are not usually used initially in the febrile neutropenic patient unless the patient has evidence of fungal infection or fails to respond to antibacterial agents. Treating the fever with acetaminophen and considering the possibility of tumor lysis should be done as soon as possible, but they are not your first priority in this patient.

52-4. A. This patient's demographic and clinical characteristics (female, white, WBC count <10,000, normal platelet count, and ALL type) are all favorable, except for her age. Children younger than 2 or older than 10 are considered high risk. Age and initial WBC count at presentation are the two most important prognostic factors for outcome of ALL. Non-T, non-B cell ALL is the most common type and carries the most favorable prognosis.

 SUGGESTED ADDITIONAL READING

Haslam DB. Managing the child with fever and neutropenia in an era of increasing microbial resistance. *J Pediatr.* 2002;140(1):5–7.
Pearce, JM, Sills RH. Consultation with the specialist: childhood leukemia. *Pediatr Rev.* 2005;26:96–104.

Small Infant

CC/ID: 4-month-old boy noted to have poor weight gain at a well-child visit.

HPI: Mother was told that D.M. was "not gaining weight" at a sick visit 2 weeks ago, and she is concerned that he looks "skinny." The baby is formula-fed; he "eats great but spits up all the time." He has bowel movements three to four times per day, and his stool is greenish or yellow, seedy, and nonbloody. He urinates approximately four times per day. D.M. cries only when he is hungry, and sleeps well, usually through the whole night. The infant had a mild cold 2 weeks ago, but otherwise has not had fever, cough, respiratory distress, vomiting, or diarrhea.

PMHx: Normal birth history; full-term delivery without complications. Birth weight: 7 lb, 10 oz (3,460 grams, 60%). No hospitalizations or illnesses.

Chart review: *At birth:* length = 50 cm (50%), head circ = 36.5 cm (70%). *At 2-month visit:* wt = 4.6 kg (20%), length = 58 cm (50%), head circ = 41 cm (75%). *At clinic visit 2 weeks ago:* wt = 5.2 kg (10%).

Meds: None

All: NKDA

Immun: UTD (4-month shots due today)

VS: Temp 36.8°C (98.2°F), HR 130, RR 38; Po₂ 99% on RA; Weight 5.2 kg (3%), length 63 cm (50%), head circumference 43 cm (75%)

PE: *Gen:* somewhat fussy but consolable infant, who appears small for age. *HEENT:* nondysmorphic. Anterior fontanelle slightly sunken and soft. Mucous membranes moist; oropharynx clear without thrush; palate intact. *Lungs:* clear. *CV:* RR&R without murmur; pulses and capillary refill brisk. *Abdomen:* flat, soft, and nontender with NABS; no hepatosplenomegaly. *Skin:* slightly dry;

no rashes. Ribs visible through skin. *Neuro/Dev:* deep tendon reflexes and tone are normal. The infant tracks, smiles, reaches, grabs, and can push chest off table with good head control; unable to sit unassisted.

THOUGHT QUESTIONS

- Plot this infant on the appropriate growth chart. What are possible causes of poor growth in this infant?
- What additional information will you seek on history or examination, and what further workup would you like to obtain on this infant?

DISCUSSION

This child is not gaining weight as expected for his age, a condition known as failure to thrive (FTT) (Fig. 53-1). FTT is defined as a fall in weight to below the third percentile for age, or a deceleration of growth crossing two major percentiles on a standard growth chart. Causes of

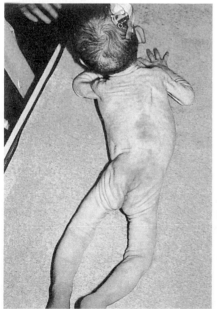

FIGURE 53-1.
A child with severe failure to thrive, illustrating loss of subcutaneous fat, muscle wasting, and skin breakdown.

FTT can be organic (internal), nonorganic (external), or a combination of the two. The differential diagnosis for FTT is extensive, so it may be helpful to divide it into causes of decreased intake or increased output. Decreased intake is usually an environmental issue, such as poverty, abuse or neglect, inexperienced parents, or poor bonding between infant and parent. Disease processes that can cause feeding difficulties must also be considered, especially neurologic disorders and malformations of the mouth and palate. Causes of increased output are more likely to be organic in nature. These include malabsorption, metabolic disease, cardiac or pulmonary disease, malignancy, chronic or acute infection, and endocrine disturbances.

The evaluation for failure to thrive should start with a careful history and physical examination. Details of feeding and output, as well as information on recent illnesses, developmental history, and family history of small stature or growth delay, should be elicited. A detailed social history is essential, including the infant's home environment, temperament, and any recent financial or social stressors present in the family. Laboratory studies should be ordered based on the likely cause of the FTT, and whenever metabolic derangements as a result of poor nutrition or intrinsic disease are suspected. Appropriate screening tests to consider include a CBC, electrolyte panel, and stool studies. Stool studies for infection include Hemoccult, white cells, culture, and ova/parasite. Stool studies for malabsorption include fecal fat, pH, and reducing substances. Carbohydrate malabsorption results in low stool pH (due to bacterial fermentation) and the presence of reducing substances (undigested sugars).

 CASE CONTINUED

On further history, you find that the mother is 16 years old, lives with her parents and six siblings, and attends a high school that allows her to bring the baby to school. The baby's father is "helpful, but busy with his job." She is part of a teen parent group, but has felt "pretty overwhelmed" by taking care of the baby. D.M. takes a 4- to 6-oz bottle of formula about four times during the day. Mom says he often spits up after feeds, and a friend told her this was due to "overfeeding," so if he is still thirsty afterward she gives him water. He sleeps for 8 hours at night, and if he wakes up, he goes back to sleep with a pacifier. You decide to observe the child feeding, and give his mother a bottle of formula, which the infant takes vigorously, then spits up a small amount and still seems hungry. Stool guaiac, pH, and reducing substances are all within normal limits.

THOUGHT QUESTION

■ How would you manage this patient?

DISCUSSION

Based on D.M.'s normal physical examination, stool studies, and the history suggesting inadequate caloric intake due to infrequent feeds and supplementation with water, you suspect a nonorganic cause for his failure to thrive. There are several ways to manage this infant, and the proper management depends on the physician's impression of the caretaker's ability and motivation to comply with outpatient treatment. Although hospitalization is necessary in cases of obvious or suspected neglect, in this case it might be reasonable to educate the mother on proper feeding of an infant this age, and if possible involve the grandparents as well in the education. Close follow-up with weekly weight checks should be performed. If the infant fails to gain weight with adequate intake as an outpatient, he should be admitted to undergo observed feeding and any further testing as needed.

QUESTIONS

53-1. Assuming that D.M. is a healthy 4-month-old child with no medical illness, at his current weight his caloric needs for adequate growth should be met by which of the following?
  A. 15 to 20 ounces of formula per day
  B. 25 to 30 ounces of formula per day
  C. 40 to 45 ounces of formula per day
  D. 55 to 60 ounces of formula per day

53-2. D.M.'s mother asks you what the best food is for him to eat in order to gain weight. The appropriate diet for a 4-month-old such as this one should include
  A. Starchy foods such as rice cereal added to formula
  B. Rich foods such as cheese and butter in addition to formula
  C. Water between feeds in order to maintain hydration
  D. Breast milk or formula only

53-3. D.M. is followed for 2 months as an outpatient, and shows improvement in weight gain. You conclude that D.M. suffered from inadequate intake, a nonorganic form of failure to thrive. You are giving a presentation about FTT to some other medical students, and one of them asks whether D.M. is ever going to be a normal size. The best statement regarding the prognosis for infants and children with FTT is that in the majority of cases

A. The cause is organic, and the child never attains a normal weight.

B. The cause is nonorganic, and the child never attains a normal weight.

C. The cause is organic, and a normal weight is attained.

D. The cause is nonorganic, and a normal weight is attained.

53-4. You have been following a child for FTT, and you plot the child's recent growth on a growth chart. Which of the following patterns is *most* consistent with an organic cause of FTT?

A. Increased weight gain is achieved during observed feeding in the hospital.

B. Weight, head circumference, and length are all equally decreased.

C. Head circumference and length are preserved relative to weight.

D. The infant's weight is in the third percentile for age.

ANSWERS

53-1. B. During the first year of life, a growing infant requires 100 to 120 calories/kg per day for proper growth. Breast milk and formula contain about 20 calories per ounce, so the recommended quantity would be 5 to 6 ounces/kg per day, or 25 to 30 ounces per day for this 5-kg infant. After the first year of life, growth velocity decreases, as do the child's caloric needs. The resultant decrease in appetite, which occurs during early toddlerhood, is a common concern among parents.

53-2. D. The nutritional needs of a healthy 4-month-old infant are met adequately by sufficient quantities of breast milk or formula alone. Additional fluids, such as water or supplements, are unnecessary. Solid foods should not be introduced until the infant has enough head control and swallowing coordination to safely swallow these foods. Rice cereal is the first solid food to be introduced, usually around 4 to 6 months of age, followed by cooked, pureed vegetables ("baby foods") at around 6 months of age. Although parents sometimes want to add rice cereal to make formula or breast milk more "nutritious," this practice actually decreases the nutritional density of formula or breast milk and is contraindicated in an infant with failure to thrive. High-calorie formulas and breast milk "fortifiers" are safe options for infants who need food of increased caloric density. Because of the risk for allergies, cow's milk and eggs are not recommended until 1 year of age, and highly allergenic foods such as nuts and shellfish should be introduced as late as possible.

53-3. D. In most cases of FTT, the cause is primarily nonorganic. About one fourth of cases involve a combination of organic and nonorganic factors. Most children with FTT have a good prognosis with respect to weight gain and growth. However, approximately one fourth of these patients remain small. Cognitive function may be impaired, and behavioral problems are more common in patients with severe or long-standing FTT.

53-4. B. Symmetric decrease in all of the growth parameters (height, weight, and head circumference) should suggest an organic or internal cause of poor growth. In the infant or child with nonorganic failure to thrive, as in this case, head circumference and length are usually relatively preserved in relation to weight. Successful weight gain with refeeding, normal laboratory tests, and normal physical examination all support a nonorganic cause of FTT.

 ## SUGGESTED ADDITIONAL READING

Krugman SD. Failure to thrive. *Am Fam Physician*. 2003;68(5): 879–884.

CASE **54**

The Shortest Kid in the Class

 CC/ID: 6-year-old boy brought in because he is "not growing."

HPI: R.T.'s mother is concerned that R.T. does not seem to be growing as fast as the other kids at school. Since she and R.T.'s father are "normal height," she is worried that he may have a vitamin deficiency, and notes that he "won't eat vegetables." R.T. has a history of asthma, which has been well controlled, and is otherwise a healthy, active boy. R.T. says he feels like he is "the shortest kid in his class." He's tired of being "a shrimp," and he wants to know if he can get some medicine to make him taller so he can play basketball.

PMHx: Asthma, as noted. No hospitalizations.

Meds: Beclomethasone inhaler, 40 μg twice daily; albuterol inhaler as needed, last used 6 months ago.

All: Eggs (hives)

Immun: UTD

SHx: Father is a sports broadcaster; mother is an organic chef. No siblings.

VS: Temp 37°C (98.6°F), HR 95, RR 22, BP 100/75; Weight 17 kg, height 108 cm

THOUGHT QUESTIONS

- Plot this child's height and weight on a growth chart. How would you characterize his growth abnormality?
- What are some possible causes of this pattern of growth abnormality, and how can you distinguish between them?

DISCUSSION

This child's height and weight are both near the fifth percentile for age. Therefore, R.T. has short stature, defined as height more than 2 standard deviations below the mean. Normal height velocity decreases after the first year of life, then increases again around puberty. Multiple patterns of aberrant growth may result in short stature, including normal velocity remaining below the fifth percentile, decreased growth velocity, or normal velocity followed by a decrease in velocity. Eighty percent of children with short stature have a normal cause, such as familial short stature or constitutional delay. These conditions have a classic pattern of growth, which can be elicited by plotting previous measurements on the growth chart.

Pathologic causes of short stature include chromosomal abnormalities (Turner's syndrome, trisomy 21), chronic disease, malnutrition, psychosocial deprivation, drugs and endocrine disorders (growth hormone deficiency, glucocorticoid excess, hypothyroidism). In these disorders, the pattern of growth delay as well as the child's history or appearance should suggest a pathologic cause. Historical factors of importance include familial growth and timing of puberty, associated systemic symptoms or chronic illness, nutrition, social stressors, and use of medications.

On physical examination, the child should be evaluated for signs of illness or malnutrition; stigmata of endocrine conditions that can affect growth, such as Cushing's syndrome or hypothyroidism; and findings suggestive of genetic syndromes such as Prader-Willi or Turner's syndrome. Previous growth records should be sought to further characterize the pattern of growth abnormality. A bone age is helpful in cases of suspected constitutional growth delay. Additional workup, such as growth hormone or insulin growth factor 1 (IGF-1) levels, karyotype, and head MRI, should be guided by the results of the history and physical exam.

 CASE CONTINUED

On further history, R.T. was a "normal-sized" infant, but he has been shorter than his peers since he was a toddler. His parents deny any chronic health conditions, and report that things at home have been stable. R.T.'s mother recalls that his father is especially concerned because he too was a short child and suffered from low self-esteem as a result until he hit his growth spurt in his teenage years.

Although mom is concerned that R.T. doesn't eat enough vegetables, he eats a varied diet that includes fish, dairy, and fruit.

PE: *Gen:* healthy-appearing, active boy in no acute distress. *HEENT:* normal facies; TMs clear bilaterally; clear oropharynx; no adenopathy. *Lungs:* clear to auscultation bilaterally. *CV:* RR&R; no murmur. *Ext:* symmetric in strength and tone; proportional limb length. *Skin:* no bruises, rashes, or birthmarks. *Neuro:* nonfocal. Remainder of exam is within normal limits. The growth record from R.T.'s chart is as follows:

    Birth: weight 4 kg, length 51 cm
    1 year: weight 10.4 kg, length 75 cm
    2 years: weight 12 kg, height 84 cm
    3 years: weight 12.5 kg, height 90 cm
    4 years: weight 14.5 kg, height 96 cm

THOUGHT QUESTIONS

- Plot R.T.'s growth on the appropriate growth chart. Based on this pattern, what is the most likely cause of this child's short stature?

- What should be your next step in diagnosis and/or management?

DISCUSSION

R.T.'s growth chart shows a pattern that is typical of children with constitutional growth delay (Fig. 54-1). A bone age is performed by obtaining a radiograph of the left wrist, and this is read as 4 years, confirming the diagnosis. The typical growth pattern of children with constitutional growth delay shows a normal size at birth, followed by a decrease in both height and weight velocity in the first few years of life, and then by normal velocity following a lower percentile. Height and weight are usually similarly affected. Familial short stature can show a similar pattern early in life. Constitutional growth delay can be differentiated from familial short stature by the use of a bone age and pubertal staging. Children with constitutional short stature are delayed in bone age as well as puberty, and usually attain normal final adult height. Children with familial short stature have normal pubertal timing and a bone age that is the same as their chronologic age, and their final height is decreased from

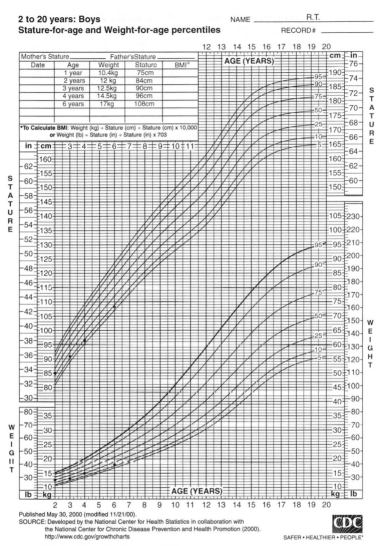

FIGURE 54-1. Growth chart for R.T.

normal. A growth pattern showing significant decrease in growth
velocity in later childhood, or weight affected significantly more or
less than height, should suggest a pathologic cause of short stature,
such as nutritional deficiency or endocrine/genetic abnormality.

Although R.T. is expected to reach a normal adult height, he is likely to remain short during childhood and to have delayed puberty. Children with short stature are at higher risk for rejection by peers, and are subject to more social and economic disadvantages as adults. Counseling parents on anticipating and responding to these feelings is an essential part of treating the child with short stature.

QUESTIONS

54-1. R.T.'s mother asks if the use of his inhaled steroid for asthma could be "stunting his growth." The most accurate statement regarding the existing data about the effect of properly administered inhaled steroids for asthmatic children on height is the following:

    A. Inhaled steroids do not affect height velocity or final height.

    B. Inhaled steroids decrease height velocity in the first year of their use, but catch-up growth seems to occur.

    C. Inhaled steroids decrease height velocity in the first year of use, and catch-up growth does not occur.

    D. Inhaled steroids result in decreased height velocity throughout the duration of their use.

54-2. R.T.'s father calls during the visit and wants to know if growth hormone could be used to enhance his son's growth. What is the best answer regarding the use of growth hormone for this child with constitutional growth delay?

    A. Growth hormone is not approved for use in children.

    B. Growth hormone is only approved for use in children with proven growth hormone deficiency.

    C. Growth hormone is approved for use in children with multiple pathologic causes of growth delay, but not for those with normal variations in growth.

    D. Growth hormone is approved for use in children with constitutional growth delay, but would not be recommended in this case.

54-3. A 10-year-old girl is being evaluated for short stature. Her height is in the 3rd percentile for her age. Her weight is normal for her height, and she is prepubertal; her exam is otherwise unremarkable. Although her length and weight at birth were in the 50th percentile, her height and weight have been following the 3rd percentile since she was 2 years old. A radiographic bone age is performed. What result for her bone age is most consistent with a diagnosis of constitutional growth delay?

    A. Bone age of 7 years old
    B. Bone age of 10 years old
    C. Bone age of 14 years old
    D. Bone age of 18 years old

54-4. A 6-year-old boy is being evaluated for short stature in the endocrine clinic. His length and weight at birth were normal. His growth velocity for height and weight were both in the 60th percentile for age until age 4, when his height velocity decreased and his weight velocity increased. His current height is 105 cm (<3rd percentile), and his weight is 25 kg (90th percentile). On exam, he is obese, prepubertal, with a very round face and purplish bands of rough skin along his abdomen. His exam is otherwise normal. Of the following diagnoses, which is most likely given this pattern of growth?

    A. Turner's syndrome
    B. Growth hormone deficiency
    C. Constitutional growth delay
    D. Glucocorticoid excess

ANSWERS

54-1. B. Multiple long-term studies of inhaled steroids for children with persistent asthma have established their efficacy and safety for this common condition. As a result, inhaled steroids are the first-line medication recommended by the National Heart, Lung, and Blood Institute in its most recent guidelines for treatment of persistent asthma in children. However, inhaled steroids are not without systemic effects. In children followed over various periods of time on inhaled steroids, a small decrease in growth velocity in comparison with that expected for age is consistently seen during the first year of therapy. Growth velocity then returns to normal, and some catch-up growth usually occurs, because final adult height in most studies is the same as that found in healthy controls. However, studies have not compared the final height attained in children on appropriate doses of inhaled steroids with untreated controls with persistent asthma, because these children are likely to have decreased final adult height due to chronic illness as well as frequent courses of systemic corticosteroids. Therefore, the consensus is that even if there is a small decrease in final adult height in children on inhaled steroids, it is likely to be similar to or less than that incurred by untreated or undertreated persistent asthma. Studies have not demonstrated long-term effects of inhaled steroids on immune function, bone density, or adrenal function in children.

54-2. C. Recombinant human growth hormone (rhGH) is approved by the Food and Drug Administration (FDA) for use in children with short stature as a result of growth hormone (GH) deficiency as well as five non-GH-deficient conditions: Turner's syndrome, chronic renal failure, Prader-Willi syndrome, children born small for gestational age, and, most recently, idiopathic short stature (ISS). Normal variations in growth, such as constitutional growth delay, are *not* considered indications for GH supplementation. However, familial short stature may have a number of different causes, and may be considered a form of ISS.

GH acts at the liver and the growth plate to promote linear growth. The response to rhGH in children is greatest in the first year of therapy; with continued therapy, growth typically proceeds at the normal velocity for age until puberty. Side effects are rare in children when GH is used at appropriate doses, and include edema, gynecomastia, arthralgia, myalgia, scoliosis, and benign intracranial hypertension. Sudden death has been reported in patients with Prader-Willi syndrome treated with growth hormone, so careful screening for risk factors for respiratory compromise is recommended in these patients being considered for growth hormone therapy. Although considered relatively safe and effective, treatment with recombinant growth hormone is still very expensive.

54-3. A. A delayed bone age of 7 years would be consistent with a diagnosis of constitutional growth delay. Children with this normal pattern of growth have delayed bone age and delayed puberty, and therefore have a later growth spurt than other children, attaining a final height that is in the normal range. A bone age that is the same as the child's chronologic age would be consistent with familial short stature, whereas a more advanced bone age is seen in precocious puberty.

54-4. D. The pattern of growth described in this case (late childhood onset of decreased height velocity with simultaneous increase in weight) is typical of certain endocrine causes of short stature. Of the listed options, glucocorticoid excess would be the most likely cause, given the growth pattern and physical exam findings. Turner's syndrome does not occur in boys, and the other options, although all causes of short stature, would not typically result in this pattern of growth abnormality. Cushing's disease, or bilateral adrenal hyperplasia, is the most common cause of endogenous glucocorticoid excess in childhood. The cause is usually a pituitary adenoma that causes hypersecretion of adrenocorticotropic hormone (ACTH). When high cortisol levels are found, the etiology of glucocorticoid excess can be differentiated with the use of a dexamethasone suppression test. Since ACTH secretion is subject to negative feedback by corticosteroids, patients with glucocorticoid excess due to increased pituitary secretion of ACTH will respond to high-dose dexamethasone with a decrease in ACTH production, and therefore a decrease in cortisol. However, patients with an ectopic or adrenal source of ACTH or cortisol will not respond to dexamethasone.

 SUGGESTED ADDITIONAL READING

Leschek EW, et al., for the National Institute of Child Health and Human Development-Eli Lilly and Company Growth Hormone Collaborative Group 2004. Effect of growth hormone treatment on adult height in peripubertal children with idiopathic short stature: a randomized, double-blind, placebo-controlled trial. *J Clin Endocrinol Metab*. 2004;89:3140–3148.

National Asthma Education and Prevention Program. Expert panel report: guidelines for the diagnosis and management of asthma—update on selected topics 2002. *J Allergy Clin Immunol*. 2002;110(5 suppl):S141–S219.

Rose SR, Vogiatzi MG, Copeland KC. A general pediatric approach to evaluating a short child. *Pediatr Rev*. 2005;26(11):410–420.

Infant with Poor Weight Gain and Fatigue

CC/ID: 15-month-old boy brought in by his mother for fatigue.

HPI: J.H. is a 15-month-old male who presents with a 1-month history of increasing fatigue, which was first brought to the mother's attention by a day-care provider. She notes that he was normally quite active, but now seems to tire easily and doesn't seem to be as active as the other children. He has not had any fever, vomiting, diarrhea, or rash. He has also been noted to be increasingly irritable, with a decreased appetite, which the mother has attributed to recent bouts of teething and upper respiratory illnesses that have now almost resolved. She reports that he seems less interested in solids, but has been taking in fluids quite adequately.

PMHx: Normal delivery at term; no complications. Hospitalized for RSV infection at 7 months.

PSHx: None

Meds: Oral topical anesthetic (Orajel) for teething; OTC cold/cough medicine

Immun: Needs DTaP no. 4; otherwise UTD.

Allergies: None reported

**Growth/
DevHx:** Poor weight gain by report since 12-month visit; can say three to four words; "mama/dada" is specific; has just started walking; plays with blocks and a "pretend" phone.

FHx: Paternal grandfather with coronary heart disease at age 45.

SHx: Lives with parents and dog; no smokers; multiple ill contacts in day care; no recent travel.

ROS: As above; clear rhinorrhea; no respiratory difficulty; no urinary changes; no constipation.

VS: Temp: 37°C (98.6°F), HR 130, RR 22, BP 95/45; Weight 10.2 kg (25%), height 79 cm (50%), head circumference 47.5 cm (50%)

PE: *Gen:* comfortable but somewhat tired-appearing; in no acute distress. *HEENT:* normocephalic; atraumatic; EOMI; PERRL; nares with clear discharge; oropharynx without lesions. Primary teeth emerging. *Neck:* supple; shotty anterior cervical lymphadenopathy. *Chest:* clear to auscultation; no crackles or wheeze. *CV:* RR&R; mild tachycardia; normal S_1S_2; grade 2–3/6 systolic ejection murmur at left sternal border; pulses normal in all areas; capillary refill time <2 seconds. *Abdomen:* positive bowel sounds; soft, nondistended, nontender; no visceromegaly. *GU:* normal external genitalia. *Neuro:* grossly nonfocal; cranial nerves intact; no noted sensorimotor deficits; no deficits in reflexes, tone, or strength.

THOUGHT QUESTIONS

- What additional elements of the history and/or physical exam would you pursue?
- What is your initial differential diagnosis?
- What initial evaluations would you include in your workup?

DISCUSSION

Evaluating the child with easy fatigability and irritability should start with a thorough history and physical exam. The differential diagnosis is wide and includes infectious etiologies (EBV, CMV, Lyme disease, tuberculosis), anemia, congenital heart disease, metabolic and endocrine disorders (causes of acidosis/ketosis, hypothyroidism), leukemia and other oncologic processes, rheumatologic causes, and neurologic causes (encephalitis, CNS degenerative disorders). It is equally as important to identify sleep disorders, environmental issues (lead poisoning, toxic ingestions/ exposures), and signs of child abuse or neglect. An initial evaluation should also include a thorough assessment of growth and development, diet history, sleep history, and a psychosocial evaluation of the family. An initial workup may also include a CBC with manual differential, electrolyte panel, urinalysis, thyroid function studies, and lead level.

Other studies should be obtained as guided by your history and physical examination.

 CASE CONTINUED

An environmental history was obtained that did not show any concerns, and the infant was not noted to have any sleep-related issues. The growth curve, when compared with his weight from a 12-month visit, demonstrated only minimal weight gain. Because of the murmur and suspicions of congenital heart disease, an echocardiogram was obtained and was normal. Results of a urinalysis, serum lead level, and chemistry panel were all normal. Careful evaluation of his conjunctiva and mucous membranes revealed marked pallor. A screening CBC revealed a WBC count of 9.5 with a normal differential, a platelet count of 580,000, and a hemoglobin of 6.2 g/dL. The mean corpuscular volume (MCV) was 65.

A diet history was obtained, and it was revealed that the child had been placed on a diet of whole cow's milk at age 11 months. He has been taking in nearly 30 ounces per day since then, even through his bouts of teething and upper respiratory tract illnesses. His parents and providers had been reassured through these episodes that he had been "taking in adequate liquids." A serum ferritin level was low, and the red blood cell distribution width (RDW) was increased, confirming, along with the above, a diagnosis of iron deficiency anemia. The child was placed on elemental iron, and diet modification was made, with full improvement clinically that was confirmed by laboratory values.

 DISCUSSION

Iron deficiency anemia is the most common anemia of infancy and childhood. It is most common between 9 and 24 months of age, but can also occur in adolescence. It is usually due to consumption of large quantities of iron-poor nutritional sources, namely cow's milk. Clinical manifestations may range from asymptomatic (mild iron deficiency) to irritability, poor weight gain, fatigue, pallor, lethargy, systolic ejection or flow murmur, and tachycardia. Splenomegaly can occur (10% to 15% of cases), as well as alterations in cognition and koilonychias (spoon nails). A CBC usually reveals a hypochromic, microcytic anemia, with an elevated RDW. Serum ferritin values are usually low, but normal or high values may also reflect ferritin's role as an acute-phase reactant during illness or stress. Transferrin is usually increased, transferrin saturation is generally decreased, and free erythrocyte protoporphyrin is increased. A reticulocyte count is usually normal, reflecting a healthy marrow. Management with elemental iron and dietary modification usually results in improvement, but in severe cases, transfusion may be required. Causes of iron loss from bleeding or anemia of other etiologies must be considered in the patient who is unresponsive to these therapies.

QUESTIONS

55-1. You suspect anemia in a 1-year-old with poor growth. His exam is significant for pallor, frontal bossing, maxillary hyperplasia, and splenomegaly. His hemoglobin is low, and his peripheral smear reveals marked hypochromia, microcytosis, and target cells. Which of the following evaluations are consistent with his likely diagnosis?
- A. Decreased serum iron levels
- B. Decreased vitamin B_{12} levels
- C. Increased serum lead levels
- D. Abnormal hemoglobin electrophoresis results with elevated hemoglobin F (HbF)
- E. Positive osmotic fragility test

55-2. Which of the following is a characteristic of iron deficiency anemia?
- A. It is most common in exclusively breastfed infants younger than 6 months.
- B. Congestive heart failure is an early sign.
- C. It can occur during the adolescent growth spurt with suboptimal dietary iron.
- D. It is common in infants who are exclusively fed goat's milk.
- E. Treatment often involves chronic transfusion therapy.

55-3. You are evaluating a 2-year-old child with microcytic anemia who has not responded well to iron therapy. The child has been thriving, and aside from some mild pallor, has a normal physical exam. After ensuring that the child has no occult sources of bleeding and evaluating the child's home environment, a hemoglobin electrophoresis is shown to be normal. Parental testing reveals microcytosis and confirms the diagnosis. What is the likely diagnosis in this child?
- A. Alpha thalassemia trait
- B. Beta thalassemia minor
- C. Alpha thalassemia hemoglobin H disease
- D. Beta thalassemia major
- E. Alpha thalassemia hemoglobin Bart's disease

55-4. A 9-month-old boy presents with failure to thrive, macrocytic nonmegaloblastic anemia, and low reticulocyte count. His WBC and platelet counts are normal. His physical examination is significant for a cleft lip, short stature, and triphalangeal thumb. What is the most likely diagnosis?

   A. Vitamin B_{12} deficiency
   B. Folate deficiency
   C. Diamond-Blackfan syndrome
   D. Transient erythroblastopenia of childhood
   E. Fanconi's anemia

ANSWERS

55-1. **D.** Along with iron deficiency anemia, there are several other causes of microcytic anemia, including thalassemia, sideroblastic anemia, lead poisoning, and copper poisoning. This child's presentation is most consistent with beta thalassemia major (Table 55-1). Although most children will present with severe hemolytic anemia and splenomegaly during the first year, marrow hyperplasia and extramedullary hematopoiesis can lead to features such as frontal bossing, maxillary hypertrophy with prominent cheekbones, and a tower skull if left untreated. Poor growth is quite common, and the diagnosis can be made by noting an elevated HbF level on electrophoresis. Vitamin B_{12} deficiency presents as a macrocytic anemia, and a positive osmotic fragility test is significant in hereditary spherocytosis.

55-2. **C.** Nutritional iron deficiency can occur during adolescence, when often a rapid growth spurt may coincide with poor iron content in the diet. However, it is *most* common in children aged 9–24 months whose diets include consumption of large amounts of whole cow's milk. Infants younger than 6 months who are exclusively breastfed are not at risk because the iron present in breast milk is much more bioavailable than that in cow's milk. However, it is recommended that these infants receive some supplemental iron sources after 6 months of age. Infants who are exclusively fed goat's milk are at high risk for folate deficiency, causing a macrocytic anemia. Congestive heart failure is generally a later sign with moderate to severe anemia. Beta thalassemia major patients are treated with chronic transfusions, but this is not a common treatment for patients with iron-deficiency anemia.

55-3. **A.** A child with a microcytic anemia who does not respond to iron therapy should be evaluated for other causes. Generally, once lead poisoning and bleeding sources have been ruled

TABLE 55-1 Laboratory Findings for the Common Microcytic Anemias

	Iron Deficiency	Thalassemia Trait	Thalassemia Major	Plumbism	Chronic Disease
RDW	↑	NL	↑	↑	NL
MCV	↓	↓	↓	↓	NL ↓
RBC no.	↓	NL	↓	↓	↓
FEP	↑	NL	NL	↑↑	↑
HbA₂	↓	β: ↑ α: NL	β: ↑ α: NL	NL	NL
Iron	↓	NL	↑	NL	↓
TIBC	NL ↑	NL	NL ↑	NL	NL ↓
% saturation	↓	NL	↑	NL	↓
Ferritin	↓	NL	↑	NL	NL ↑

RDW, red blood cell distribution width; MCV, mean corpuscular value; FEP, free erythrocyte protoporphyrin; TIBC, total iron-binding capacity; ↑, increased; ↓, decreased; NL, normal.
From Marino B, Snead K, McMillan J. *Blueprints in Pediatrics*. 3rd ed. Malden, MA: Blackwell Science; 2003:107, with permission.

out, the thalassemia syndromes should be considered. Normally, hemoglobin electrophoresis reveals >90% hemoglobin A (HbA), 2% to 3% hemoglobin A_2 (HbA$_2$), and 2% to 3% HbF. Alpha thalassemia minor (deletion of two α-globin genes) is often confused with iron deficiency anemia. Electrophoresis results are generally normal, and the diagnosis can be confirmed by examining for microcytosis in the parents. Beta thalassemia minor also may present similarly, but will show an elevated HbA$_2$ and HbF on electrophoresis (Table 55-1). Hemoglobin Bart's disease is a homozygous form of alpha thalassemia that results in failure to produce any α-globin chains; it results in death in utero due to hydrops fetalis.

55-4. C. Macrocytic anemias are divided according to the presence or absence of megaloblastosis (ineffective DNA synthesis within an RBC precursor). Megaloblastic macrocytic anemia can be caused by vitamin B_{12} and folate deficiency. Nonmegaloblastic macrocytic anemia can be caused by Diamond-Blackfan syndrome, idiopathic aplastic anemia, or Fanconi's anemia. Diamond-Blackfan syndrome generally is a pure red cell aplasia, and nearly one fourth of patients will present with associated congenital anomalies. Transient erythroblastopenia of childhood is an acquired pure red cell aplasia, but generally presents in toddlers; it is usually associated with a normocytic anemia, and the associated anomalies are usually absent.

 ## SUGGESTED ADDITIONAL READING

Segel GB, Hirsh MG, Feig SA. Managing anemia in pediatric office practice: part 1. *Pediatr Rev.* 2002;23:75–84.

Segel GB, Hirsh MG, Feig SA. Managing anemia in pediatric office practice: part 2. *Pediatr Rev.* 2002;23:111–122.

X

Cases Presenting with a Rash

Itchy Rash with Fever

CC/ID: 7-year-old girl is brought to the clinic complaining of an itchy rash for 3 days.

HPI: K.B.'s rash is rough, dry, and itchy and is located on her trunk, neck, back, arms, and upper thighs. Her mother has applied calamine lotion with some relief. K.B. has stayed home from school for the last 2 days with fever and headache, which improved with acetaminophen. Mom is concerned because K.B. refused to eat breakfast, saying she had a stomachache. There is no history of runny nose or cough, joint pain, chest pain, or dysuria. She has never had a rash like this before.

PMHx: No hospitalizations or surgeries

Meds: Calamine lotion; acetaminophen for fever

All: NKDA

Immun: UTD

SHx: 5-year-old brother, mother, and mother's girlfriend at home. Plays goalie in soccer; has a new kitten.

THOUGHT QUESTIONS

- What is your differential diagnosis for this child with fever and an itchy rash?
- What findings will you look for on physical examination, and which laboratory tests would you consider to help with your diagnosis?

DISCUSSION

The differential diagnosis should include infectious and noninfectious conditions. A variety of bacterial and viral syndromes can cause fever and rash, including adenovirus, enterovirus, mononucleosis, scarlet fever (due to group A streptococcal [GAS] pharyngitis), toxic shock syndrome, and sepsis. Noninfectious causes of a diffuse, itchy rash include eczema, contact dermatitis, urticaria (hives), and scabies. Other causes of rash and fever, such as acute rheumatic fever, Kawasaki disease, and Lyme disease, should be considered as well.

Your first priority, as always, should be to ensure that the patient is hemodynamically stable. Serious conditions such as toxic shock syndrome, sepsis, and anaphylaxis may present with a rash, and can cause life-threatening hypotension and airway compromise. The rest of the evaluation should be geared toward narrowing the differential. Further history should clarify the progression of the rash, as well as the patient's general health and other systemic symptoms, travel, contacts, and recent illness. Physical examination should include careful documentation of the distribution and appearance of the rash. Other characteristic features of the conditions in the differential diagnosis should be sought, such as conjunctivitis, exudative pharyngitis, adenopathy, or arthritis. The use of laboratory tests should be guided by the findings on examination and the additional history. Specific tests for mononucleosis and GAS pharyngitis may be helpful, or more general tests for infection and inflammation may be indicated (e.g., CBC, blood culture, ESR).

CASE CONTINUED

Additional history: K.B.'s rash started 2 days ago on her trunk, and has spread to her neck and limbs. She has been healthy aside from the current illness, and has not traveled or had any unusual contacts recently. Her brother was treated with antibiotics for a sore throat 2 weeks ago. When asked specifically if her throat hurts, K.B. says it hurts to swallow.

VS: Temp 39.5°C (103.2°F), BP 100/70, HR 120, RR 21; Weight 22 kg (40%)

PE: *Gen:* itchy but nontoxic, healthy-appearing girl. *HEENT:* tongue has a whitish coating, with prominent papillae visible. Oropharynx remarkable for enlarged, erythematous tonsils with exudate, and petechia on soft palate. No conjunctivitis or rhinorrhea. Enlarged, tender cervical lymph nodes are palpable bilaterally. *CV:* RR&R; no murmur; pulses equal; capillary refill brisk. *Skin:* diffuse, erythematous, blanching, dry, finely papular rash covering trunk, back, arms, and thighs. Creases in the skin folds of the arms and groin appear enhanced. *Musculoskeletal:* full ROM of all extremities; no joint swelling or pain.

Labs: Rapid GAS throat swab is positive.

THOUGHT QUESTIONS

- What is the most likely diagnosis?
- How would you treat this patient, and what long-term consequences are you attempting to prevent by treating her?

DISCUSSION

This patient has scarlet fever, a syndrome consisting of GAS pharyngitis with a characteristic rash. The rash of scarlet fever is caused by toxins produced by certain strains of GAS. The rash is typically a diffuse, dry, blanching, finely papular, sandpaperlike pruritic rash that starts on the trunk or neck and spreads to the extremities. It is more pronounced in skin creases, a finding known as Pastia's lines, and often desquamates after 10 to 14 days (Fig. 56-1). Management of scarlet fever is identical to that of GAS pharyngitis.

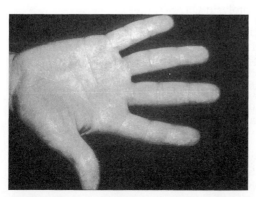

FIGURE 56-1.
Desquamation of skin from fingertips, which occurs during the convalescent phase of scarlet fever.

GAS pharyngitis consists of the triad of pharyngitis, lymphadenopathy, and fever. Upper respiratory infection symptoms are notably absent. In younger children, abdominal pain or headache are common presenting complaints, and sore throat may be less prominent, as in this patient. Clinical diagnosis alone has been found to be unreliable, except when the identifiable rash of scarlet fever is present. Therefore, diagnosis should be confirmed by rapid antigen test or throat culture before treatment.

In addition to the pharynx, GAS may infect the skin, the urine, or the lymph nodes (adenitis). Although usually self-limited, GAS infections can result in both suppurative and nonsuppurative complications. Nonsuppurative complications include acute rheumatic fever (ARF) and poststreptococcal glomerulonephritis (PSGN). Treatment with penicillin is universally recommended to prevent ARF, and also prevents suppurative complications (such as peritonsillar or retropharyngeal abscess), but has not been shown to prevent PSGN. The effect of antibiotics on the course and severity of symptoms is minimal.

 QUESTIONS

56-1. You are seeing a 6-year-old girl with pharyngitis who has a history of four episodes of "strep throat" in the last 2 years. Her parents are considering tonsillectomy. Before referring the family to a surgeon for evaluation, you wish to be sure that her current episode of pharyngitis is in fact due to GAS. What is the *most specific* diagnostic test for acute GAS infection in this case?
- A. Presence of tonsillar exudate on clinical exam
- B. Positive rapid GAS antigen test
- C. Positive throat culture for GAS
- D. High anti-streptolysin-O (ASO) titer

56-2. The Jones criteria for diagnosis of acute rheumatic fever include both major and minor criteria. The major criteria include polyarthritis, carditis, Sydenham's chorea, erythema marginatum, and
- A. Fever
- B. Subcutaneous nodules
- C. Recent episode of exudative pharyngitis
- D. Positive throat culture for group A streptococcus

56-3. You are treating a 6-year-old boy with fever and pharyngitis whose rapid GAS test is positive. He had an anaphylactic reaction to penicillin as an infant. The most appropriate management of this patient would include

   A. No antibiotics, because acute rheumatic fever is rare
   B. Amoxicillin
   C. A macrolide, such as azithromycin or clindamycin
   D. An intramuscular injection of ceftriaxone

56-4. A 12-year-old girl is brought by ambulance to the emergency room unconscious, with a high fever. She is found to be hypotensive, with poor perfusion, and is immediately intubated and given fluid resuscitation. On further examination, she has a diffusely erythematous sunburnlike rash, erythema of her mouth and conjunctivae, and a red, swollen infected insect bite on her right arm. Cultures of the infected area are most likely to grow which of the following?

   A. Group A streptococcus
   B. *Neisseria meningitidis*
   C. *Staphylococcus aureus*
   D. *Staphylococcus epidermidis*

 ANSWERS

56-1. D. The *most* specific test for an acute GAS infection in this case is an elevated ASO titer. Although a positive throat culture and rapid antigen test are very specific for the *presence* of GAS in the throat (>95%), these tests may also be positive in an individual who is *colonized* with GAS. Since it is important to differentiate between colonization and acute infection in this case (because medical management of colonization should be tried before tonsillectomy), the ASO titer is the most specific test to order. However, this test is *not* recommended for diagnosing routine cases of GAS pharyngitis. Although many physicians feel confident making the diagnosis of an acute GAS pharyngitis clinically, based on history and physical findings, studies show that it is more accurate *and* cost-effective to use laboratory tests such as the rapid antigen test and throat culture to confirm the diagnosis and guide therapy. Both of these tests rely on the quality of the sample for adequate sensitivity. The rapid antigen test is highly specific, but its sensitivity varies from institution to institution. Therefore, a throat culture is usually sent when the rapid test is negative to catch possible false negative results. Prevention of ARF is achieved if treatment is begun within 10 days of the start of the infection, so treatment can be held until throat culture results are obtained. Some physicians prefer to start therapy based on clinical suspicion, and stop treatment if the rapid test and culture are negative. Treatment is effective in preventing ARF as well as suppurative complications, and may produce a slight decrease in duration of symptoms.

56-2. B. Subcutaneous nodules is the fifth of the major criteria (Table 56-1). Fever is a minor criterion, and evidence of a recent GAS infection, such as recent pharyngitis or positive GAS culture, is considered supportive of the diagnosis. The revised Jones criteria for diagnosis of ARF are listed in Table 56-1. ARF is an immune-mediated condition that occurs 3 to 4 weeks after an infection with particular "rheumatogenic strains" of GAS, and involves the tissues

TABLE 56-1   Revised Jones Criteria for the Diagnosis of Acute Rheumatic Fever

Major Manifestations

Carditis

Polyarthritis

Chorea

Erythema marginatum

Subcutaneous nodules

Minor Manifestations

Clinical

Fever

Arthralgia

Previous rheumatic fever/rheumatic heart disease

Laboratory

Acute-phase reaction[a]

Prolonged PR interval

Additional Criteria

Supporting evidence of preceding streptococcal infection (increased ASO or other streptococcal antibodies), *or*

Positive throat culture for group A streptococci, *or*

Recent scarlet fever

[a]Elevated serum erythrocyte sedimentation rate (ESR), C-reactive protein (CRP); leukocytosis.
From Marino B, Snead K, McMillan J. *Blueprints in Pediatrics.* 2nd ed. Malden, MA: Blackwell Science; 2001:155, with permission.

of the heart, joints, skin, and brain. Its prevention is an important reason to treat acute GAS pharyngitis. Although rheumatic fever has declined greatly in prevalence since the initiation of wide-spread use of penicillin to treat GAS infections, it still exists; thus, it should be kept in mind as part of the differential diagnosis in a case such as this one. Treatment of ARF includes antibiotics, anti-inflammatory drugs, and cardiac management. Patients with ARF should also be treated with prophylactic penicillin to prevent sub-sequent GAS infections, which are associated with recurrence.

56-3. C. A 10-day course of an oral macrolide is the current recommended treatment for GAS pharyngitis in penicillin-allergic patients. Although rheumatic fever is rare, treatment is still recommended in all cases of documented GAS pharyngitis to reduce the risk of this serious complication. In an individual with a previous anaphylactic reaction to penicillin, amoxicillin or a penicillin-related antibiotic such as a cephalosporin would be contraindicated, because there is a 10% to 15% chance of a serious reaction to this closely related class of antibiotics. Patients with a history of a mild reaction to a penicillin antibiotic could be given a cephalosporin with close observation.

56-4. C. This patient shows the signs and symptoms of toxic shock syndrome, a life-threatening toxin-mediated condition that usually results from a toxin produced by strains of *S. aureus*. A similar syndrome can result from streptococcal toxins as well. The rash of toxic shock syndrome is a diffuse sunburnlike erythema, and is accompanied by hypotension (shock), high fever, conjunctival and oral erythema, and multiple organ system involvement. Although historically associated with tampon use, the syndrome can also occur as a result of staphylococcal infection in other locations, such as bone or skin. Treatment consists of supportive care as well as appropriate antibiotic therapy.

 SUGGESTED ADDITIONAL READING

Bisno AL, Gerber MA, Gwaltney JM, et al. Practice guidelines for the diagnosis and management of group A streptococcal pharyngitis. Infectious Diseases Society of America. *Clin Infect Dis.* 2002;35(2):113–125.

Hahn RG, et al. Evaluation of poststreptococcal illness. *Am Fam Physician.* 2005;71(10):1949–1954.

Painless Dots

CC/ID: 7-year-old boy is brought in by his father for a rash.

HPI: J.S.'s rash started 2 days ago with some red dots around the eyes. It has now spread to the chest and back, and is starting to appear on his arms and legs as well. The rash is not itchy or painful, and J.S. has never had a rash like this before. Aside from a recent cold, J.S. has been feeling completely well, without fever, cough, sore throat, headache, neck stiffness, nausea, or vomiting. In fact, he is mad at his father for making him come to see the doctor, because he is missing soccer practice.

PMHx: None

Meds: None

All: NKDA

Immun: UTD

SHx: Lives with father; parents are divorced. No siblings. No significant family illnesses.

VS: Temp 37.2°C (98.9°F), BP 100/65, HR 92, RR 19; Weight 25 kg (65%)

PE: *Gen:* sullen but cooperative boy in no acute distress, wearing a Coldplay T-shirt. *HEENT:* good dentition; clear oropharynx except for a small amount of oozing blood around the gums. Nares are clear. No nuchal rigidity or photophobia. No lymphadenopathy. *Abdomen:* soft, nontender; no masses; no hepatosplenomegaly. *Skin:* multiple discrete, nonblanching pinpoint (1- to 2-mm) red-purple macules densely cover the face, chest, and back, with a few seen on the arms and legs. There is no scale or excoriation on the rash. Several 3- to 4-cm areas of subcutaneous purplish discoloration are noted on the child's shins and knees. Remainder of exam is within normal limits.

THOUGHT QUESTIONS

- What is the name of this type of rash, and what are some of its likely causes?
- What further history would you like to obtain, and what laboratory tests would you request to help with the diagnosis?

DISCUSSION

This well-appearing patient has a diffuse petechial rash, characterized by tiny subcutaneous microhemorrhages, appearing as scattered discrete purple or red nonblanching pinpoint macules. Focal petechiae may occur after trauma (e.g., petechiae around the eyes after vomiting or choking), whereas a more diffuse pattern suggests impaired coagulation. Some causes of petechiae are benign; others are immediately life threatening. If at any time a patient with a petechial rash appears toxic or hemodynamically unstable, the patient should be presumed septic and stabilized with fluid resuscitation and antibiotics immediately. In the nontoxic, stable child, a more leisurely search for the likely cause can be performed.

Diffuse petechiae are often caused by an alteration in the number or function of platelets. In general, platelets can be affected by infection, malignancy, drugs, autoimmune processes, and consumption by the spleen. Because the differential diagnosis is so wide, the history and physical examination are key in identifying accompanying symptoms such as fever, headache, irritability, other types of bleeding (especially mucosal bleeding, epistaxis, or hematuria), organomegaly, joint swelling or pain, malaise, weight loss, and recent medication use. The most important screening lab test in evaluating a petechial rash is the CBC, which enumerates platelets as well as other cell lines that may be altered in infection or bone marrow failure. Coagulation studies, such as PT and PTT, may also be helpful, especially when the CBC reveals a normal platelet number. A blood culture should be sent if infection is suspected. Additional studies may be indicated based on the results of the history and physical exam.

CASE CONTINUED

J.S. and his dad deny recent prolonged bleeding, joint pain, or swelling. There is no recent use of antibiotics, aspirin, or other medications. When asked about the bruising, Dad says that J.S. is an active boy who "always has bruises." When asked directly, J.S. admits that his gums bled when he brushed his teeth this morning, but it didn't hurt, so he didn't tell anybody.

Labs: *CBC:* WBC 7.6 with normal differential, Hct 38, platelets 12,000/mm³. Smear reveals giant platelets (megakaryocytes); otherwise normal cell morphology. *Coagulation studies:* PT 13.6, PTT 37.5.

THOUGHT QUESTION

■ What is your diagnosis, based on the history, examination, and laboratory findings?

DISCUSSION

Given this patient's well appearance and thrombocytopenia (defined as platelet count <150,000) without additional laboratory abnormalities, he is given a likely diagnosis of idiopathic thrombocytopenic purpura (ITP). ITP, also known as immune thrombocytopenic purpura, is the most common cause of thrombocytopenia in children. The incidence is around 5 per 100,000 children per year, just less than that of leukemia. It often occurs several weeks after a viral illness, and results from the binding of antiplatelet antibodies to platelet membranes, followed by their destruction by the reticuloendothelial system. Patients appear completely well, and aside from an often profound thrombocytopenia, other laboratory tests, including CBC, coagulation studies, and blood culture, should all be normal. The platelets found in patients with ITP tend to be large and "sticky" (since they are recently produced), so they are well functioning despite their small number. Perhaps because of this, serious complications, such as internal or intracranial hemorrhage, are very rare, occurring in 0.1% to 0.5% of patients.

QUESTIONS

57-1. After discussion with your attending physician, you decide to admit J.S. since his platelet count is less than 20,000. J.S.'s father wants to know what you can do if his son begins to have more bleeding from his gums. In the hemodynamically stable ITP patient with clinically significant bleeding, the most appropriate first intervention would be

   A. Whole blood transfusion
   B. Platelet transfusion and administration of fresh frozen plasma (FFP)
   C. High-dose steroids and/or intravenous immunoglobulin (IVIG)
   D. Splenectomy

57-2. J.S. wants to know when he can go back to soccer practice, where he plays center halfback. What are the most appropriate instructions regarding the safe participation in contact sports for patients with ITP?

   A. Contact sports are safe as long as a helmet is used.
   B. Contact sports should be avoided for 6 months.
   C. Contact sports can be reinstituted after treatment.
   D. Contact sports should be avoided until the platelet count is higher than 70,000.

57-3. J.S.'s dad wants to know what the likely course of this illness is. What is the best statement regarding the prognosis for ITP in otherwise healthy children?

   A. Eighty percent of cases resolve spontaneously within 6 months.
   B. Eighty percent of cases become recurrent or chronic.
   C. The chance of complete recovery is higher with appropriate therapy.
   D. Patients who develop ITP are at increased risk of leukemia.

57-4. You are taking care of a patient who has hemolytic uremic syndrome (HUS) as the result of an enteral infection with *Escherichia coli* (type 0157). In addition to anemia, hyperuricemia, and acute renal failure, the patient has profound thrombocytopenia, with a platelet count of $22,000/mm^3$. What is the major cause of this patient's thrombocytopenia?

   A. Decreased production of platelets by the bone marrow
   B. Microangiopathic destruction of platelets
   C. Increased adhesion of platelets to damaged endothelium
   D. Consumption of platelets by an overactive spleen

ANSWERS

57-1. C. High-dose steroids, IVIG, and anti-D immunoglobulin would all be effective at temporarily increasing the platelet count in an ITP patient with clinically significant bleeding. In general, the management of ITP is directed toward avoiding the rare but serious complications of internal or cerebral hemorrhage. Management therefore should always include avoiding trauma and providing supportive care, and may also include medical or surgical measures to slow the destruction of platelets. High-dose steroids, IVIG, and intravenous anti-D immunoglobulin have all been shown to temporarily raise platelet counts due to decreased clearance of antibody-coated platelets, but they do not shorten the duration of antibody production or the long-term outcome of ITP. The exact role of medical treatment in management of ITP is controversial, but most providers agree that it is indicated if clinically significant bleeding is present. Some physicians also treat for platelet counts below 20,000. Because of this patient's low platelet count but lack of clinically significant bleeding, some physicians would treat him initially with steroids or immunoglobulin, whereas others would treat only for clinically significant bleeding. When the platelet count is >20,000, outpatient management could be initiated, with regular checks of platelet count to document recovery. Blood and/or platelet transfusion might be indicated to restore intravascular volume and control bleeding in the patient with acute, hemodynamically significant hemorrhage, but would not be indicated in this case. With platelet transfusion in particular, any effect is very short-lived, because the transfused platelets are rapidly destroyed by antibodies. FFP would not be significantly helpful in controlling bleeding in the ITP patient.

57-2. D. Patients with ITP should be advised to avoid contact sports and activities that may result in trauma, such as bike riding or rollerblading, until the platelet count is at least 70,000. This recommendation can be challenging to implement in young children, and occasionally young children may be admitted to the hospital for closer supervision during their recovery.

57-3. A. The majority (80%) of cases of ITP resolve spontaneously by 6 months, and never recur. No treatment has been shown to affect the long-term outcome of ITP. Chronic ITP is more common in older children (>10 years), and is defined as thrombocytopenia persisting for longer than 6 months. It is treated with repeated doses of IVIG or with splenectomy, which induces remission in 70% to 80% of cases. In refractory cases with uncontrolled bleeding, immunosuppressive drugs, plasmapheresis, or drugs that inhibit fibrinolysis have been used. Rarely, ITP may be the presenting symptom of HIV infection or an autoimmune disease such as systemic lupus erythematosus (SLE). The risk of leukemia in patients with ITP is no higher than in the general population.

57-4. C. Thrombocytopenia in HUS is caused by increased platelet activation and adhesion to vascular endothelial cells due to endothelial injury. HUS is caused by immune-mediated damage to endothelial cells in the vascular and renal systems, which results in microangiopathic hemolytic anemia and renal failure. It is primarily associated with enteritis due to *E. coli*, particularly type 0157, but can occur after other infections as well. Most children survive the acute phase, although the majority (60%–80%) require transient dialysis. The prognosis is better in children with diarrhea-associated HUS than in those without diarrhea.

 SUGGESTED ADDITIONAL READING

Buchanan GR. Thrombocytopenia during childhood: what the pediatrician needs to know. *Pediatr Rev.* 2005;26(11):401–409.

Journeycake JM, Buchanan GR. Coagulation disorders. *Pediatr Rev.* 2003;24:83–91.

Kaplan RN. Differential diagnosis and management of thrombocytopenia in childhood. *Pediatr Clin North Am.* 2004;51(4): 1109–1140, xi.

Periorbital Redness

CC/ID: 5-year-old boy is brought in by his father for redness and swelling around his left eye.

HPI: A.K.'s eye seemed "puffy" this morning before school, and this afternoon it seemed to be getting worse. A.K. complains of itching and discomfort around the eye, but has not complained of changes in vision. He has no fever, runny nose, or malaise. Both A.K. and his dad deny trauma to the eye, but Dad notes that A.K. had a mosquito bite on his left cheek a few days ago, and he is worried that it might have become infected. He says, "I told him to stop scratching it."

PMHx: No hospitalizations; gets "hayfever" in the spring.

Meds: None

All: NKDA

Immun: UTD

SHx: Lives with his two fathers. A.K. is in kindergarten, plays third base for his T-ball team.

THOUGHT QUESTIONS

- What diagnosis are you most concerned about in this patient?
- What examination findings will you specifically look for, and which, if any, laboratory tests would you consider?

DISCUSSION

A careful examination of the eye and vision is essential with any eyelid swelling to guide further investigation. The most important diagnosis to exclude in a case of swelling around the eye is orbital cellulitis. This serious infection is located posterior to the orbital septum, which separates the space behind the eye from the more anterior tissues of the eyelids and face. It is characterized by an abrupt onset of severe eye swelling with proptosis, limitation of extraocular movements (EOMs), and visual impairment. Orbital cellulitis endangers vision and is a medical emergency. Systemic toxicity is common in infants in whom the cause is usually hematogenous. In older children, it is often associated with underlying sinus, dental, or bony infection. If orbital cellulitis is suspected, blood cultures should be drawn and the child should be admitted for close observation and IV antibiotics to cover the most likely organisms, including *Haemophilus influenzae* type b and *Streptococcus pneumoniae*. Both of these organisms are vaccinated against as part of the routine childhood vaccinations, but may still occur, especially in immunocompromised or unimmunized children. Imaging, such as a CT scan of the orbit and face, should be performed to delineate involvement of the orbital tissues or sinuses and to rule out complications such as orbital abscess or osteomyelitis (Fig. 58-1). Ophthalmology consultation should be obtained whenever possible, to help with assessment and preservation of vision.

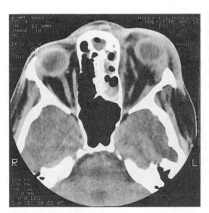

FIGURE 58-1.
Computed tomographic scan showing pansinusitis and diffuse orbital swelling and proptosis on the left side, consistent with orbital cellulitis.

A much more common but less serious infectious cause of eyelid redness and swelling is periorbital or preseptal cellulitis. This condition is usually a limited and easily treatable infection involving the skin around the eye, which does not result in findings of proptosis, visual change, and limited EOMs. Noninfectious causes of periorbital swelling include angioedema, allergic conjunctivitis, trauma, and local irritation.

CASE CONTINUED

VS: Temp 37.1°C (98.7°F), BP 110/70, HR 110, RR 20; Weight 18 kg (50%)

PE: *Gen:* alert, nontoxic-appearing, well-developed boy in no acute distress. *HEENT:* left upper eyelid mildly swollen and slightly erythematous, with extension of pink color to left upper cheekbone and around a yellow-crusted pustule. The skin is mildly tender to palpation around the crusted lesion, and slightly warm to the touch. EOMs are intact without pain, and no proptosis, conjunctivitis, or injection is noted. Visual acuity is 20/20 in both eyes. There is no sinus tenderness, TMs are normal bilaterally, oropharynx is clear, and no lymphadenopathy is noted. The teeth appear healthy; no cavities are visible. Remainder of exam within normal limits.

 ## THOUGHT QUESTIONS

- What is your differential and most likely diagnosis?
- How would you manage this patient?

 ## DISCUSSION

The differential diagnosis for this well-appearing boy with periorbital swelling and a nearby crusted lesion, without evidence of orbital involvement, includes periorbital cellulitis, conjunctivitis, an allergic reaction, angioedema, varicella or HSV infection, or cellulitis extending from infection of the sinuses, teeth, or other facial structures. Of these, the most likely diagnosis is mild periorbital cellulitis extending from a superinfection, or impetigo, of his insect bite.

Cellulitis is a bacterial infection of the skin characterized by redness, warmth, swelling, and tenderness. It is usually caused by the skin's normal flora (e.g., group A streptococci, *Staphylococcus aureus*), which gain access to the dermis and epidermis through a break in the integument. Cellulitis may also occur from the spread of bacteria from other underlying infections, such as dental infection or sinusitis, mastoiditis, osteomyelitis, or septic arthritis.

Treatment of localized cellulitis in a nontoxic-appearing child can be accomplished with an appropriate oral antibiotic active against staphylococcal and streptococcal species (such as cephalexin or amoxicillin/clavulanate). Recently, strains of community-acquired methicillin-resistant *Staphylococcus aureus* (CA-MRSA) have become prevalent in certain areas, so local sensitivities should dictate antibiotic choice. These strains are usually sensitive to clindamycin or trimethoprim-sulfamethoxazole. An oral pain reliever will help with discomfort, and an antihistamine with itching, if present. To help monitor for further spread of infection, it may be helpful to draw a line around the edge of the indurated or erythematous area in the clinic. A patient with cellulitis that is associated with high fever, toxicity, rapid spread, or lymphangitic streaking should be admitted for treatment with intravenous antibiotics and close observation. Blood cultures may be obtained to rule out bacteremia.

QUESTIONS

58-1. Culture of this child's insect bite is most likely to grow
A. *Staphylococcus* species
B. *Streptococcus* species
C. Gram-negative organisms
D. *Pseudomonas* species

58-2. A 5-year-old girl presents with a "spider bite" on her cheek that her mother is worried has become infected. On exam, you note a 2-cm erythematous, raised, tender lesion on the skin with a 1-mm clear vesicle in the center. You would like to distinguish between an allergic reaction to the insect bite and cellulitis. The physical finding that is most suggestive of cellulitis in this case is
A. Erythema
B. Induration
C. Pain
D. Vesicle

58-3. A 10-year-old girl presents to the urgent care clinic with sudden onset of bilateral eye swelling and itchiness. As you begin to get her history, she develops erythema and swelling of her lips and the rest of her face, begins to cough with a harsh sound, and becomes progressively somnolent. Her temperature is 36.7°C (98°F), HR is 160, RR is 20, and BP is 80/45; her O_2 saturation is 94%. What is the most likely diagnosis?
A. Sepsis
B. Anaphylaxis
C. Orbital cellulitis
D. Croup

58-4. A 16-month-old boy is being seen for a "pimple" on his left buttock. On exam, you see a raised, erythematous swelling 4 cm wide on the lateral left buttock, which is tender to palpation. There is a yellow pustule in the center, with a 2-cm surrounding firm induration and a central area of fluctuance. The child is afebrile, with normal vital signs, and appears vigorous and well. He has no significant PMHx, but his mother has recently completed her third course of oral antibiotics for "boils." She reports that she was told she had "resistant bacteria." What is the intervention that is *most* likely to be effective in treating this infant's infection?

    A. Warm compresses applied three times daily to encourage drainage

    B. Administration of IV antibiotics effective against MRSA

    C. Administration of oral antibiotics effective against MRSA

    D. Incision and drainage of the abscess

ANSWERS

58-1. A. Impetigo is a superficial infection of the skin. It is most commonly caused by staphylococcal species, but streptococcal species may also be present. Impetigo occurs in two forms: bullous and nonbullous. Bullous impetigo, most common in newborns, is always caused by *S. aureus*, and produces thin-walled bullae over an erythematous base that produce a clear, thin coating when they rupture. Nonbullous impetigo is a common and relatively benign infection of the skin that may be caused by staphylococcal *or* streptococcal species, and typically involves painless, small (5-mm) vesicles and pustules that rupture, producing a golden crusted coating over an ulcerated base (Fig. 58-2). Limited nonbullous impetigo can be treated with topical mupirocin ointment, whereas bullous or extensive nonbullous impetigo is treated with an oral antibiotic effective against *Staphylococcus* and *Streptococcus*, such as a first-generation cephalosporin.

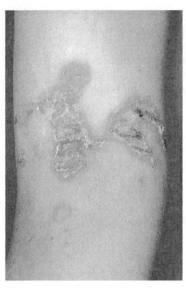

FIGURE **58-2.**
Typical appearance of impetigo.
(*From Rudolf M, Levene M.*
Paediatrics and Child Health. Oxford:
Blackwell Science; 1999:209, with
permission.)

58-2. C. Pain is one of the hallmarks of cellulitis and is the most suggestive sign of an infectious rather than an allergic process. Both cellulitis and allergic reactions will cause erythema, induration, and warmth. Allergic reactions are commonly pruritic rather than painful. Clear vesicles are often seen at the site of insect bites. A yellow crusting exudate is suggestive of bacterial superinfection of the skin (impetigo).

58-3. B. This child shows the signs and symptoms of anaphylaxis, which is a rapid and life-threatening systemic allergic reaction. Impending airway compromise may be heralded by lip or tongue swelling, wheeze, dry cough, or difficulty speaking. Hypotension is an early sign of the circulatory effects of anaphylaxis, which may progress to shock if not identified and treated early. Urticaria, abdominal pain, and diarrhea are other signs of anaphylaxis. Any suspicion of airway inflammation in a patient with an allergic reaction should be treated immediately with subcutaneous epinephrine, and the patient should be taken to an area where the airway can be secured if necessary. Circulatory complications should be managed as necessary with fluid resuscitation and cardiovascular support. Intravenous steroids and antihistamines should be administered as soon as possible.

58-4. D. Incision and drainage is the most effective therapy for abscesses, even those due to MRSA. Although this infant has cellulitis visible on the surface of the skin, the presence of an area of firm induration with a fluctuant center suggests the presence of a collection of pus below the skin. Oral and IV antibiotics do not effectively penetrate collections of pus, and therefore drainage is the only effective treatment. Sometimes after drainage a child may be placed on oral or IV antibiotics to complete healing of the infection, but studies have shown that with effective drainage, the majority of these infections will resolve on their own. The mother's history is highly suggestive of MRSA, and therefore the antibiotic choice, if indicated, should be based on suspected MRSA, and modified based on the results of culture of fluid obtained from the wound.

 ## SUGGESTED ADDITIONAL READING

Buescher ES. Community-acquired methicillin-resistant *Staphylococcus aureus* in pediatrics. *Curr Opin Pediatr.* 2005;17(1):67–70.

Wald ER. Periorbital and orbital infections. *Pediatr Rev.* 2004;25(9): 312–320.

Itchy Rash

CC/ID: A $2^1/_2$-year-old girl is brought in by her father for an itchy rash for 2 weeks.

HPI: The rash first appeared on B.J.'s neck, and now has spread to her face, hands, and trunk. Recently, B.J. has been awake and scratching at night, making the rash worse, and her father is worried that it has become infected on one of her hands. She has always had dry, sensitive skin, which has been worse this winter. She developed a similar rash a few months ago after playing on a neighbor's lawn, but has been otherwise well, without fever or malaise.

PMHx: B.J. tends to wheeze when she gets a cold, and her father was told she had something called "reactive airway disease." Never hospitalized; no surgeries; no recent illnesses.

Meds: None

All: NKDA

Immun: UTD

FHx: 6-year-old brother has asthma. Mother has "dry skin" on her eyelids and hands, is allergic to strawberries, and gets "hayfever" in the spring. Newborn baby sister is 4 weeks old.

THOUGHT QUESTIONS

- What is the differential diagnosis?
- What details about the rash will you ask about in further history, and what will you look for when you examine the child to help in your diagnosis?

DISCUSSION

The differential diagnosis in this case includes a variety of allergic and infectious rashes, including atopic dermatitis, contact dermatitis, rhus dermatitis (poison oak or poison ivy), psoriasis, urticaria (hives), ringworm, scabies, and impetigo. With most dermatologic conditions, the history and examination are the keys to diagnosis. You should determine the physical and temporal pattern of the rash, as well as its relation to any possible infectious or environmental triggers such as insects, plants or pollen, food, pets, stress, sunlight, household chemicals, or other allergens. Important associated findings include fever and other signs and symptoms of illness or allergy. On exam, describe the color, distribution, texture, and pattern of the rash.

CASE CONTINUED

On further history, the rash does not seem to be related to any particular foods, although B.J. eats "everything." There have not been any new detergents, soaps, or lotions used on the child or her clothes. The family lives in an apartment in the city, and they have a 2-year-old dog and a new parakeet. There are no smokers at home, although several of the parents' friends smoke. The family has not traveled out of the state and has not been hiking or camping recently.

VS: Temp 36.9°C (98.4°F), HR 120, RR 28; Weight 15 kg (85%)

PE: *Gen:* well-appearing and playful little girl, scratching at her left hand and belly. *HEENT:* mild rhinorrhea; pale nasal mucosa; otherwise normal. *Skin:* patches of dry, cracked, erythematous skin are noted behind the ears, at the nape of the neck, and behind the knees (Fig. 59-1). Areas of red, papular, excoriated skin are present on both wrists, the cheeks, and the trunk. There are no vesicles or burrows seen, and the diaper area is notably free of rash. The left dorsal wrist has several deep excoriations, some coated with a golden crust. Remainder of exam is within normal limits.

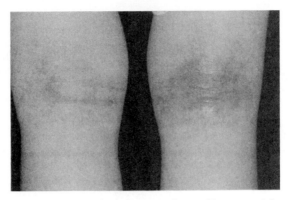

FIGURE 59-1. Rash on flexor surfaces of legs, as might be seen on the patient in this case. (*From Rudolf M, Levene M. Paediatrics and Child Health. Oxford: Blackwell Science; 1999:203, with permission.*)

THOUGHT QUESTIONS

- What is your diagnosis?
- How would you manage this patient?

DISCUSSION

This child has the classic rash of atopic dermatitis, commonly called eczema. Atopic dermatitis (AD) is a chronic allergic skin condition that affects about 5% of children before the age of 5, with the majority (60%) developing the condition before the age of 1 year. The morphology and distribution of the rash change with age: Infants aged 2 months to 2 years have dry or weeping pruritic patches on the face, scalp, trunk, and extremities (Fig. 59-2); older children have erythematous, excoriated papular patches on the flexor surfaces of extremities and the dorsa of hands and feet (Fig. 59-3); and adolescents and adults have dry, papular patches on the dorsal surfaces of the hands and feet, flexor surfaces, and eyelids. AD can also appear in a nummular form, with coinlike patches of dry, papular skin, or a dyshidrotic form, which appears as a dry, vesicular eruption on the fingers, palms, and soles.

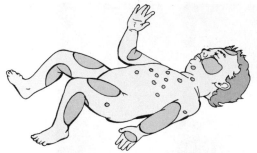

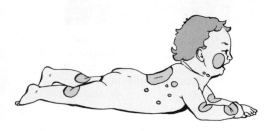

FIGURE 59-2.
In the infant, atopic dermatitis occurs primarily on the face, but may develop on symmetric areas of the body. Diaper areas are usually clear.

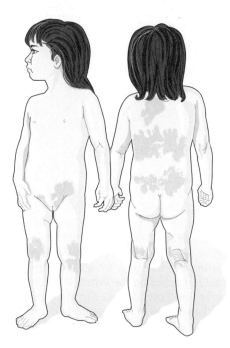

FIGURE 59-3.
Image of toddler showing common areas of atopic dermatitis on the skin.

AD has a waxing and waning course. Treatment involves aggressive management of acute flares and prevention of subsequent flares. Management of acute flares should include intense moisturization of the skin, application of topical steroids, and other itch-control measures to prevent scratching, which increases the risk of infection and permanent scarring. Superficial infection with *Staphylococcus* is common, and topical or oral antibiotics may be indicated, depending on severity. Prevention of flares includes frequent moisturization, low-potency topical steroids when indicated, and identification and avoidance of allergens. Typical triggers include foods, pets, soaps, lotions, makeup, and detergents. Referral to a dermatologist or allergist may be necessary in severe or refractory cases.

 QUESTIONS

59-1. B.J.'s father wants to know whether he can bathe B.J., since she seems to enjoy the feeling of the water on her skin. What is the most appropriate recommendation about bathing children with AD?

A. Bathing in hot water and scrubbing vigorously will help with itching.

B. The child should be bathed twice daily with soap and warm water to decrease risk of skin infection.

C. Baths should be avoided, because they will exacerbate the rash and dryness.

D. Brief, tepid baths without soap, when followed immediately by emollient, are hydrating for the skin.

59-2. B.J.'s father wants to know if she will develop asthma, like her brother. What is the most accurate statement regarding the risk of asthma in children with AD?

A. All children with AD eventually develop asthma as well.

B. Asthma is more common among children with AD than in the general population.

C. Development of asthma is no more common in children with AD than those without AD.

D. Because B.J. has not yet been diagnosed with asthma at this age, she will not develop it.

59-3. B.J.'s father is concerned about B.J.'s infant sister's risk of developing asthma and AD. He and his wife have heard that breast-feeding can prevent the development of these allergic (atopic) conditions. What is the best statement regarding the etiology of atopy and the role of breastfeeding?

 A. Atopic conditions are related to prenatal exposures, not postnatal exposures.
 B. Atopy is inherited, so the infant's risk is predetermined and cannot be modified.
 C. Breastfeeding has been associated with decreased atopy in infants, especially those with risk factors.
 D. Atopic conditions can be prevented by early exposure to a variety of foods, rather than exclusive breastfeeding.

59-4. B.J.'s father is concerned when you mention the possibility of using a topical corticosteroid to help control B.J.'s acute eczema flare. What is the most accurate statement about the risks of appropriate use of topical steroids in children with mild or moderate eczema?

 A. Growth retardation occurs in the majority of patients with chronic use.
 B. Symptoms of glucocorticoid excess (Cushing's syndrome) are common, but tend to be mild.
 C. Significant side effects are rare.
 D. Topical corticosteroids should never be used in children younger than 2 years.

ANSWERS

59-1. D. Bathing in hot water and scrubbing with soap will actually exacerbate dryness and itchiness of the skin. Tepid water baths are recommended, and additives such as oatmeal may be helpful for additional relief. An oral antihistamine such as diphenhydramine can help reduce itching, but may cause drowsiness during the day. Trimming fingernails short prevents excoriation of the skin, and the use of cotton gloves at night may further reduce damage from scratching. Regular moisturization, especially immediately after bathing, hydrates and heals the skin.

59-2. B. The exact relationship between asthma and AD as well as other atopic conditions is unclear. However, infants and children with AD have a higher incidence of asthma than the general population. Most children have shown some signs of asthma (such as this child's history of recurrent wheezing with upper respiratory infections) by the time they are diagnosed with AD. Asthma may develop at any age.

59-3. C. Breastfeeding has a number of proven benefits for newborn infants. In terms of its role in preventing development of atopy, multiple studies have resulted in somewhat disparate findings. The overall trend is one of protection from atopy, and the protective effect, if any, seems to be greatest in infants with risk factors for development of atopy. Therefore, the consensus is to recommend breastfeeding in all infants; those with risk factors for atopy are most likely to benefit from the additional protective effects of breastfeeding against development of atopy.

59-4. C. When used properly, topical steroids rarely cause significant side effects in patients with mild or moderate eczema. Low to high potencies of topical steroids are available, and should be selected based on the location and severity of the rash. In general, the lowest-potency agent that controls the patient's symptoms should be employed, and prolonged use or use on extensive areas of skin should be avoided. Higher-potency steroids should not be applied to the eyelids and other areas of delicate skin. Children with severe eczema or those who use moderate- or high-potency topical steroids for prolonged periods of time may have some systemic side effects. The most common side effect is thinning or sensitivity of the skin. Very rarely, systemic symptoms of glucocorticoid excess have been reported with prolonged use of high-potency topical steroids over large areas of the body.

SUGGESTED ADDITIONAL READING

Friedman NJ. The role of breast-feeding in the development of allergies and asthma. *J Allergy Clin Immunol.* 2005;115(6): 1238–1248.

Pink Eye

CC/ID: 5-year-old girl sent home from school for "pink eye."

HPI: N.J. is a spunky 5-year-old girl who woke up this morning with her right eye crusted shut. Her foster mother washed it off and noticed that the white part of the eye was pink; the child seemed fine, however, so she sent her to school. N.J. was sent home from school by her teacher, who said she needed to see the doctor because she might be contagious. N.J. has had a recent runny nose and has been coughing and sneezing for a few days, just like most of the kids in her classroom. Mother says that N.J. has been rubbing her eye, but has not been complaining of pain or itching.

PMHx: Seasonal allergies

SHx: Lives with foster parents, two rabbits, and a lizard.

Meds: None

All: NKDA

Immun: UTD

THOUGHT QUESTIONS

- What are possible causes of a pink eye in a child this age?
- What will you look for on further history or physical exam to help you make a diagnosis?

DISCUSSION

The appearance of pink color, or "injection," on the surface of the eye is most often caused by inflammation of the conjunctiva, the mucosal surface of the eye. Infection, allergy, and trauma are all possible causes of conjunctivitis. Other obstructive or inflammatory conditions of the eye, such as glaucoma or uveitis (inflammation of the middle part of the eye, including the iris, vitreous, and choroid), can also cause an injected eye and should be especially considered when pain or visual change is a prominent symptom. In neonates, an injected eye can be a sign of neonatal conjunctivitis (termed "ophthalmia neonatorum") or may be caused by complications from an obstructed tear duct (dacryostenosis), chemical sensitivity, or birth trauma.

The history should focus on eliciting associated local symptoms (pain, itching, visual change, discharge), systemic symptoms, and recent illness or trauma. On physical exam, describe the anatomic location of the injection or inflammation (conjunctiva, eyelid, iris, sclera); other findings, such as edema, exudate, or tearing; and function, such as extraocular movements and vision. An examination with a Wood's lamp and fluorescein (a fluorescent dye) or with a slit lamp may be indicated when a foreign body, abrasion, or ulceration of the surface of the eye is suspected, or when infection or inflammation inside the eye is considered.

 ## CASE CONTINUED

On further history, N.J. has never had these symptoms before. She denies changes in vision, and states that her eye feels "sticky." Mother and daughter both deny recent eye trauma.

VS: Temp 36.8°C (98.5°F), HR 110, RR 22; Weight 18 kg (35%)

PE: *Gen:* alert, playful, well-appearing child in no acute distress, with a pink right eye. *HEENT:* The right eyelid is mildly erythematous and puffy above and below the eye, but nontender. The right bulbar and palpebral conjunctivae are injected and edematous. A yellowish exudate is seen pooling in the corners of the eye. The left conjunctiva is mildly injected. EOMs are full without pain, and pupillary reflexes are intact and symmetric. Mild rhinorrhea is noted, and both TMs are pearly, translucent, and mobile. No adenopathy is noted. *Lungs:* clear. *CV:* RR&R; soft flow murmur at left upper sternal border. *Skin:* no rashes; pink and well perfused. Remainder of exam within normal limits.

THOUGHT QUESTIONS

- What is the most likely cause of this child's pink eye?
- How would you like to manage her condition, and when can she go back to school?

DISCUSSION

This child's physical exam is consistent with conjunctivitis, which can be caused by infection (viral, bacterial), allergy (allergic rhinitis, local allergen on surface of eye), or irritation (trauma, foreign body, chemical irritation) (Fig. 60-1). The presence of a "sticky" sensation, yellow exudate, and mild lid swelling is consistent with infectious conjunctivitis. Although infectious conjunctivitis is usually viral in adults and older children, pathologic bacteria (most commonly *Streptococcus pneumoniae* and nontypeable *Haemophilus influenza*) can be found in more than 50% of cases of infectious

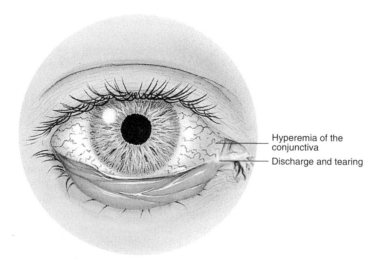

Hyperemia of the conjunctiva

Discharge and tearing

FIGURE **60-1.** Findings in conjunctivitis.

conjunctivitis in children younger than 6. Because the condition is highly contagious, treatment with antibiotic ointment or drops (such as erythromycin or polymyxin B/trimethoprim) is usually recommended. In older children, or those in whom a clear viral syndrome is present, supportive care alone may be used.

When ipsilateral otitis media is seen, systemic antibiotics effective against *H. influenzae*, a common cause of conjunctivitis-otitis syndrome, are recommended. For allergic conjunctivitis, known allergens should be avoided, and systemic or ophthalmic antihistamines may be used for symptomatic relief. Chemical or traumatic conjunctivitis should be treated with avoidance of the offending agent, and patching of the eye for comfort. An ophthalmologic exam may be indicated to rule out damage to the surface of the eye.

QUESTIONS

60-1. A 6-year-old girl presents to the clinic with an acutely painful, mildly injected eye. The conjunctiva is clear, and on slit-lamp examination she is found to have acute inflammation of the iris and evidence of chronic inflammation in the anterior vitreous, consistent with uveitis. What condition is most likely to be associated with chronic uveitis in children?

    A. Acute lymphocytic leukemia
    B. Kawasaki syndrome
    C. Juvenile rheumatoid arthritis
    D. Henoch-Schönlein purpura

60-2. You are examining a 4-day-old newborn in the nursery and note that the infant's left eyelid is swollen, with a yellow crust on the eyelashes. The conjunctiva is markedly injected and thickened, and yellow-green exudate is seen pooling in the palpebral fissure. The infant was born vaginally without difficulty to a mother without prenatal care. What organisms should be considered likely causes of this infant's ophthalmia neonatorum?

    A. Group B streptococci and *Escherichia coli*
    B. *Staphylococcus aureus* and *Streptococcus pneumoniae*
    C. *Neisseria gonorrhoeae* and *Chlamydia trachomatis*
    D. *Haemophilus influenzae* and *Pseudomonas aeruginosa*

60-3. A 4-year-old child is brought in after he developed acute pain and inability to open his eye while playing in the park. Anesthetic eye drops are administered, and a 1-mm fragment of pine needle is removed from the surface of his eye. Fluorescein is used to stain the surface of the eye, which pools in a small corneal abrasion under the upper lid. When the anesthetic wears off, the boy states that he feels better and is able to open his eye, but he feels like "something is still in there." Vision and extraocular movements are normal. What should the appropriate management of this child include at this point?

A. Referral to an ophthalmologist
B. Patching of the affected eye for comfort
C. Vasoconstricting eye drops to reduce redness
D. A slit-lamp examination for internal foreign body

60-4. The medical student you are working with mentions that she has seen ophthalmologists use corticosteroid eye drops to treat viral conjunctivitis. What is the major contraindication to the use of topical steroids for symptomatic relief in viral conjunctivitis?

A. Suspected HSV infection
B. Suspected uveitis
C. Suspected allergic conjunctivitis
D. History of glaucoma in the family

ANSWERS

60-1. C. Uveitis refers to inflammation of the middle part of the eye, from the iris to the choroid. Uveitis is rare overall in children, who account for around 6% of cases. Juvenile rheumatoid arthritis (JRA) is the most frequent cause of chronic uveitis among children. Of the three types of JRA (pauciarticular, polyarticular, and systemic), the pauciarticular type is the most likely to be associated with uveitis. Pauciarticular onset is the most common type of JRA, and is five times as common in girls. The cause of uveitis and arthritis in JRA remains unknown. About 10% of JRA patients develop uveitis. The involved eyes are often asymptomatic, but 30% to 40% of patients with JRA-associated uveitis experience severe loss of vision as a consequence of their condition. Most patients respond to topical corticosteroids; a minority require the use of systemic immunomodulatory agents to control their condition.

60-2. C. This neonate has ophthalmia neonatorum, which refers to conjunctivitis within the first month of life. It may be chemical or infectious in cause. This infant's unilateral presentation, including injected, thickened conjunctiva and purulent discharge, suggests an infectious cause. For infection that presents in the first few days of life, such as in this infant, the most common causes are organisms acquired through the birth canal, such as *N. gonorrhoeae* and *C. trachomatis*. Less common causes, which usually present after the first week of life, include HSV, *S. aureus*, *H. influenzae*, and *P. aeruginosa*. *Chlamydia trachomatis* may cause conjunctivitis up to 8 weeks after birth, and is often associated with concurrent pneumonia. Chemical conjunctivitis in the neonate may be caused by birth trauma or by sensitivity to topical agents applied to the skin or eye. It is usually bilateral, with a serous rather than purulent discharge.

60-3. B. This child has evidence of a corneal abrasion after a foreign body. The sensation of there being "something still in the eye" is common with mild corneal abrasions. Severe pain, inability to open or move the eye, or change in vision suggests a more significant injury and should be investigated with additional examinations. The management of mild corneal abrasions is supportive, and may include patching the eye for comfort. For some children, patching the eye is distracting, and may be deferred. Bacterial conjunctival superinfection may occur after a foreign body is removed from the eye, and may be managed with topical antibiotic ointment or drops if evidence of conjunctivitis develops.

60-4. A. The absolute contraindication to topical corticosteroids for symptomatic relief in viral conjunctivitis is suspected or proven HSV infection. When used in this instance, topical steroids can lead to further spread of this potentially dangerous ocular infection. Immunocompetent children with suspected HSV infection of or near the eye should be started on systemic acyclovir and referred urgently to an ophthalmologist for evaluation. Glaucoma or cataracts are considered possible complications of long-term use of topical corticosteroids, but a family history of glaucoma would not preclude their use for a brief period for symptomatic relief. Uveitis is usually treated with topical corticosteroids. Allergic conjunctivitis is not a contraindication for the use of topical corticosteroids.

SUGGESTED ADDITIONAL READING

Greenberg MF. The red eye in childhood. *Pediatr Clin North Am.* 2003;50(1):105–124.
Leibowitz HM. The red eye. *N Engl J Med.* 2000;343(5):345–351.

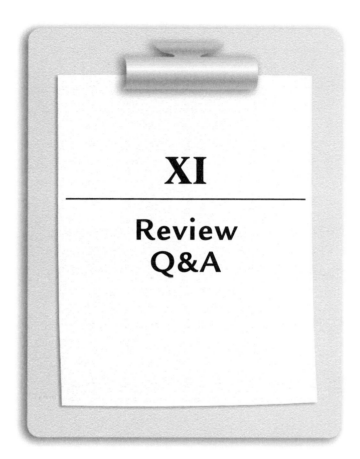

XI

Review
Q&A

Questions

1. A 2-year-old toddler is brought in to the clinic for fever and refusing to drink. Her exam is significant for a red oropharynx and a distinct 3-cm, very tender, erythematous, warm mass anterior to the sternocleidomastoid. She has been otherwise healthy. Vital signs are normal except for a temperature of 38.9°C (102°F). The toddler is smiling and appears well hydrated, but will not turn her head. The rest of the exam is within normal limits. What is the most likely cause of this child's neck mass?
   A. Reactive adenopathy
   B. Infected thyroglossal duct cyst
   C. Infectious mononucleosis
   D. Acute suppurative adenitis
   E. Epiglottitis

2. A 16-month-old girl is being evaluated for the acute presentation of a neck mass. The mass is warm, tender, and red. It is located 2 cm below the chin, at the midline of the neck, and is noted to be draining milky white fluid. What is the most likely diagnosis?
   A. Reactive adenopathy
   B. Infected thyroglossal duct cyst
   C. Infectious mononucleosis
   D. Acute suppurative adenitis
   E. Epiglottitis

Questions 3–5
An 8-month-old girl is brought to the clinic with 3 days of fever. Her parents deny runny nose, cough, rash, vomiting, or diarrhea. She has been refusing solids but drinking well, and her urine output has been adequate. Her past medical history is unremarkable, and she is up to date on her immunizations. Her older brother is sick with a cold. Her vital signs include T of 39.5°C (103°F), HR of 160–180, and normal RR and BP. She is fussy but quite consolable, drinks from her bottle, smiles, and appears well hydrated, with a moist mouth and brisk capillary refill. Her exam is completely within normal limits.

3. What is the *most likely* cause of her fever?
   A. A viral infection
   B. Kawasaki disease
   C. Occult bacteremia
   D. Pyelonephritis
   E. Teething

4. The patient's mother wants to know why her heart is beating so quickly. What is the most appropriate next step at this point regarding the child's tachycardia?
   A. Administer adenosine.
   B. Start an IV and give a bolus of normal saline.
   C. Treat her fever.
   D. Perform carotid massage.
   E. Order an EKG.

5. Your preceptor asks if you would like to perform any labs on this well-appearing infant with fever without a source. You confirm that the infant's immunizations are up to date, including three doses of the pneumococcal vaccine. What is the most appropriate approach to this child at this time?
   A. No labs, because she appears well and is fully immunized.
   B. Send a CBC and blood culture.
   C. Send a urine sample for urinalysis and culture.
   D. Send CBC, blood culture, and urine sample for urinalysis and culture.
   E. Send CBC, blood culture, and urine and perform a lumbar puncture.

Questions 6–8
You are examining a newborn on the third day of life in the nursery and note that the infant appears jaundiced. The exam is otherwise normal. The infant was born at term to a G2, P1 mother with good prenatal care, by C-section for failure to progress. The infant was vigorous at delivery, with Apgar scores of 8 and 9 at 1 and 5 minutes, respectively. Prenatal labs were unremarkable. Mother's blood type is O+, and the baby's is A+. The baby has been at the breast every 1 to 2 hours, and the mother's milk came in last night. The infant is urinating every 6 hours, and has passed meconium four times since birth. Birth weight was 3,420 g; today's weight is 3,390 g.

6. A visiting medical student asks you why you are interested in knowing about the ABO and Rh blood types of the mother and infant. What is the most accurate statement regarding the results of the blood typing of this mother and infant?

A. The blood types are matched.
B. The mother's serum has antibodies against the baby's red cell type.
C. The baby's serum has antibodies against the mother's red cell type.
D. The baby's red cells may attack the mother's red cells.
E. The mother's red cells may attack the baby's red cells.

7. You order a total and direct bilirubin, and the results show a total bilirubin of 12.6 and a direct bilirubin of 8.2. What is your interpretation of these results?
A. These lab results are normal in the newborn.
B. This infant has an unconjugated hyperbilirubinemia, which is likely physiologic.
C. This infant has an unconjugated hyperbilirubinemia, which is likely pathologic.
D. This infant has a conjugated hyperbilirubinemia, which is likely physiologic.
E. This infant has a conjugated hyperbilirubinemia, which is likely pathologic.

8. The infant appears well and has normal vital signs. What should your next step be regarding the management of this infant?
A. Reassure the mother that this is physiologic jaundice.
B. Switch from breast milk to formula.
C. Start phototherapy.
D. Perform exchange transfusion.
E. Investigate the etiology of the hyperbilirubinemia.

Questions 9–11
A 4-year-old boy is brought into the clinic for "looking tired." His mother is concerned that he has not been sleeping well, because there is swelling around his eyes. Mom also notes that her son's ankles looked swollen at the end of the day yesterday. On further history, he has had a decrease in appetite and in urine output, but no change in color of the urine. He had an upper respiratory infection 3 weeks ago. Growth parameters and vital signs are within normal limits for age, including a normal blood pressure. The exam shows a tired-appearing, pale young boy, with periorbital edema. The exam is otherwise noncontributory. A CBC and electrolyte panel (including BUN and creatinine) are within normal limits, and a urinalysis reveals 1–5 RBCs, no WBCs, small ketones, and large (4+) protein; otherwise, it is negative. His albumin level is 2.1.

9. You suspect a renal process. What is the most likely explanation for this patient's symptoms and lab results?
A. Poststreptococcal glomerulonephritis
B. Nephrotic syndrome
C. Acute renal failure
D. Pyelonephritis
E. Vesicoureteral reflux

10. To confirm the diagnosis, the most appropriate test would be
A. 24-hour urine collection
B. Urine culture
C. Renal ultrasound
D. Renal biopsy
E. Voiding cystourethrogram (VCUG)

11. After confirming the diagnosis, what would be your next step in management?
A. Admit him for dialysis.
B. Treat with antibiotics.
C. Treat with steroids and salt restriction.
D. Perform a renal biopsy.
E. Start maintenance IV fluids.

Questions 12–18
Match each rash description with one of the infectious organisms or conditions in the following list:
A. Measles
B. Herpes simplex virus
C. *Candida*
D. Roseola
E. Parvovirus
F. Varicella
G. Impetigo
H. Rocky Mountain spotted fever
I. Meningococcemia
J. Lyme disease
K. Coxsackie virus
L. Tinea corporis
M. Toxic shock syndrome

12. Distinct, pruritic clear vesicles on an erythematous base, appearing in crops on the trunk, extremities, and face.

13. Blanching, maculopapular exanthem starting on the trunk and spreading up to the face, in a well-appearing infant who had 2 days of fever prior to the onset of the rash.

14. Painful cluster of milky vesicles on an erythematous base on the finger of a toddler.

15. Palpable, nonblanching purpura appearing rapidly on the limbs of an ill-appearing, febrile teen.

16. Beefy red, well-demarcated, confluent papular rash in the creases of the diaper area in an infant.

17. Oozing, honey-crusted, ruptured vesicles around the mouth of a drooling toddler.

18. Annular patch with thickened, scaly border and central clearing on the cheek of a school-aged child.

19. You are performing a school physical on a 14-year-old boy. His physical exam, including hearing and vision screens, are normal for age, and he has no known illnesses. His growth and development have been appropriate for age. His mother mentions that she is concerned that all of his grades have been falling for the last 2 years, and he is currently at risk of failing math and being kicked off the basketball team. After talking further with the teen and his parents, you elicit information that suggests that this teen may have a learning disability. Under what circumstances would this teen's public school be required to perform a learning assessment and provide an individualized education plan (IEP)?
   A. After neurologic causes for school failure have been ruled out
   B. At the request of his primary care physician
   C. At the request of his teacher
   D. At the request of his parents
   E. Public schools are not required to perform a learning assessment unless they believe it to be necessary.

20. You are seeing a 14-year-old teenage girl for an asthma exacerbation, and decide to perform an assessment of health risk factors. When you talk to the teen alone, she reveals that she smokes marijuana with her friends about once a week and wonders if this could be contributing to her asthma. Suddenly she looks scared, and asks you whether you are going to tell her parents about her marijuana use. What is your most appropriate response regarding the confidentiality of this information?

    A. You are obligated to tell her parents about her drug use, since it affects her health.

    B. You are not allowed to repeat any information relayed to you in confidence by a teen.

    C. You are obligated to respect her confidentiality, unless the information presents a significant danger to her or to others.

    D. You will only tell her parents about her drug use if they ask you about it directly.

    E. You can respect her confidentiality if she signs a confidentiality agreement.

21. A 5-year-old boy presents to the ED with difficulty breathing that has been getting worse since leaving a picnic today where he was playing with balloons. He has a past history of myelomeningocele repair and has required frequent bladder catheterization. His mother notes no drug allergies. His vital signs show a RR of 50/min, BP of 75/45, and HR of 140/min. His physical exam shows severe respiratory distress and wheezing, and diffuse urticarial lesions on his trunk and extremities. What is the most appropriate initial step?

    A. CBC and blood culture

    B. Epinephrine

    C. Systemic corticosteroids and antihistamines

    D. Neuroimaging

    E. Beta-adrenergic agonists and inhaled corticosteroids

Questions 22–25

Select the answer that best reflects the most likely etiology from the following choices:

    A. *Mycoplasma pneumoniae*

    B. *Bordatella pertussis*

    C. *Streptococcus pneumoniae*

    D. *Chlamydia trachomatis*

    E. *Chlamydia pneumoniae*

    F. Respiratory syncytial virus

    G. Parainfluenza virus

22. A 5-week-old infant boy presents with cough and respiratory distress. He is afebrile and has mild tachypnea and wheezing on exam. His chest x-ray shows bilateral interstitial infiltrates. His mother notes that his only past medical problem was a bout of "eye infection" after he was born.

23. A 2-year-old girl presents to the ED with a 2-day history of fever, worsening cough, and shortness of breath. She is ill appearing, tachypneic, and has decreased breath sounds unilaterally with crackles. Her CXR shows a lobar consolidation, and a CBC reveals an elevated WBC count.

24. A parent in your clinic is concerned about her 6-week-old infant girl. She has had almost 1 week of congestion and rhinorrhea, which has now progressed to uncontrollable coughing episodes that are accompanied by choking and gagging. She is afebrile and seems to be well when not coughing. This morning, she had an episode of "turning blue" while coughing.

25. A now 6-month-old infant boy who was born prematurely at 25 weeks' GA presents with respiratory distress and rapid breathing. He is wheezing on exam, with fine crackles bilaterally and chest wall retractions. His oxygen saturation is 88% on room air. His parents note that everyone in his day care is sick, and that he has had a low-grade fever and rhinorrhea for the past several days.

26. A 14-year-old boy presents to the ED with scrotal pain over the last 2 to 3 days. He is afebrile and has no nausea or vomiting. He denies any trauma and is not sexually active. His exam reveals unilateral pain limited to the upper testicular pole and an accompanying "blue dot" visible through the scrotum. His cremasteric reflex is present. What is the most appropriate next step in management?
   A. Immediate surgical management
   B. Surgery, radiation, and chemotherapy with counseling
   C. Reassurance, rest, and analgesia
   D. Prompt antibiotic therapy
   E. Transillumination and surgery

27. An 11-year-old girl presents with a 3-day history of abdominal pain. She has had nausea, nonbloody and nonbilious vomiting, and fever. She denies any cough, rash, or diarrhea. Her pain, which was initially centered around the umbilicus, was worse yesterday on her right lower side, and today is diffuse throughout her abdomen. She appears ill and dehydrated, and refuses to move during the examination. Her exam reflects guarding, rigidity, rebound, and diffuse tenderness. What is the most likely diagnosis?
   A. Intussusception
   B. Appendicitis with perforation
   C. Appendicitis
   D. Pancreatitis
   E. Right lower lobe pneumonia

28. A 15-year-old boy presents with unilateral knee pain that has been bothering him for the last several months. He is an active athlete and has attributed the pain to sports-related injury. His parents are concerned because he seems more fatigued lately, with low-grade fevers and some noted weight loss, all of which he attributes to ill contacts at school and his active lifestyle. His exam reveals a unilaterally painful, swollen knee with a palpable soft tissue mass. You obtain a plain x-ray, which reveals diffuse, lytic lesions affecting the femoral diaphysis, with an "onion-skin" appearance of the cortex. Empiric antibiotic therapy for her acute illness should be targeted against which organisms?

- A. *Streptococcus pneumonia* and *Moraxella catarrhalis*
- B. *Staphylococcus aureus* and *Pseudomonas aeruginosa*
- C. *Aspergillus* and *Candida* spp
- D. *Mycobacterium avium-complex*
- E. *Escherichia coli* and *Proteus* spp

29. A 5-month-old girl is suspected of having seizures. She is noted to have flexor-extensor episodes that the parents say appear like "abdominal crunches" lasting a few seconds each. Her EEG is notable for hypsarrhythmia. Which of the following may represent an appropriate next step in therapy?

- A. Therapy with antipyretics and fever avoidance
- B. Therapy with ACTH and corticosteroids
- C. Therapy with ethosuximide
- D. Therapy with stimulants
- E. Reassurance and education

30. The parents of a 3-year-old girl are concerned about an abdominal mass that was noted on a routine examination. She appears healthy but complains of mild abdominal pain. Her blood pressure is elevated, and she is noted to have hematuria on a screening urinalysis. An MRI confirms a completely intrarenal mass that does not cross the midline, and a tissue biopsy shows embryonic renal cells. When counseling the parents, which of the following statements is appropriate to include in your discussion about the diagnosis?

- A. Watchful waiting is indicated.
- B. The overall prognosis is poor.
- C. Therapy involves surgery and chemotherapy.
- D. Diagnosis is confirmed by urine catecholamine studies.
- E. This disorder has an infantile autosomal recessive form.

31. At a well-child exam, you are examining a patient who is able to sit alone without support, is starting to pull to stand, uses "mama" and "dada" nonspecifically, has an immature pincer grasp, and has a noticeable parachute postural reaction. Assuming average development, what age is this child most likely to be?

- A. 2 months
- B. 4 months
- C. 6 months

D. 9 months
E. 12 months

32. An 8-year-old girl with cystic fibrosis is admitted to the hospital for bronchopneumonia and respiratory distress. Which of the following antibiotics is appropriate to use empirically in her treatment?

A. Amoxicillin and clavulanic acid
B. Tobramycin and ceftazidime
C. Ampicillin and metronidazole (Flagyl)
D. Azithromycin
E. Amphotericin B

33. You are seeing a patient with suspected Prader-Willi syndrome. In describing this disease, which of the following is an appropriate statement to include in a discussion with the parents?

A. Affected patients have hypotonia, hypogonadism, and mild mental retardation.
B. Affected patients have a karyotype of 45XO.
C. Affected patients have symptoms caused by teratogenic exposures.
D. Affected patients appear to have a "happy-puppet"-like syndrome.
E. Affected patients usually have a trinucleotide repeat causing a detectable breakage on the affected chromosome.

34. A 15-month-old boy has a history of recurrent pneumonia, sinusitis, and otitis episodes, often requiring hospitalization. His previous illnesses have been slow to respond to conventional antibiotic therapy, even though *Streptococcus pneumoniae* and *Haemophilus influenzae* were identified as causative organisms. You suspect a primary humoral immunodeficiency. Which of the following laboratory tests is most likely to support your diagnosis?

A. Mitogen stimulation response test
B. Flow cytometry
C. Nitroblue tetrazolium test
D. Delayed hypersensitivity skin testing
E. Quantitative and qualitative immunoglobulin tests

Questions 35–37
Select the answer that best reflects the most likely etiology from the following choices.

A. Viral laryngotracheobronchitis
B. Bacterial tracheitis
C. Epiglottitis
D. Foreign body aspiration
E. Retropharyngeal abscess
F. Viral tonsillopharyngitis

35. A 5-year-old girl presents with respiratory distress, stridor, lethargy, and fever of sudden onset. She is toxic appearing, drooling, has marked retractions, and is leaning forward in a "tripod" position for comfort. Her immunization status is unknown.

36. A 3-year-old boy presents with a 3-day history of fever, and progressive refusal to drink or eat. There is minimal respiratory distress, no stridor, and mild torticollis. The throat exam reveals a bulging posterior pharyngeal wall.

37. A 15-year-old boy presents with a 10-day history of rhinorrhea, headache, fever, and throat pain. He was seen a week ago and prescribed amoxicillin. He appears dehydrated, and his exam reveals marked cervical lymphadenopathy, a maculopapular rash, and grayish exudates bilaterally on his tonsils. His symptoms are unchanged since the administration of amoxicillin, and the rash appeared 2 days ago.

38. You are assessing a child during a routine well-child visit. The parents report that their daughter can copy a circle, uses three-word sentences, can kick a ball, and enjoys riding a tricycle. Upon questioning her, she can report her full name, age, and sex. If this child is developmentally normal for age, what is her likely age?
- A. 24 months
- B. 30 months
- C. 3 years
- D. 4 years
- E. 5 years

39. An 18-month-old girl presents with nearly 2 days of emesis and intermittent bouts of abdominal pain. The parents report that the emesis is nonbloody and that yesterday, when not in pain, she was quite playful. Her physical examination now reveals a lethargic, moderately to severely dehydrated child with a palpable tubular mass in her right abdomen without peritoneal signs. The parents report no rashes, but say that she has had reduced urine output, and that her latest diaper had mucus and blood-tinged stool. After fluid resuscitation, which of the following is the most appropriate next step in the management of this patient?
- A. Stool culture for ova and parasites
- B. Oral rehydration therapy
- C. Emergent dialysis
- D. Contrast or air enema
- E. Technetium-99 pertechnetate scan

40. A 12-year-old girl is evaluated for a 3-month history of diarrhea and abdominal pain. Her physical examination reveals perianal skin tags and tender nodules on her shins. Which of the following is correct regarding her likely diagnosis?

    A. Lower endoscopy likely reveals skip lesions and transmural involvement.

    B. She may have a significantly increased risk of developing colon cancer.

    C. Antineutrophil cytoplasmic antibody is nearly 80% positive.

    D. A history of camping near mountain streams is likely.

    E. Symptoms resolve with a gluten-free diet.

41. You are counseling the family of a newborn child with Down syndrome. When reviewing associated findings and increased risk of disease, which of the following statements is appropriate to include in your discussion?

    A. Rockerbottom feet are common.

    B. Mortality is nearly 50% within the first 4 to 6 weeks.

    C. Risk of leukemia is similar to the general population.

    D. Clinodactyly will improve over time.

    E. Radiographic screening for atlantoaxial instability will be indicated later in life.

42. A 15-month-old boy presents this morning to the ED with an acute onset of bloody emesis and diarrhea that started 2 hours ago. He was noted earlier to be well, but his caregiver suspects an ingestion because her prenatal vitamin bottle was found to be open, with several tablets missing. After initial stabilization, which of the following best describes the appropriate management of this child?

    A. Administration of activated charcoal and whole-bowel irrigation

    B. Supportive management and family safety education

    C. Administration of ipecac syrup and D-penicillamine

    D. Examination of serum iron levels and administration of deferoxamine

    E. Examination of liver function tests and administration of pyridoxine

43. A 15-year-old girl presents with delayed onset of puberty. Along with no breast tissue and no menarche, she is short for her age, and her exam is notable for a webbed neck with mild kyphoscoliosis. She is also noted to have increased levels of follicle-stimulating hormone (FSH) and luteinizing hormone (LH), but low estradiol levels. Her past medical history is notable for a horseshoe kidney and a repaired coarctation of the aorta. Which of the following is characteristic of her most likely diagnosis?

A. Further evaluation may reveal anosmia.

B. Management with L-thyroxine provides a full clinical resolution.

C. Inheritance pattern is autosomal dominant.

D. Southern blot and PCR analysis show CGG repeats on the FMR-1 gene.

E. Newborns may present with congenital lymphedema of the hands and feet.

44. A 9-year-old boy with asthma, on no current medications, presents for a follow-up visit. His mother reports that he has wheezing or coughing episodes at least twice a week, but not daily. This past month, he also has had three episodes of coughing and respiratory difficulty at night. Which of the following best describes an appropriate course of long-term management for this patient?

A. Daily rescue therapy with inhaled albuterol

B. Daily low-dose inhaled corticosteroid

C. Staying inside to avoid potential allergens

D. Daily inhaled long-acting beta-agonist

E. Daily inhaled anticholinergics

45. A 16-year-old girl presents with persistence of epistaxis over the past few weeks. Upon further history, she reports menorrhagia and reveals that she bruises easily and that she had excessive bleeding after a recent wisdom tooth extraction. She denies any joint complaints and has otherwise been healthy. Laboratory results indicate that her PT is normal, an activated PTT is prolonged, and her bleeding time is prolonged. What is the most likely diagnosis?

A. von Willebrand's disease

B. Hemophilia A

C. Vitamin K deficiency

D. Idiopathic thrombocytopenia

E. Wiskott-Aldrich syndrome

46. A 10-day-old girl presents with jaundice, poor feeding, and emesis for the past few days. She had been born at home and is exclusively breastfed. She had been initially well appearing, but was noted to be somewhat lethargic over the past few days. Physical exam now reveals an ill-appearing infant with jaundice and hepatomegaly. Lab results show evidence of hypoglycemia, hepatic failure, acidosis, and a blood culture that is positive for *Escherichia coli*. Which of the following is the most likely diagnosis?

A. Hereditary fructose intolerance

B. Galactosemia

    C. Gaucher's disease
    D. Phenylketonuria
    E. Ornithine transcarbamylase deficiency

47. A term newborn boy is being evaluated in the NICU. He is small for his gestational age and appears ill. His physical exam is significant for congenital cataracts, a patent ductus arteriosus, hepatosplenomegaly, and a "blueberry muffin" type of purpuric rash. Which of the following congenital infections is most likely?
    A. Rubella
    B. Toxoplasmosis
    C. Cytomegalovirus
    D. Herpes simplex virus
    E. Syphilis

48. You are evaluating an 18-month-old boy for trauma. He had been brought in by his caregiver after he tripped and fell. Which of the following fractures would be the most suggestive of nonaccidental trauma in this patient?
    A. Tibial spiral fracture with fibula intact
    B. Salter-Harris grade V physeal fracture
    C. Metaphyseal chip fracture of the femur
    D. Clavicular fracture
    E. Supracondylar fracture of the humerus

49. A 9-year-old boy presents with severe respiratory distress from an acute asthma exacerbation. After his ABCs are secured, he is administered oxygen and continuous inhaled albuterol, and intravenous access is established. Which of the following therapies is best suited to treat the underlying inflammatory process?
    A. Magnesium sulfate
    B. Montelukast
    C. Theophylline
    D. Epinephrine
    E. Methylprednisolone

50. You are reviewing immunizations with a family in your office. In reviewing the risks and benefits of immunizations, which of the following would be an absolute contraindication to vaccine administration?
    A. Varicella vaccine in patients with egg allergy
    B. MMR in a leukemia patient receiving chemotherapy
    C. DTaP in a patient with rhinorrhea and fever to 38.2°C (100.8°F)
    D. Inactivated polio vaccine (IPV) in a patient with a household contact with HIV
    E. Meningococcal conjugate vaccine in patients receiving chemotherapy

51. A 15-year-old girl with cystic fibrosis presents with respiratory distress and hypoxia. You suspect a bacterial pulmonary infection and start empiric therapy. Which of the following is the most appropriate parenteral antibiotic regimen for this patient?

A. Azithromycin and ampicillin
B. Cefotetan and metronidazole
C. Ampicillin/sulbactam and clindamycin
D. Piperacillin/tazobactam and tobramycin
E. Cefazolin and oxacillin

52. You are evaluating a 15-month-old boy with feeding difficulty and intermittent emesis. The parents report that he has been having frequent episodes of nonbloody, nonbilious emesis, generally after feeding. Occasionally during a feed, he also appears to be uncomfortable and tends to arch backward and position his neck to one side. Poor weight gain is noted, and the physical exam is notable for mild wheezing. Which of the following statements best fits the most likely diagnosis?

A. Chest x-ray and antibiotics are indicated.
B. Point tenderness at the costochondral junction is likely.
C. pH probe is likely to reveal the diagnosis.
D. Screening for metabolic disease is indicated.
E. Bronchodilators and steroids provide complete resolution.

53. A 6-year-old girl presents to your office with fatigue, low-grade fever, and anorexia over the past few weeks. Her physical exam is significant for a violaceous periorbital heliotropic rash that also covers her nasal bridge, hypertrophic and erythematous skin lesions over her knuckles, and proximal muscle weakness. There have been no preceding illnesses, and she has been taking no medications. Which of the following statements best reflects her likely diagnosis?

A. Corticosteroids are contraindicated.
B. There is a high association of malignancy.
C. Calcium deposition in the skin, muscle, and fascia is common.
D. Positive anti–double-stranded DNA titers suggest the diagnosis.
E. Creatine kinase levels are generally normal.

54. A 1-hour-old baby boy born at 33 weeks' gestational age becomes increasingly tachypneic with an increased Fio_2 requirement (>60% Fio_2) to maintain blood oxygen saturations above 90%. A CXR was obtained, which showed low lung volumes and a diffusely hazy appearance throughout the lung fields with no free air. An ABG revealed a Pco_2 value of 90 torr. What is the most appropriate immediate management step?

A. Intubate and place a chest tube.
B. Intubate and give a bolus of normal saline.
C. Intubate and give exogenous surfactant.
D. Place umbilical arterial and venous lines and repeat an arterial blood gas.
E. Determine the amniotic fluid lecithin/sphingomyelin (L/S) ratio to determine if the infant has RDS.

55. The labor and delivery service contacts the pediatrics team covering high-risk deliveries regarding a 16-year-old pregnant girl with gestational diabetes who is in preterm labor at 33 weeks. She had an amniocentesis earlier that day to determine the extent of fetal lung maturity. Which of the following is the best predictor of fetal lung maturation in this clinical scenario?
A. Maternal age
B. Gestational age
C. L/S ratio of amniotic fluid
D. Presence of phosphatidylglycerol (PG) in amniotic fluid
E. Prenatal ultrasound showing fetal breathing movements

56. A 1-day-old full-term baby boy is admitted to the NICU for central cyanosis after his mother reported that his color did not seem right during breastfeeding. Physical exam showed a loud pansystolic murmur heard loudest at the left lower sternal border, with bounding peripheral pulses. Over the next few hours the lung exam also revealed crackles bilaterally, and the baby became more tachypneic and had worsening color. An echocardiogram confirmed the diagnosis of the congenital heart disease truncus arteriosus. What is the most likely cause of this baby's worsening condition?
A. Systemic overcirculation
B. Pulmonary overcirculation
C. Patent ductus arteriosus
D. Left ventricular failure
E. Respiratory distress syndrome

57. A full-term newborn infant diagnosed with a hypoplastic left ventricle is admitted to the NICU for management of his congenital heart defect. He is started on a prostaglandin E_1 (PGE_1) infusion in order to maintain patency of his ductus arteriosus to allow systemic perfusion. The bedside nurse reports that he has had three episodes of apnea with marked desaturation requiring moderate stimulation to resume breathing. What is the most likely cause of his apnea?
A. Intraventricular hemorrhage
B. Increased intracranial pressure
C. Pulmonary edema
D. Apnea of prematurity
E. PGE_1 infusion

58. A 2-year-old boy with failure to thrive is being evaluated by a pediatric gastroenterologist. A detailed history reveals that he only passes stools once every 3 to 5 days and had initially failed to pass meconium until nearly 36 hours of age. He has had sporadic bouts of feeding intolerance that included abdominal distension and bilious vomiting, which were always self-resolved. What test will most likely confirm this toddler's underlying diagnosis?

    A. Digital rectal exam
    B. Barium enema showing transition zone
    C. Upper GI series
    D. Rectal biopsy
    E. Anal manometry

59. A newborn infant with Down syndrome is noted to have bilious vomiting following the first feeding. Additional history revealed that there was polyhydramnios in utero. Radiographic studies of the abdomen are most likely to show which of the following findings?

    A. Isolated enlarged gaseous stomach
    B. Barium enema showing transition zone
    C. "Double-bubble" sign
    D. "Corkscrew" appearance of bowel
    E. Pneumatosis intestinalis

60. A full-term newborn infant is noted to have signs of hydrops fetalis demonstrated by mild generalized edema. Further examination reveals he has a low ventricular heart rate of 58 bpm, with no rashes. A chest x-ray reveals no cardiomegaly, and the mother reports having no acute illnesses during her pregnancy. Which of the following laboratory tests from his *mother* could best explain his findings?

    A. Rubella IgM and IgG positive
    B. CMV IgM and IgG positive
    C. Rapid plasma reagent (RPR) positive reactivity
    D. Maternal O+ blood type
    E. ANA positive

61. A 1-month old baby girl is brought into the emergency department via ambulance and breathing 100% oxygen via a face mask after her mother dialed 911 because of the infant's worsening color and respiratory distress. The infant is immediately placed on a cardiorespiratory monitor, which reveals a wide-complex tachycardia consistent with ventricular tachycardia, and a low mean blood pressure of 25 mm Hg. What is the most appropriate next management step?

    A. Synchronized cardioversion
    B. Nonsynchronized defibrillation
    C. Intubation
    D. IV lidocaine infusion
    E. IV procainamide infusion

62. A newborn infant is born with ambiguous genitalia. In the delivery room, the parents are appropriately advised that immediate actions will be taken to determine the sex of their baby. A physical exam reveals no palpable gonads. Which of the following statements is true regarding the key points of congenital adrenal hyperplasia (CAH)?

- A. 17-hydroxylase deficiency accounts for 90% of the cases of CAH.
- B. In 21-hydroxylase deficiency, female infants are born with ambiguous genitalia, whereas male infants have no genital abnormalities.
- C. In salt-wasting 21-hydroxylase deficiency, symptoms of emesis, salt wasting, dehydration, and shock develop on the first day of life.
- D. The diagnosis of CAH is made by documenting elevated levels of 21-hydroxyprogesterone in the serum.
- E. Therapy for 21-hydroxylase deficiency includes estrogen therapy.

63. A full-term infant is born to a mother with gestational diabetes. At 1 hour of age, the infant is noted to be jittery, and a serum blood glucose level is measured at 20 mg/dL. Which of the following statements best describes the most likely cause of this newborn's hypoglycemia?

- A. Maternal hyperinsulinism
- B. Transient hyperinsulinism in the infant
- C. Type 1 diabetes in the infant
- D. Type 2 diabetes in the infant
- E. Islet cell adenoma of the infant's pancreas

64. A 2-month old boy has had diarrhea during the past week. His mother brings him to the urgent care clinic, where she reports that he weighed 10 kg a week earlier using the same weighing scale during a well-child visit. She has been able to keep up with most of his fluid losses but is concerned that his illness has continued for over 5 days. Which of the following clinical findings is most consistent with this child's level of dehydration?

- A. Dry mucosa of the mouth
- B. No urine in last 12 hours
- C. Sunken eyes and fontanelle
- D. Low blood pressure
- E. Reduced skin turgor

65. A 4-month old boy has had diarrhea during the past week. His mother brings him to the urgent care clinic, where he is noted to have an approximately 10% weight loss since his well-child visit 1 week ago.

The mother is reliable and is ready to follow an oral rehydration therapy protocol at home. An acceptable oral rehydration solution should contain K^+ 15 mEq/L, Cl^- 75 mEq/L, HCO_3^- 30 mEq/L, glucose 2 g/dL, and which of the following Na concentrations?

A. Na^+ 10 mEq/L
B. Na^+ 25 mEq/L
C. Na^+ 90 mEq/L
D. Na^+ 150 mEq/L
E. Na^+ 200 mEq/L

66. A 6-month old girl has had diarrhea during the past week. Her mother reports that the symptoms began a couple of days after they were visiting a neighborhood gym for children. The diagnosis is most consistent with acute viral gastroenteritis, and the mother asks whether antidiarrheal medications would be appropriate to give her daughter. She is advised against antidiarrheal use during gastroenteritis by her general pediatrician. Which of the following complications is the most likely reason for advising against antidiarrheal medications?

A. Hyponatremia
B. Hypernatremia
C. Intussusception
D. Toxic megacolon
E. Hemolytic-uremic syndrome (HUS)

67. A 3-year-old boy is brought to a well-child visit, during which the mother reports that they have begun toilet training over the past 6 months. She reports that her son has had sporadic success but that more commonly his stools are hard, difficult to pass, and infrequent. He also occasionally complains of diffuse abdominal pain but does not have any bouts of diarrhea. What is the most appropriate next management step?

A. Reassuring the mother that the most likely diagnosis is intentional withholding of stool (functional constipation) and advising dietary changes initially with close follow-up
B. Consultation with a pediatric surgeon to arrange rectal biopsy to rule out Hirschsprung's disease
C. Obtaining a serum lead level to rule out plumbism (lead poisoning)
D. Performing a sweat chloride test to rule out cystic fibrosis
E. Obtaining thyroid function tests to rule out hypothyroidism

68. A 4-year-old boy is brought to a well-child visit, during which the mother reports she is concerned about his long history of constipation since 6 months of age. She reports that her son has hard, difficult to pass, and infrequent stools produced every 3 to 4 days. An otherwise normal physical exam reveals poor sphincter tone and stool in the rectal vault on rectal exam. What is the most likely diagnosis?

    A. Hirschsprung's disease

    B. Hypocalcemia

    C. Chronic intestinal obstruction

    D. Intussusception

    E. Intentional withholding of stools (functional constipation)

69. A 4-year-old boy is brought to the emergency department with a history of profuse watery diarrhea over the past 2 days. Of the following serum electrolyte lab results (mEq/L), which abnormal set of values requires rapid correction?

    A. Na^+ 170, K^+ 4, CO_2 14

    B. Na^+ 140, K^+ 5, CO_2 20

    C. Na^+ 135, K^+ 5, CO_2 4

    D. Na^+ 120, K^+ 5, CO_2 10

    E. Na^+ 170, K^+ 4, CO_2 26

70. A 4-year old boy is brought to the emergency department with a history of profuse watery diarrhea over the past 2 days. His serum electrolytes reveal a CO_2 level of 10 mEq/L. The decision is made to administer a normal saline bolus of 20 mL/kg to begin fluid resuscitation for the moderate acidosis. Which of the following is an appropriate time period over which to administer the fluid?

    A. 5 minutes

    B. 30 minutes

    C. 60 minutes

    D. 120 minutes

    E. 180 minutes

71. A full-term baby girl is born via spontaneous vaginal delivery to a mother with insulin-dependent diabetes mellitus who had received good prenatal care and had good control of her blood sugar levels throughout pregnancy. The infant is large for gestational age (LGA) with a birth weight of 4,250 grams and is noted to have an initial serum glucose level of 25 mg/dL. What is the most appropriate next management step?

    A. Feed the infant formula via nipple.

    B. Feed the infant formula via gavage tube.

    C. Start a peripheral IV and administer 40 cc D10W via IV push.

    D. Start a peripheral IV and administer 10 cc D10W via IV push.

    E. Start a peripheral IV and administer 10 cc D25W via IV push.

Answers and Explanations

1. D	**19.** D	**37.** F	**55.** D
2. B	**20.** C	**38.** C	**56.** B
3. A	**21.** B	**39.** D	**57.** E
4. C	**22.** D	**40.** A	**58.** D
5. C	**23.** C	**41.** E	**59.** C
6. B	**24.** B	**42.** D	**60.** E
7. E	**25.** F	**43.** E	**61.** C
8. E	**26.** C	**44.** B	**62.** B
9. B	**27.** C	**45.** A	**63.** B
10. A	**28.** D	**46.** B	**64.** A
11. C	**29.** B	**47.** A	**65.** C
12. F	**30.** C	**48.** C	**66.** D
13. D	**31.** D	**49.** E	**67.** A
14. B	**32.** B	**50.** B	**68.** E
15. I	**33.** A	**51.** D	**69.** C
16. C	**34.** E	**52.** C	**70.** B
17. G	**35.** C	**53.** C	**71.** D
18. L	**36.** E	**54.** C	

1. D. Acute suppurative adenitis is the most common cause of an acutely inflamed lateral neck mass in a toddler. The most common bacterial causes are gram-positive cocci, such as group A streptococci and *Staphylococcus aureus*. Other less likely causes of an acutely inflamed lateral neck mass in a toddler include tuberculosis (scrofula), catscratch disease, and an infected branchial cleft cyst. A retropharyngeal abscess can present with neck swelling, but is less likely to be a distinct mass, as described in this child. Reactive adenopathy and infectious mononucleosis can cause a lateral neck mass, but should not be as red, warm, and painful as this mass is. A thyroglossal duct cyst is midline, and would not present in this manner. Epiglottitis does not usually present with a neck mass, but rather with signs of upper airway obstruction and drooling in a toxic-appearing toddler.

2. B. The location of this mass, midline under the chin, is classic for an infected thyroglossal duct cyst. Reactive adenopathy, infectious mononucleosis, and acute suppurative adenitis are causes of lateral neck masses, not midline neck masses. Epiglottitis would not cause a midline neck mass.

3. A. This infant has a fever without a source. About 20% of infants and young children with fever present without an apparent source after thorough history and physical exam. The *most likely* cause of this infant's fever is a viral infection. Although the other causes must be considered and in some cases ruled out by physical exam or lab tests, viral infection is still the most common cause of fever without a source in infants and young children beyond the neonatal period. Teething occasionally causes low-grade fever in infants this age, but should not cause such a high or prolonged fever as in this infant.

4. C. Common causes of tachycardia in sick infants include fever, pain, distress, and dehydration/hypovolemia. This infant's tachycardia is most likely due to her fever, since she does not have evidence of the other etiologies. An infant's heart rate is quite dynamic, and sinus heart rates as high as 200 beats per minute are commonly seen in infants who are crying or in distress from illness or procedures. Although supraventricular tachycardia (SVT) is one cause of tachycardia to consider, a heart rate that varies, as this infant's does, and is less than 200 beats per minute is unlikely to be caused by SVT. Attempts to identify and correct the more common causes of sinus tachycardia should be undertaken before ordering an EKG or treating for SVT in this case. Carotid massage is not recommended in infants with SVT, and adenosine should not be given until an EKG has documented the presence of SVT.

5. C. The most appropriate next step in this infant would be a urinalysis and culture to detect possible UTI or pyelonephritis. Although she appears well, she still has an appreciable risk (5%–10%) of having pyelonephritis. Since she is immunized against *Haemophilus influenzae* and *Streptococcus pneumoniae*, her risk of serious bacterial illness (bacteremia, meningitis) is very low (<1%), and therefore a CBC is unlikely to change management. Immunizations do not protect against UTI, which is usually caused by *Escherichia coli* and other gram-negative bacteria.

6. B. This infant and mother are matched by Rh positivity, but there is potential ABO incompatibility. When a mother is blood type O, she has no A or B antigen on her red cells, and therefore has both anti-A and anti-B antibodies in her serum. These antibodies can cross the placenta and cause hemolysis in an infant who has A or B antigen on his or her red blood cells. Therefore, this mother's serum contains antibodies that could potentially attack her infant's red cells. The degree of hemolysis that occurs depends on the quantity of antibody that crossed the placenta during gestation and delivery.

7. E. This infant has a primarily conjugated hyperbilirubinemia, which is nearly always pathologic. Unconjugated hyperbilirubinemia is usually due to physiologic causes, such as impaired liver conjugation of bilirubin and decreased gut motility. Breastfeeding and dehydration are factors that commonly exaggerate this physiologic jaundice in the newborn. Conjugated hyperbilirubinemia, on the other hand, occurs when there is impaired passage of bile through the biliary system, and various causes of cholestasis must be considered.

8. E. The next step in this well-appearing infant is to seek the cause of the conjugated hyperbilirubinemia. The cause will dictate the most effective intervention strategy. Phototherapy will not help this infant, because this intervention serves to convert unconjugated bilirubin into a water-soluble form that can be excreted in urine and stool. There is no indication to stop breastfeeding in this infant who is feeding well and has lost only a minimal amount of weight (up to 10% of body weight can be lost in the first few days of life in normal, healthy newborns).

9. B. This child has physical findings and lab results consistent with nephrotic syndrome. Nephrotic syndrome is defined by the presence of edema, hypoalbuminemia, massive proteinuria (>40 mg/m^2/hr over 24 hours) and hyperlipidemia. Although this patient has not had lipid studies or a 24-hour urine collection, nephrotic syndrome is highly suggested by the presentation and lab results. Glomerulonephritis is characterized by hematuria rather than proteinuria, and edema is absent or very mild. Renal failure is unlikely since electrolytes, BUN, creatinine, and blood pressure are normal. Pyelonephritis would present with fever, flank pain, dysuria, and the presence of white cells, nitrites, and bacteria in the urine, none of which are seen in this patient. Vesicoureteral reflux is a cause of recurrent UTI, which can occasionally lead to renal scarring and renal failure in children.

10. A. The diagnosis of nephrotic syndrome can be made with a 24-hour urine collection to quantify urine protein loss. An average protein loss of >4 mg/m²/hr is diagnostic of nephrotic syndrome.

11. C. The next step in management for this stable patient with nephrotic syndrome should be steroids and salt restriction. Minimal change disease (MCD) is by far the most common cause of nephrotic syndrome in children aged 2 to 6 years, and most of these patients respond well to outpatient therapy. Prognosis for MCD is excellent. Although up to 80% of patients may experience a relapse, very few progress to renal insufficiency. Renal biopsy is not indicated for children likely to have minimal change disease, unless they do not respond to steroids. The other options are not indicated based on this patient's adequate presentation and lack of evidence of renal failure.

12. F. This description is classic for varicella, or chickenpox (Table A-1). The pruritic, clear vesicles are distinct and appear in crops, so that lesions in several different stages of evolution are present at one time. Although much less common now that varicella is part of the recommended immunization schedule, both wild-type and vaccine-related disease can still occur.

TABLE A-1   Infectious Exanthems of Childhood

Organism or Syndrome	Description of Exanthem	Other Clinical Features
Measles	Confluent, erythematous, blanching maculopapular rash. Starts at hairline, spreads caudally. May appear on hands or feet, or both.	Cough, coryza, and conjunctivitis usually present. Koplik's spots may be seen on buccal mucosa.
Herpes simplex virus	*Primary gingivostomatitis:* painful, clustered vesicles on erythematous base on gingiva, buccal membranes, tongue, lips. *Herpetic whitlow:* cluster of milky vesicles on an erythematous base, usually on fingers.	Treatment of gingivostomatitis is most likely to be effective if started within 72 hr of symptoms. Systemic treatment is recommended for herpetic whitlow, eczema herpeticum, or if lesions are near eye.

(*Continued*)

TABLE A-1   Infectious Exanthems of Childhood (*continued*)

Organism or Syndrome	Description of Exanthem	Other Clinical Features
Candida	Diaper dermatitis: beefy red, papular, and confluent patch with separate "satellite lesions" located in creases of groin and diaper area.	May also occur in moist creases of neck, or in mouth as thrush. Topical antifungal treatment is usually effective.
Roseola (human herpesvirus 6)	Blanching, erythematous papules/macules start on trunk as fever resolves, and spread up to face.	Self-limited virus; fever usually resolves as rash appears.
Parvovirus (fifth disease)	"Slapped-cheek" rash (slightly raised, blanching, erythematous patches on cheeks) followed by reticular, blanching pattern on limbs.	Usually self-limited in children, although can cause transient bone marrow suppression. Primary infection during pregnancy may result in fetal hydrops. Patients with hemoglobinopathy may experience aplastic crisis.
Varicella (chickenpox)	Distinct, pruritic papules that progress to clear vesicles on erythematous base ("dewdrop on rose petal") and later rupture and crust over. Lesions in several different stages of evolution are present at one time.	Fever, systemic illness common in wild-type infection. Vaccinated children may get attenuated infection with few vesicles.
Impetigo	Oozing, honey-crusted, ruptured clusters of vesicles at sites of trauma or moist skin.	Commonly caused by *Staphylococcus* or *Streptococcus* species. Topical treatment if mild; systemic treatment if widespread.
Rocky Mountain spotted fever (*Rickettsia rickettsiae*)	Small, erythematous, blanching macules on wrists, forearms, and ankles 2 to 5 days after onset of fever. Later spreads and evolves to nonblanching petechiae and/or purpura that may involve palms and/or soles.	Tick-borne; found throughout continental United States, as well as southern Canada, Central America, Mexico, and parts of South America. Treatment with doxycycline is effective.
Meningococcemia	Rapidly progressive appearance of nonblanching petechiae and/or purpura in febrile, systemically ill patient.	May not be accompanied by meningitis. Rapidly progressive to death if untreated. Immediate resuscitation and treatment with broad-spectrum antibiotics.

(Continued)

TABLE A-1   Infectious Exanthems of Childhood (*continued*)

Organism or Syndrome	Description of Exanthem	Other Clinical Features
Lyme disease (*Borrelia burgdorferi*)	Erythema migrans: large, annular blanching erythematous area with central clearing. Occurs at site of tick bite, 7 to 10 days later.	Tick-borne. Primarily found in Northeastern US. Initial appearance of rash is often accompanied by fever, malaise, arthralgias.
Coxsackie virus (hand-foot-mouth syndrome)	Painful, nonclustered vesicles on posterior oropharynx. Also gray, linear vesicles on palms, soles, and/or perineum.	Usually accompanied by high fever in infants and toddlers. Dehydration is primary morbidity.
Tinea corporis	Mildly pruritic, dry, scaly, annular patches with heaped-up borders and central clearing.	Topical antifungal is usually effective. For lesions on scalp (tinea corporis), systemic treatment is needed.
Toxic shock syndrome (*S. aureus*)	Sunburnlike rash (erythroderma) in setting of patient with signs of shock and systemic illness.	Immediate stabilization with airway support and fluid resuscitation is key to survival. Antibiotics.

13. D. Roseola is one of the most common viral exanthems of infancy. The rash classically begins with resolution of fever in a relatively well-appearing infant. It typically starts on the chest, and climbs up to the face (hence the name "exanthem subitum"). Roseola is usually asymptomatic, but can be quite dramatic in its appearance.

14. B. This description is classic for herpetic whitlow, an infection with HSV on the finger of a toddler or infant. The infection is usually caused by HSV-1, and can be transmitted from an adult with active oral HSV, or from the toddler's own mouth. It should be treated with oral or IV acyclovir.

15. I. Rapidly appearing palpable purpura in a toxic, febrile patient is meningococcemia until proven otherwise. A patient with these findings should be stabilized immediately with control of airway, breathing, and circulation. Cultures of blood and CSF should be obtained, and broad-spectrum antibiotics active against meningococcus should be administered as soon as possible.

16. C. The location and appearance of this rash are typical of a candidal diaper rash. The rash is often described as beefy red, papular, and confluent, with separate "satellite lesions" seen outside of the confluent area. It occurs in moist areas, such as the creases of the groin or neck.

17. G. Impetigo is superinfection of the skin with either *Staphylococcus* or *Streptococcus* species. Impetigo can be bullous or nonbullous.

The nonbullous type is more common, consists of ruptured, honey-crusted vesicles at sites of trauma or moist skin (such as around a drooling toddler's mouth), and can be caused by either staphylococci or streptococci. The bullous type consists of thin-walled bullae that rupture, leaving a denuded base with clear exudate. It is more common in neonates, and is always caused by staphylococci. Both can be treated with an oral first-generation cephalosporin, or another antibiotic with staphylococcal and streptococcal coverage.

18. L. The rash described here is ringworm, or tinea corporis. The lesions are classically mildly pruritic, dry, scaly, annular patches with heaped-up borders and central clearing. Tinea corporis usually responds to a topical antifungal, such as clotrimazole. When similar lesions occur on the scalp, they are called tinea capitis. Tinea capitis is associated with alopecia, and should be treated with a systemic antifungal, such as griseofulvin or terbinafine.

19. D. Public schools must perform a learning assessment and provide an IEP for any student whose parents request such an assessment.

20. C. Patient-provider confidentiality must be protected under all circumstances *except* when the provider feels that the information revealed presents a direct threat to the patient or to others. For example, suicidal ideations or plans, an expressed desire to harm others, or the presence of a firearm or other weapon on the patient's person should be reported to the appropriate services or authorities in order to protect both patient and provider. In this patient's case, the patient's marijuana use does not represent a direct threat to the patient or to others, so her request for the information to remain confidential should be honored. However, you may encourage the patient to discuss these issues with her parents, offer to help her talk to her parents, or help her to obtain support services if desired.

21. B. This patient's presentation is most consistent with anaphylaxis, and immediate administration of epinephrine would be the most appropriate initial treatment. Anaphylaxis is an acute, life-threatening, IgE-mediated phenomenon that can be associated with hypotension, wheezing, and acute respiratory distress. Corticosteroids, antihistamines, and beta-adrenergic agonists are helpful adjunctive therapies. Patients with myelomeningocele are more prone to developing latex allergy because of repeated exposure.

22. D. *Chlamydia trachomatis* can be a common cause of pneumonia in the neonate. Often presenting between 1 and 3 months after birth, symptoms include a staccatolike cough and respiratory difficulty. Fever is usually absent, and a history of conjunctivitis after birth may be present. CXR findings of bilateral interstitial infiltrates and a CBC with eosinophilia may suggest the diagnosis.

23. C. *Streptococcus pneumoniae* is the most common cause of bacterial pneumonia in children in this age group. Rapid onset of symptoms, ill appearance, crackles on exam with respiratory distress, and lobar consolidation on CXR are all suggestive of bacterial pneumonia. The CBC usually shows an elevated WBC count with neutrophil predominance. Other causes of bacterial pneumonia in this age group are usually *Haemophilus influenzae* species, and *Moraxella catarrhalis*. In older children, *Mycoplasma pneumoniae* and *Chlamydia pneumoniae* are increasingly common, along with the previously mentioned organisms.

24. B. This infant has signs and symptoms consistent with pertussis, or whooping cough, which is caused by *Bordatella pertussis* is the most common pathogen involved. Young, unimmunized infants are at the highest risk for severe illness, and adolescents and adults with waning immunity are usually major sources of infection. This infant is likely in the paroxysmal phase of the illness. Diagnosis can usually be made via clinical suspicion and can be confirmed by culture or direct fluorescent antibody testing.

25. F. RSV (respiratory syncytial virus) is the major pathogen involved in bronchiolitis. Premature infants are particularly susceptible to more severe illness. Along with the symptoms described, it is important to note that apnea may also occur in young infants.

26. C. This patient is likely experiencing torsion of the appendix testis, which must be differentiated from torsion of the spermatic cord. Pain is usually more gradual in onset. Examination may reveal a "blue-dot" sign, representing the cyanotic appendix testis at the upper pole of the hemiscrotum. Also, unlike torsion of the spermatic cord, the cremasteric reflex is usually present. Imaging studies usually are normal, and management generally includes rest and analgesics. Epididymitis, testicular neoplasms, hydrocele, and varicocele must also be considered in the differential diagnosis.

27. C. Appendicitis generally peaks in the pediatric population at this age and is the most common cause of acute surgery in childhood. Perforation and peritonitis are usually present after 36 to 40 hours of symptom progression, but can be difficult to determine clinically in the younger child (<4 years). Pancreatitis and right lower lobe pneumonia must also be considered in the diagnosis. Intussusception is generally found in children aged 3 or younger, and peaks around 6 to 9 months of age.

28. D. This patient likely has an Ewing's sarcoma, based on his clinical history and imaging findings. Osteogenic sarcoma generally presents with metaphyseal findings and periosteal findings with a "sunburst" appearance on x-ray. Systemic symptoms are generally less common.

29. B. This patient is likely having infantile spasms. They are characterized by a series of brief myoclonic jerking movements, which can consist of sudden arm extension followed by flexion of the head and trunk. Infantile spasms peak between 3 and 7 months of age and may be associated with several identifiable causes. Hypsarrhythmias can be found characteristically on EEG. Adrenocorticotropic hormone (ACTH) and corticosteroids can be used to treat infantile spasms.

30. C. Wilms' tumor must be identified and treated promptly with surgery and chemotherapy. A Wilms' tumor reflects primary nephroblastoma and is an intrarenal process, unlike neuroblastoma. Diagnosis of neuroblastoma can be achieved via urine catecholamine studies as well as imaging and biopsy. Wilms' tumor generally carries a favorable prognosis based on histology (nearly 88% overall survival).

31. D. The developmental milestones achieved by this patient are most consistent with that of a 9-month-old child.

32. B. The most likely pathogens in acute bacterial infection in a CF patient such as this one include *S. aureus* and *P. aeruginosa*. *Burkholderia cepacia* is becoming increasingly common. Empiric therapy should be directed towards these pathogens. Fungal pathogens, as well as the other organisms listed, can occur, but are much less common. These organisms should be suspected if the patient does not respond as expected to empiric therapy.

33. A. Prader-Willi syndrome and Angelman's syndrome are examples of imprinting, both with deletions on chromosome 15. Angelman's syndrome is described as dysmorphisms, severe mental retardation, and jerking arm movements and ataxia (leading to its description as the "happy puppet" syndrome). 45XO is the karyotype of patients with Turner's syndrome. There are no known teratogenic exposures associated with Prader-Willi syndrome. The trinucleotide repeat sequence describes the fragile X syndrome.

34. E. Primary humoral immunity is much more common than disorders of cell-mediated immunity. Quantifying and qualifying immunoglobulin levels can aid in the diagnosis. Mitogen stimulation testing and delayed hypersensitivity testing can aid in detecting disorders of T-cell function. The nitroblue tetrazolium test can aid in testing phagocytic function. Flow cytometry can be an alternative to the nitroblue tetrazolium test to demonstrate the poor oxidative burst seen in chronic granulomatous disease.

35. C. The patient is demonstrating signs and symptoms consistent with an acute epiglottitis episode. Acute onset, ill appearance, and stridor in the context of impending obstruction are the hallmarks of this disease.

36. E. The clinical history and physical exam in this patient are most consistent with a retropharyngeal abscess.

37. F. This patient is likely to have EBV-mediated tonsillopharyngitis. Although symptoms can also include a primary rash in some patients, the rash described is generally secondary to amoxicillin administration. Typically it is a diffuse, maculopapular rash that erupts nearly 1 week after starting amoxicillin.

38. C. The child described is likely 3 years old, reflected by the various developmental milestones that have been achieved. An assessment involves parental reporting as well as demonstration. It is important to recognize that premature infants require age-adjusted parameters when assessing their development until they are 2 years old.

39. D. The likely diagnosis for the child described in this vignette is intussusception. A sausage-shaped tubular mass is present in nearly 75% of patients. Although it is a relatively late finding, it is important to note rectal bleeding, which can occur in nearly 80% of patients. Contrast or air enema administration can be both diagnostic and therapeutic. Other causes of rectal bleeding may include Meckel's diverticula, which can be identified by a technetium-99 pertechnetate scan and generally involves painless rectal bleeding. Stool studies for ova and parasites can identify causes of enterocolitis that generally present with chronic symptoms. Emergent dialysis may be indicated in severe cases of hemolytic uremic syndrome associated with *Escherichia coli* O157:H7 or dehydration causing acute renal failure. Oral rehydration is best clinically indicated in cases of mild to moderate dehydration.

40. A. Inflammatory bowel disease may present with a multitude of extraintestinal manifestations. Perianal disease can occur frequently with Crohn's disease. The nodules described in this patient may also reflect erythema nodosum, which may also be present in patients with Crohn's disease. Skip lesions and transmural involvement are associated with Crohn's disease upon endoscopic evaluation. Antineutrophil cytoplasmic antibody evaluation may be helpful in establishing the diagnosis of ulcerative colitis, which is also associated with a significantly increased risk of colon cancer. A gluten-free diet is involved in celiac disease, which often presents earlier in life. Giardiasis may be associated strongly with a preceding history of exposure to mountain stream water, but is not associated with perianal skin tags or erythema nodosum.

41. E. Atlantoaxial instability can occur in nearly 25% of children with Down syndrome, and radiographic screening is generally indicated by 3 to 5 years of age. Down syndrome is also associated with clinodactyly, among many other physical findings, and an increased risk of leukemia (nearly 20 times that of the general population). Unlike trisomy 18 or trisomy 13, Down syndrome (trisomy 21) is not generally associated with increased mortality in the first year of life. Rockerbottom feet are one of the characteristic physical findings in patients with trisomy 18.

42. D. Iron ingestion is one of the most common childhood poisonings, and prenatal vitamins are a common source. Examination of serum iron levels within 2 to 6 hours after an ingestion can help identify the need for administration of deferoxamine, an iron binding agent. Deferoxamine should also be given if severe gastrointestinal symptoms are present, as in the child described in the clinical vignette. Activated charcoal is not recommended in suspected iron ingestion because it does not bind to iron, and whole-bowel irrigation has no proven benefit in this situation. The management should always be supplemented by supportive care and education. Ipecac syrup is not likely to be effective 2 hours after an ingestion, and D-penicillamine is an agent that is useful in lead and mercury poisoning. Poisoning with isoniazid (INH) can be treated with pyridoxine.

43. E. The patient described in the clinical vignette demonstrates a clinical picture that is consistent with Turner's syndrome, a sex chromosome disorder in which part or all of one X chromosome is missing. These patients often have delayed onset of puberty due to gonadal dysgenesis, resulting in hypergonadotropic lab values. Newborns with Turner's syndrome often present with lymphedema and swelling of the hands and feet. Anosmia is characteristic of Kallmann's syndrome, an isolated gonadotropin deficiency. Multiple CGG repeats are the hallmark of the fragile X syndrome. Hypothyroidism as a result of Hashimoto's thyroiditis may also cause delayed puberty, but generally presents with different clinical manifestations.

44. B. The child described likely can be assessed as having mild persistent asthma (Table A-2). Because of the role of inflammation in persistent asthma, long-term control of symptoms can often accomplished with the use of a daily inhaled anti-inflammatory medication. The single safest and most effective option is an inhaled corticosteroid. Cromolyn sodium and leukotriene modifiers are safe, but not as effective at controlling persistent asthma. Rescue therapy with albuterol is appropriate as needed, but would not contribute to

TABLE A-2 Classification and Maintenance Treatment of Asthma

Severity	Symptoms	Maintenance Medications, Age ≤5 Years		Maintenance Medications, Age >5 Years	
		Preferred	Alternative	Preferred	Alternative
Mild intermittent	≤2 d/wk and/or ≤2 nights/mo	None	None	None	None
Mild persistent	≥2 d/wk and/ or ≥2 nights/mo	Low-dose inhaled corticosteroid	Cromolyn or leukotriene receptor antagonist	Low-dose inhaled corticosteroid	Cromolyn, leukotriene receptor antagonist, nedocromil, or sustained-release theophylline
Moderate persistent	Daily and/or >1 night/wk	Low-dose inhaled corticosteroid and long-acting inhaled β_2-agonist or medium-dose inhaled corticosteroid	Low-dose inhaled corticosteroid and either leukotriene receptor antagonist or theophylline	Low- to medium-dose inhaled corticosteroid and long-acting inhaled β_2-agonist	Low- to medium-dose inhaled corticosteroid and either leukotriene receptor antagonist or theophylline
Severe persistent	Continual daily, and frequent nightly	High-dose inhaled corticosteroid and long-acting inhaled β_2-agonist and (if needed) oral corticosteroid	None accepted	High-dose inhaled corticosteroid and long-acting inhaled β_2-agonist and (if needed) oral corticosteroid	None accepted

long-term control. Although environmental allergen control is an important principle of long-term asthma control, staying inside would not be an appropriate way to meet this goal. Long-acting beta-agonists may be helpful in patients with more severe, frequent symptoms, but are not approved in children <4 and should be prescribed with caution due to recent studies suggesting an increased risk of death in patients on these medications. Anticholinergic medication may be used as adjuncts to relieve acute bronchospasm, but are not indicated for long-term control.

45. A. The patient described exhibits signs and symptoms that are consistent with von Willebrand's disease. Patients with hemophilia generally tend to have bleeding into their joints, and generally are male. Bleeding time in von Willebrand's patients is prolonged, whereas it is generally normal in patients with hemophilia or vitamin K deficiency. Patients with Wiskott-Aldrich syndrome tend to have thrombocytopenia along with other clinical findings, such as eczema. Thrombocytopenic patients tend to have normal activated PTT values.

46. B. Galactosemia is an autosomal recessive disorder that is caused by a deficiency in galactose-1-phosphate uridyltransferase. Symptoms generally follow the introduction of breast milk or cow's milk, and may include vomiting, diarrhea, and poor feeding. Hepatomegaly and cataracts are also prominent physical findings. Lab values may show hepatic dysfunction, hypoglycemia, and acidosis. Sepsis, as a result of *Escherichia coli*, is typically associated with galactosemia. Newborn screening can often aid in the diagnosis. Hereditary fructose intolerance generally follows the introduction of fruit or fruit juices, and tends to be later in infancy. Gaucher's disease is a lysosomal storage disease that is characterized by neurodegeneration and typical bony changes. Phenylketonuria generally does not present in the newborn period. Ornithine transcarbamylase deficiency, although it may be clinically similar to galactosemia, is an X-linked recessive disorder of the urea cycle that causes severe symptoms in newborn males upon introduction of protein.

47. A. This patient's clinical presentation is most consistent with congenital rubella syndrome (Table A-3). Congenital syphilis may manifest with fever, maculopapular rash on the palms/soles and trunk, and evidence of anemia, thrombocytopenia, leukopenia, and hepatitis.

48. C. Any fracture can be due to abuse, if not consistent with the mechanism of injury. However, metaphyseal chip fractures of the long bones are considered nearly pathognomonic of abuse. These fractures are the result of torsional and twisting forces on the long bones and often will result in a chipping that can appear like a bucket

TABLE A-3 Differentiating and Evaluating Some Congenital Infections

Agent	Specific Clinical Features	Laboratory Evaluation
Toxoplasma gondii	Hydrocephalus with generalized calcifications; chorioretinitis	Toxoplasmosis IgG antibody followed by IgM, which is more specific.
Treponema pallidum	Osteochondritis and periostitis; eczematoid skin rash; snuffles	Nontreponemal test such as RPR or VDRL, supported by a treponemal test such as IgM FTA-ABS.
Rubella	Eye: cataracts, cloudy cornea, pigmented retina Skin: "blueberry muffin" spots Bone: vertical striation Heart: patent ductus, pulmonary stenosis	Maternal rubella immune status. If immune, send infant's IgG and the more specific IgM. If IgM is negative but IgG is positive, viral cultures from urine, cerebrospinal fluid, and throat swabs may isolate the virus.
Cytomegalovirus	Microcephaly with periventricular calcifications; hepatosplenomegaly; chorioretinitis; inguinal hernias; thrombocytopenia (in males)	Urine for cytomegalovirus culture or rapid CMV early antigen test.
Herpes simplex	Skin vesicles or denuded skin; keratoconjunctivitis; acute central nervous system findings such as seizures	Viral cultures from CSF, skin lesions, conjunctivae, urine, blood, rectum, and nasopharynx should grow within 2 to 3 days. PCR of CSF. Direct fluorescent antibody staining of scraping from skin lesion is specific but not sensitive.

CMV, cytomegalovirus; CSF, cerebral spinal fluid; FTA-ABS, fluorescent treponemal antibody absorption test; PCR, polymerase chain reaction test; RPR, rapid plasma reagent test; VDRL, Venereal Disease Research Laboratory test.

handle. Posterior rib fractures, fractures in multiple stages of healing, scapular fractures, sternal fractures, and vertebral fractures are others which are suggestive of abuse. A spiral fracture of the tibia sparing the fibula is known as a "toddler's fracture" because it can occur as the result of a young child's fall while ambulating. Its occurrence in a pre-ambulatory child should be concerning for abuse. Falls on an outstretched arm can produce supracondylar fractures of the elbow as well as clavicular fractures, both of which are common in childhood. The Salter-Harris classification refers to fractures involving growth plate, and does not reflect fractures more specific for abuse.

49. E. Corticosteroids are the mainstay of therapy for addressing the inflammatory process that accompanies airway constriction in acute episodes of asthma exacerbation, generally acting 3 to 6 hours after administration. Theophylline, magnesium sulfate, salmeterol, and epinephrine are all medications that play a role in bronchodilation, but do not assist in anti-inflammatory therapy. Montelukast is a leukotriene-modifying agent that does not have a role in acute asthma management.

50. B. MMR (measles, mumps, rubella) and varicella are live vaccines and should not be administered to immunocompromised patients. Because IPV and meningococcal conjugate vaccine are both nonlive vaccines, they are considered safe in immunocompromised patients. Mild illness with rhinorrhea and fever is not considered a contraindication. Egg allergy is not a precaution for varicella vaccine, because the vaccine is not developed with egg protein.

51. D. Cystic fibrosis patients frequently present with respiratory distress due to bronchopulmonary exacerbations. Infections are often the source, and common pathogens include *Staphylococcus aureus, Pseudomonas aeruginosa,* and *Burkholderia cepacia.* Piperacillin/tazobactam and tobramycin offer a viable choice for empiric antibiotic coverage.

52. C. Gastroesophageal reflux disease (GERD) may present with emesis and poor feeding. Sandifer syndrome describes the characteristic posturing that may reflect the accompanying painful esophageal irritation. Poor weight gain and irritability can often be associated with GERD. Although clinical presentation is highly suggestive, pH probe studies are the gold standard for making the diagnosis of GERD. Wheezing can often accompany GERD, because esophageal irritation and microaspiration of gastric contents can cause bronchospasm.

53. C. The patient in this clinical vignette has signs and symptoms that are suggestive of dermatomyositis. Along with the constitutional, cutaneous, and muscle weakness findings that are described, calcium deposition is commonly found. Creatine kinase levels are markedly elevated, and corticosteroids are the mainstay of therapy. Unlike in adults, pediatric patients exhibit virtually no increased risk for malignancy. Anti–double-stranded DNA antibodies are generally a more specific marker for SLE.

54. C. This infant is suffering from respiratory distress syndrome (RDS), based on his clinical presentation and CXR findings. Once the diagnosis of RDS is made based on clinical grounds or via radiologic confirmation, if significant respiratory distress leads to hypercarbia (elevated Pco_2) requiring intubation, the treatment of choice is to administer exogenous surfactant. Chest tube placement is generally reserved for evacuation of a pneumothorax, and normal saline bolus is indicated for treatment of hypotension. Although umbilical catheters are useful in this clinical scenario, their placement should be preceded by control of the baby's ventilation. Determination of the L/S ratio is an often useful predictor of prematurity, but is of little importance in the face of a premature infant with obvious clinical and radiologic signs of RDS.

55. D. The presence of phosphatidylglycerol (PG) in amniotic fluid is the most sensitive and specific marker of lung maturity. Its detection is particularly useful in aiding decisions regarding premature delivery, especially in high-risk pregnancies such as those occurring in women with diabetes. Maternal or gestational age are often not useful to determine lung maturity, particularly at gestational ages between 32 and 36 weeks. Although there is a lower likelihood of RDS with an L/S ratio greater than 2:1, certain conditions such as hypoxia or acidosis may increase the risk despite a "mature" L/S ratio. The presence or absence of PG is thus a more sensitive and specific test for lung maturity. Fetal breathing movements do not, by themselves, reflect lung maturity.

56. B. Babies with truncus arteriosus or any mixing lesion are at risk of developing pulmonary edema secondary to pulmonary overcirculation. As the pulmonary vascular resistance falls in the first few days after birth, excessive shunting of blood to the lungs leads to desaturation and worsening of systemic perfusion. A PDA is not of concern in babies with truncus arteriosus, since there is fusion of the systemic and pulmonary outflow tracts. Left ventricular failure is generally not associated with worsening in truncus arteriosus; rather, the right ventricle is usually overloaded. RDS is unlikely in this full-term infant.

57. E. Continuous PGE_1 infusion may be associated with transient apnea even in full-term infants. This patient is otherwise not at risk for intraventricular hemorrhage or increased intracranial pressure. Although pulmonary edema may be a sequela of pulmonary over-circulation as the infant's pulmonary vascular resistance drops, it is an unlikely cause of apnea. This infant is also an unlikely candidate for apnea of prematurity given his full-term gestational age.

58. D. This toddler's presentation is most consistent with a diagnosis of Hirschsprung's disease. The definitive diagnosis can only be confirmed by rectal biopsy showing a lack of ganglion cells in Meissner's plexus and Auerbach's plexus. A barium enema showing a transition zone between a narrowed distal segment and dilated segment as well as an abnormal digital exam and anal manometry are highly suggestive but not definitive of Hirschsprung's disease. An upper GI series may not add valuable information, since this lesion is found very distally.

59. C. A diagnosis of duodenal atresia deserves consideration in a newborn infant with trisomy 21. The classic presenting sign is bilious vomiting following initiation of feeds; a possible history of polyhydramnios in utero further supports this diagnosis. A KUB is most likely to show a "double bubble" caused by distended stomach and proximal duodenum, separated by the pylorus. Management includes immediate decompression and surgical intervention. Barium enema may not be useful, since the diagnosis of Hirschsprung's disease is less likely. Similarly, although a "corkscrew" appearance of bowel is suggestive of a malrotation with volvulus, this lesion is less likely in this infant. Pneumatosis intestinalis describes intramural free air within bowel walls and is most commonly seen in infants with necrotizing enterocolitis (NEC).

60. E. This infant's hydropic presentation is most likely secondary to his low ventricular heart rate. A markedly slowed ventricular heart rate below 60 bpm is suggestive of third-degree atrioventricular block. Of the given choices, maternal systemic lupus erythematosus (SLE) is the most likely diagnosis to explain this infant's congenital complete heart block and would be demonstrated by a positive maternal ANA. Although maternal ABO incompatibility and the TORCH infections listed (rubella, CMV, and syphilis) can present with hydrops fetalis in very severe instances, the lack of cardiomegaly makes these less likely. Other diagnoses presenting with congenital complete heart block include L-transposition of great arteries, history of open heart surgery, cardiomyopathy, and Lyme disease.

61. C. The management of all unstable infants must begin with the ABCs. This infant is presenting with ventricular tachycardia and is at very high risk of developing ventricular fibrillation. The first step therefore is to intubate. Once a stable airway is established, the hypotensive infant with ventricular tachycardia must receive synchronized cardioversion. Once the rhythm is stabilized, a lidocaine infusion can be started while a more thorough diagnostic workup is performed. Nonsynchronized defibrillation is reserved for patients with ventricular fibrillation, and procainamide is often used in normotensive patients with ventricular tachycardia following IV lidocaine load.

62. B. Female infants born with 21-hydroxylase deficiency are born with ambiguous genitalia and account for 90% of the cases of CAH. Male infants with 21-hydroxylase deficiency have no genital abnormalities. Symptoms of salt-wasting 21-hydroxylase deficiency develop in the first 2 to 4 weeks of life. The diagnosis of CAH is made by documenting elevated levels of 17-hydroxyprogesterone in the serum, and treatment includes cortisol and mineralocorticoid therapy.

63. B. This infant is presenting with transient hyperinsulinism, most likely secondary to maternal hyperglycemia. Because glucose is easily transported across the placenta to the fetus, the fetal response is transient overproduction of insulin to maintain euglycemia. Once the increased glucose load is removed following delivery, insulin production will gradually decrease to normal levels. Maternal hyperinsulinism is rare and would cause hypoglycemia in the mother. If severe, maternal hyperinsulinism may adversely affect the normal nutrient delivery, affecting fetal development. Diabetes usually does not present in the newborn period; islet cell adenoma is also rare and is a diagnosis of exclusion once other causes of hypoglycemia have been ruled out.

64. A. This child is presenting with 5% dehydration based on his weight loss. Given this mild degree of dehydration, the only clinical finding that may present on examination is dry mucosa of the mouth. The other listed clinical findings are more consistent with more moderate to severe dehydration (10%–15%).

65. C. The oral rehydration solution recommended by the World Health Organization (WHO) is composed of Na^+ 90 mEq/L along with the additional electrolytes and glucose as listed. The Na^+ concentrations of 10 and 25 mEq/L are too low to replace losses and would result in hyponatremia. Solutions with excessive Na^+ would replace Na^+ too quickly and could result in hypernatremia beyond the first few hours of use.

66. D. Toxic megacolon is a potential complication of antidiarrheal use during acute diarrhea in children. Hyponatremia, hypernatremia, hemolytic-uremic syndrome (HUS), and intussusception would not be expected to occur as a result of antidiarrheal medications alone but may be associated complications due to the underlying cause of infection or diarrhea.

67. A. The most common cause (90%–95%) of constipation beyond the neonatal period is voluntary withholding (functional constipation). A history of toilet training indicates a strong suspicion that a nonorganic cause may be responsible for the symptoms. Other organic causes as listed require more elaborate or invasive investigation and should be considered once simply dietary or psychosocial adjustments have failed.

68. E. The most common cause (90%–95%) of constipation beyond the neonatal period is voluntary withholding (functional constipation). Despite the seemingly chronic nature of this child's problem, the key physical finding that is inconsistent with a diagnosis of Hirschsprung's disease is poor sphincter tone. Children with Hirschsprung's disease would be expected to always have exaggerated sphincter tone. Hypocalcemia and chronic or intermittent bowel obstruction would be accompanied by additional clinical symptoms, including tetany and bilious or bloody stools.

69. C. These lab results are suggestive of severe metabolic acidosis given the markedly low CO_2. This degree of acidosis indicates significant dehydration with poor tissue perfusion and the production of organic acid from anaerobic metabolism. A rapid correction of acidosis with appropriate fluid resuscitation is the next management step. Although the other electrolyte disturbances of hyponatremia and hypernatremia are also abnormal, they will require a much slower correction to prevent excessive rapid flux of fluid between tissue compartments.

70. B. Thirty minutes is an appropriate time period over which to administer a fluid bolus in the patient who is hemodynamically stable. A hypotensive patient may require fluid volume as rapidly as possible. The patient in this case is in need of fluid replacement secondary to dehydration in order to improve tissue perfusion and switch from anaerobic to aerobic metabolism. Improved intravascular volume will also restore intestinal function to reduce diarrhea and increase renal perfusion and function. Fluid should not be administered too rapidly, which could cause pulmonary edema.

71. D. The appropriate management of a hypoglycemic infant with serum glucose below 30 mg/dL is to start a peripheral IV and administer 2 to 3 cc/kg D10W. For glucose values greater than 30 mg/dL, it may be acceptable to initiate early feeds via nipple of gavage. In general, boluses of greater than D10W concentration are not advised due to the possibility of a rebound hypoglycemia following sudden insulin release.

Index

Page numbers followed by *f* or *t* indicate figures or tables, respectively.